BODY WISDOM

The Use and Training of the Human Body

BODY WISDOM

The Use and Training of the Human Body

Arthur Lessac

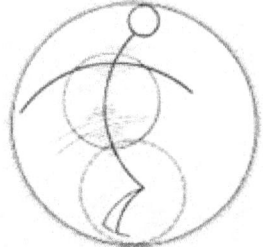

An official LTRI publication

Published in the USA by the
Lessac Training and Research Institute (LTRI)
60 Seaman Avenue #1D
New York, New York 10034
www.lessacinstitute.org

Copyright © 2019 Lessac Training and
Research Institute

All rights reserved. No part of this publication
may be reproduced without permission by the LTRI.

Cover design: Michael Mufson

ISBN: 978-0-9996164-9-9 (paperback)
Printed and bound in the United States by Ingram Spark

Contents

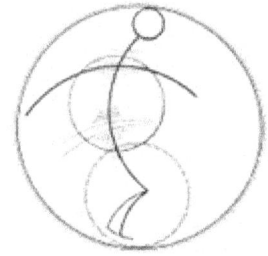

Acknowledgements i
Foreword ii
    Deborah Kinghorn
Introducing Body Wisdom 1

Part One A HUMAN ECOLOGY
ON FINDING THE WAY 5
1 MOVING BEYOND WILDNESS 11
In collaboration with Michael Lessac
    What is natural? 11
    The two environments 13
    Beyond wildness 17
2 A NEW LEARNING PROCESS 20
3 BODY ESTHETICS 26

Part Two: ENERGY AND RELAXATION
UNIFYING THE TWO OPPOSITES 32
4 THE BODY ENERGIZERS 34
5 RELAXER-ENERGIZERS 59
6 RHYTHM 67

Part Three ENERGY AND RELAXATION IN MOVEMENT

IMAGES, BALANCE-RHYTHM,
EVOLVING BODY CURVE 71

7   GETTING THE BODY INTO A COMPACT BALL 79
8   THE BODY AS A SMALL SPHERE 88
9   THE BODY AS AN EXPANDED SPHERE 108
10 THE BODY AS A CRESCENT – LYING DOWN 124
    A MIDWORD BREAK 135
11 THE BODY AS A CRESCENT – STANDING UP 139
12 THE PERCEPTION OF THE UPRIGHT 175
    POSTSCRIPT TO CHAPTERS 7 – 12 215
13 THE BODY'S PERSONAL SPACE SPHERES 226
14 IN SEARCH OF A SELF IMAGE 246

CODA

YOU AND YOUR BODY 250
    At Home
    At Work
    At Play
    In Sports
    In the Arts

INDEX 297

ACKNOWLEDGEMENTS

To my wife Birdie, who encouraged me, assisted me, and struggled through this massive project with me.

Arthur Lessac, 1978

To Michael Lessac, for his generosity, contributions, and support to the original manuscript and in providing permission for the book to be re-published.

Lessac Institute, 2019

ii

FOREWORD
By Deborah Kinghorn

Footnotes
By Marth Munro

When I attended my first Lessac Kinesensic Voice and Body Training Intensive in the summer of 1984, *Body Wisdom* had been published only six years earlier. Already trained in the vocal component of the approach, I was curious about the body work, but expected no more than an expanded version of what was already present in Arthur Lessac's first text, *The Use and Training of the Human Voice*. Happily, I was completely wrong.

Looking back over my journals from that time, my reactions were, "Where has this been?" and "I don't know how I ever taught the voice work without this!" to "This makes so much sense!" I am not the only person who has thought this. Hundreds of people who have studied Kinesensics agree that the wisdom found in *Body Wisdom* informs every other part of the training. In fact, long before "embodied training"[i] was a popular phrase, Lessac had brought together voice, movement, and behavioral training into one approach which immediately benefitted actors, and which, because of its organic roots, grew to benefit anyone who was seeking a healthy body, voice and behavior for a productive life. People from all walks of life, including athletes, clergy, speech/language pathologists and therapists, singers, educators, somatic specialists, politicians, public speakers, dancers, and even those in the diverse fields of engineering, architecture, and physics recognized the power and the potential inherent in Lessac's vision.

Simply put, that vision is that the body is a source of infinite wisdom and information, and if we will only become aware of its messaging, we can shape our world so that the body can function easily and freely, thus reducing stress, anxiety, and pain, all of which lead to dis-ease and malfunction. The present recognition of "mindfulness"[ii] reflects this same tenet; over forty years ago Lessac labelled it "habitual awareness", stating that it was the only habit we could afford to have.

Throughout his life, Lessac tested his theories on himself and used the feedback he received from his own body as a source for further evolution of his approach to voice and body training.[iii] When he was in his early 90's, he gathered a group of his certified trainers to define the means by which Kinesensic training would continue.[iv] Out of that meeting, the present Lessac Training and Research Institute was born, and it is that Institute which has continued to evolve this training, as expressly wished by Lessac. Lessac considered his experiments and writings "pre-scientific", in that science had not yet caught up with some of his findings. He had faith that it would, and in fact, in many cases, it has.[v] He had a keen sense of curiosity, continually reading about new advances in psychotherapy, somatics, and energy medicines, among other interests. Everything was tested and either embraced or rejected according to the basic principles found at the beginning of this book (see "Preface to Part One"). Embedded in those principles is a profound respect for humans, both as a species and as individuals. Also embedded is the recognition that all things evolve, including training systems. Lessac instilled in all of us the understanding that nothing remains static; that everything is always evolving, and that we must evolve Lessac Kinesensics accordingly.

It is with that in mind that I suggest that the majority of this book is still pertinent today, because it is based on principles that are derived from a common understanding of the functioning of human body and have therefore been recognized in many other methodologies, including those originating in Eastern philosophies, such as yoga and T'ai Chi.

Modern cognitive neuroscience was in its infancy when this book was first published, but Lessac's reference to "twin-brain research" (p5) is well-known now as the modern split-brain studies of Roger Sperry, Joseph Bogen and Michael Gazzaniga which gave rise to our current understanding of hemispheric specialization and integration.[vi] Although Lessac could not prove it scientifically at the time, his own research indicated that the brain was not dominant over the body,[vii] and that the body and the brain communicated via "inner body languages" (p5) which we could begin to hear and understand if we became aware of them. Lessac's belief that the body/mind was a gestalt gave rise to his way of working, in which the body, voice, emotion, and intellect were not separate, but intertwined, or embodied.[viii] Knowledge of embodied learning has grown substantially since this book was written. Researcher and Lessac Master Teacher Marth Munro has identified nine principles that are present in all systems of embodied learning, including holistic integration, organic congruencies, personal uniqueness, sensory awareness, inner and outer, continuous change, habitual patterns, re-patterning, and self-teaching.[ix] Compare these with the principles in the Preface to Part One and it is clear that Lessac employed embodied learning.

Even today, there is very little pedagogy that addresses the development of the whole human instrument, including body, voice, and emotion. To my knowledge, Lessac was the first to attempt to do so. Lessac's first book, *The Use and Training of the Human Voice*, catapulted him into the national spotlight in 1960, and it wasn't until 1978 that this book followed with the full treatment of that which had only been hinted at in the previous book. Yet, due to publishers differences (the books were published by different companies) Lessac could not integrate his voice work into this text as he wished to do. The separate existence of the books seemed to imply a separation between teaching voice and teaching body work, which was not the philosophy that Lessac promoted. When this book went out of print in the early 1990's, another blow was dealt to Lessac's vision of a comprehensive training. Although his voice book is still in print, many people no longer even know that he was a leader in the field of embodied training.

That misperception is what we hope to change with the re-introduction of this seminal text. But the training has continued to evolve since this book was written, and I would like to point out those evolutions, as I believe they will impact your reading of this book. Even though the voice training is given minimal treatment in this book, I will include its evolution as well.

Evolving word choices

If words are actions, and action creates reaction, then we can assume that our choice of words has an effect on our body's response to those words. When we teach this work, we have found it important to re-visit the terminology used to be sure it influences the body in a positive way.[x] Continuous and conscious use of the terminology is important because it creates a specific aesthetic which allows for positive responses from the body. For example, we use the words experiment and exploration rather than practice or exercise, because the former words create a sense of wonder and curiosity, drawing on mindfulness which the latter two do not. Likewise, we "tap" consonants; we do not "hit" them. Tapping is light and playful; hitting is not. When asking students to explore something again, we ask them to explore another version, which implies that the first version was not wrong, but merely different. Lessac advocated that "any effort is too much effort" and our phrasing seeks to remove any sense of force or judgement and instead allow playfulness[xi] and curiosity to lead us to discoveries.

The following phrases have evolved over time, and we feel they inspire this kind of positive response.

Posture vs. dynamic alignment

The word posture evolves from the root "to pose". People tend to think of posture as static and fixed, which is antithetical to both freedom of movement and breathing. Dynamic alignment[xii] suggests an energetic arrangement of the body's components for coordinated functioning. This follows the principle that our bodies are never completely still, but always in motion. Therefore, our alignment must be flexible and fluid. This precept leads to exploring the body as a small ball, an expanded sphere and as a cylinder, and carrying those discoveries into our perception of upright orientation. These explorations also honor the developmental movement patterns of babies, [xiii] and so help to reconnect us with our bodies as they functioned before we developed adverse habitual patterns. The idea that alignment is dynamic also increases our awareness of our ever-shifting balance, leading to better balance and reduced fear of falling.

Forward Facial Posture vs. Forward Facial Orientation

Like its body counterpart, the use of the word "posture" with the delicate and flexible extension of the levitor and zygomatic muscles led to misunderstandings which resulted in people holding their lips outward or creating awkward shapes with the mouth, thus negating the freedom and flexibility which Lessac advocated. The word "orientation" implies a general direction rather than a static placement. It also implies that one can move in any direction as long as one returns to the feeling of forward motion. Without going into too much detail, this forward motion comes from the natural movement of those muscles when we engage in the beginning of a yawn. Research has proven that the elongation of these muscles in an easy, relaxed manner creates a desirable openness inside the oral cavity which in turn positively affects the quality of tone produced. In singing, this is often introduced via the "straw exercise"[xiv], where one hums or trills into a straw. As with all of his teachings, Lessac sought natural functions of the human body to produce the desired effect, and in this case, the unforced instigation of a yawn achieves the same effect without resorting to outside mechanical intervention to induce it.

C-curve vs. upright orientation

Lessac advocates that "the longer the spine, the healthier the spine" and with this I think no one can disagree. It was the phrase "C-curve" that distorted his intentions. I remember vividly the day he said to me, "I wish I had never coined that term!" because so many had misunderstood it. In brief, he advocated for a *long spine with the smallest amount of curve possible within the framework of an individual's anatomy.* This did not belie the "natural" curves of the spine; however, it did challenge the assumption that to "stand up straight" would be beneficial to the body. In fact, when one "stands up straight", one inevitably pulls the shoulders back and thrusts the pelvis backwards, all of which throws the spine out of alignment, fighting the gravitational pull instead of finding harmonic relationship between the body and gravity. Lessac's insistence that we recognize that there is no straight line in the body, only curves,[xv] was complicated by the term "C-curve", which many took to mean curving the coccyx under and rounding the thoracic spine in order to create a single, unbroken curve, and which, indeed, is illustrated that way in this book. However, what is often forgotten is that Lessac's curve did not end at the coccyx. He asked us to imagine the spine extending from the crown of the head and then bifurcating in the pelvis and continuing down the backs of the legs into the hollows of the knees. This important image helps to release the femur joint and the groin, which then prevents tucking of the pelvis.

In our evolution of his work, we have replaced "C-curve" with "upright orientation", so as to honor the idea that the spine is not static; that it is in motion, and that the energy source from the middle of the spine upward and downwards creates an opposition which extends and releases tension in the lower back, effectively lengthening the spine, and decreasing any curve that is *not conducive* to a long and healthy spine.

Action vs. Energy

Initially, all of the different qualities of movement in the body were called "actions" because at the time, it complemented Stanislavsky's use of the word and seemed the best way to indicate the constant motion of the body. Lessac changed this to "energy" for this text, and eventually changed his voice text to utilize the word as well. This reflects the accepted physics principle that all matter is in motion, which correlates with Lessac's research indicating that the body itself is in perpetual motion. This motion is known as kinetic energy, and Lessac therefore chose to differentiate the body's energy into four different qualities, known as buoyancy, radiancy, potency, and inter-involvement. (See Chapter 4 of this book). Modern energy practitioners instantly recognize and accept this terminology, but at one time, this was considered unusual and more in line with Eastern medicine and philosophies. This is just another example of how Lessac's thinking was ahead of his time. In practice, Lessac trainers seek to encourage the uninterrupted flow of energy through the body, and hence the voice as well.

Evolutions in Teaching

Contiguous Continuity and the Teacher Within

As you will find in reading this text, the phrase "contiguous continuity" means "not moving from any one spot on the body until you experience the feel of its most proximally adjacent (closest touching) spot" (p. 91) It is also called "atom-to-atom movement" (p. 91). The evolution is that this now extends to all of the teaching of the work. From the end of every exploration, the trainer is seeking the "just noticeable difference" that will indicate where a new exploration begins. Therefore, when warming up the body, or when tuning up the voice, there is no segmentation, such as working the arms only, or only working on resonance. Everything is interconnected, and it is our job, as trainers and as learners, to find those connections in order to find the blocks or tensions that may be standing in the way of ease-ful functioning. The more I have worked with this concept, the more I understand that in our habituated, patterned states, we will unwittingly by-pass blocks of tension only because we have learned to do so. By slowing down, and truly living moment to moment with the explorations, we can discover what is holding us back from being the fully realized individuals we all can be. This is also the source of the phrase "teacher within", coined by Master Teacher Barry Kur. If we are to be effective teachers, the first person we learn to teach is ourselves.[xvi] When teaching anyone else, then, it is most effective to go inside and experience the lesson as you teach it as if you are learning it yourself for the first time. This releases you from the pressure of having to "remember" steps and sequences; rather, you learn to trust your inner sensing to guide you and your student to the next point.

Journeys

The recognition of the need to find interconnection has resulted in a process of exploration known as "journeying". It follows the sentiment of the Ursula K. Le Guin quote, "It is good to have an end to journey toward; but it is the journey that matters, in the end." (1987). Many other artists, inventors, and business people have written about the need to recognize the journey as at least as important, if not more so, than the destination. And while this is not a new concept in teaching, it is one which we have deliberately emphasized over the past two decades. It has helped trainers and participants alike to understand the importance of individual journeys and recognize that what works for one may not work for all. This honors Lessac's insistence that what he taught was not a "technique" or a "method", both of which imply an orderly, logical, and systematic way of instruction or inquiry. Lessac felt that one could begin studying his work at any point in his two books, and jump around if one wished, and still get the training one needed. What results is great freedom for the teacher and the student to investigate and explore without adhering to any particular sequence, and this is particularly potent in individual work. In group work, the addition of the more formalized journeys is to allow everyone the opportunity to experience with new awareness how concepts which have been introduced intertwine with each other; again, a recognition that the whole is greater than the sum of the parts. This is the mystery of voice and of movement. How these concepts materialize and combine within each of us is unique, and therefore the end result will always be unique to the individual, never a copy of someone else.[xvii] If one were to skip over the journey, the results would be less rich, less individual, and perhaps more an imitation of what one thinks the result should be.

Therefore, in reading this book, keep in mind that while written communication demands a linear progression, you may hop around, experiment and explore in various sections of the book, put ideas and sequences together in your own fashion, and still realize benefit from the work.

Another thing to bear in mind is that it is more important to apply the principles to your own body, at your own speed, acknowledging your own limitations, than it is to try to copy any of the illustrations in the book. These are only examples of the ways in which the work can be used; it is necessary for you to stay on your own path as you explore and experience. Not all people are or want to be the fastest runner in the world; yet, with the principles presented, anyone can run with good form and with carefreeness. Listen to your body.

Voice and Body vs. bodyvoice

Voice and body training can be studied separately, and there is much to be gained from such study. But there is also a potential loss for the student, who is usually required to figure out how the two go together. Lessac believed that there was no separation between the two; that what affected the body affected the voice and vice versa, and while there are those today who now advocate the same thing, he was ahead of his time when he began teaching that way. A strong focus of our teaching now is specific integrated body/voice explorations which provide the student with the experience of the interconnectedness of body/voice and also the disconnection that may occur when the two are combined. These disconnects are specific to each individual but normally occur from tension or holding the breath, both of which interfere with the easy functioning of the bodyvoice.[xviii] However, by identifying the spots where conflict occurs, it is possible for the trainer to help the student find the missing points of contiguous continuity, which allows the student to recognize the block or tension and approach resolving it with an atom-to-atom sense of discovery.

Continuing Evolution

Lessac felt that the principles of Kinesensics were present in all humans, in all cultures, and that therefore, it could adapt to all languages. Of course, this does not occur just from reading a book, which by its nature is finite and of a moment in time. The Lessac Institute has continued to explore the application of the basic principles of Kinesensics to other languages and cultures through workshops in South Africa, Croatia, Brazil, Puerto Rico, the Philippines, Malaysia, Thailand, Korea, Finland, Ireland, England, New Zealand and Australia. Through these journeys we have decided that the first principle (The Human Likeness Principle) needs adjustment. It is stated as "All human organisms, throughout the world, at one and the same time: are the same, vary, and are totally different. Although our dimensions vary and, experientially, each of us is unique, we are all structurally and organically precisely alike" (p. 5). We have re-stated it as, "The personal uniquenesses which we respect, embrace and celebrate are underscored by human likenesses presented in structural and organic manifestations." Does this seem like a small adjustment? I can assure you that when working in any country with a history of oppression, especially colonialist oppression, it makes a big difference to recognize our differences first and our likenesses second. One simply cannot say "We are all alike", because the experience of many has been one of marginalization and disempowerment. To recognize and celebrate our differences first leads us to the eventual discovery that those differences are underscored by some significant likenesses. Our journeying has confirmed that while our cultures and languages may seem to define and possibly differentiate us, pointing to diversity, there are organic congruencies which unite us, which when embraced contribute to inclusivity without diminishing our unique lived experiences. We embrace that we, as humans, with equal value and beauty are closer to one another than outside forces would have us believe. Respect for the interface between diversity and inclusivity is possible through moving and dancing together and through making sounds and singing together.

Body Wisdom opened my eyes to the possibility that expressive and healthy movement (and consequently voice) is not dependent on someone else's system because we all have our own, unique system. The knowledge we need is contained in our body's wisdom. We can all flourish when we learn to listen and follow its directives. It is my hope that as you read this book, you will discover how simple and effective are the solutions the body offers you. I trust that your journey will resonate with discovery, and that you will find better health and zest for life because of it.

References

Bánovčanová, Z. and Slavík, J., eds. 2014. Body in education. *Journal of Pedagogy*, 1, 5-8.

Dargin, T.C. 2016. *The Impact of Semi-Occluded Vocal Tract Exercises on Vocal Function in Singers: Straw Phonation vs. Lip Trill.* Unpublished PhD dissertation. https://kuscholarworks.ku.edu/bitstream/handle/1808/22392/Dargin_ku_0099D_14827_DATA_1.pdf?sequence=1 (accessed 15 October 2018).

Gallahue, D. L., Ozmun, J. C. & Goodway, J. D. (eds.). 2012. *Understanding motor development: infants, children, adolescents, adults.* 7th ed. New York : McGraw-Hill.

Gazzaniga, M.S. 2005. Forty-five years of split-brain research and still going strong. *Nature Reviews / Neuroscience* Vol 6, August: 653-659.

Hackney, P. 2002. *Making Connections: Total Body Connectivity through Bartenieff Fundamentals.* New York: Routledge.

Hart, S. 2018. *Brain, Attachment, Personality: An Introduction to Neuroaffective Development.* New York: Routledge.

Hocking, B., Haskell, J. and Linds, W., 2001. *Unfolding bodymind: exploring possibility through education.* Brandon, VT: Foundation for Educational Renewal.

Kabat-Zinn, J. 2005. *Full catastrophe living: Using the wisdom of your body and mind to face Stress, Pain and Illness* (15th anniversary edition). New York: Bantam Dell.

Le Guin, U.K. 1987. *The Left Hand of Darkness.* New York: The Berkley publishing Group.

Lövdén, M, Wenger, E, Mårtensson, J, Lindenberger, U & Bäckmann, L. 2013. Structural Brain Plasticity in Adult Learning and Development. *Neuroscience and Biobehavioral Reviews* 37:2296–2310.

MacLachlan, M. 2004. *Embodiment: clinical, critical and cultural perspectives on health and illness.* Berkshire: Open University Press, McGraw-Hill.

Mainemelis, C & Ronson, S. 2006. Ideas are Born in Fields of Play: Towards a Theory of Play and Creativity in Organizational Settings. *Research in Organizational Behavior* 27:81-131.

Munro, M. 2018. Principles for Embodied Learning Approaches. *South African Theatre Journal* Vol 31, Nr 1, March: 5-14.

Noland, C. 2009. *Agency and Embodiment: Performing Gestures/ Producing Culture.* Cambridge: Harvard University Press.

Robert, S. 2008. Words and their meanings: Principles of variation and stabilization. In: Martine Vanhove (ed), *From polysemy to semantic change: towards a typology of lexical semantic associations,* Studies in Language Companion Series 106, Amsterdam: John Benjamins: 55-92.

Stolz, S.A., 2015. Embodied learning. *Educational Philosophy and Theory*, 47 (5), 474–487.

Ellis, C. & Bochner, A.P. (eds.). 2002. *Ethnographically speaking: autoethnography, literature, and aesthetics.* Walnut Creek, CA: AltaMira Press.

Sparkes, A.C. 2002. Autoehtnography: self indulgence or something more? In: Ellis, C. & Bochner, A.P. (eds.), *Ethnographically speaking: autoethnography, literature, and aesthetics.* Walnut Creek, Calif: AltaMira Press.

Titze, I. R. 2000. Voice research: Phonation into a straw as a voice building exercise. *Journal of Singing – the Official Journal of the National Association of Teachers of Singing,* 57(1), 27-28.

Peterson, KL, Barkmeier, JM, Verdolini-Marston, K & Hoffman, HT. 1994. Comparison of Aerodynamic and Electroglottographic Parameters in Evaluating Clinically Relevant Voicing Patterns. *Annals of Otology, Rhinology and Laryngology* 103:335-346.

Verdolini, K, Druker, DG, DG, Palmer, PM, & Samawi, H. 1998. Laryngeal Adduction in Resonant Voice. *Journal of Voice* 12:315-327.

Verdolini-Marston, K, Burke, MK, Lessac, A, Glaze, L & Caldwell, E. 1995. Preliminary Study of Two Methods of Treatment for Laryngeal Nodules. *Journal of Voice* 9(1):74-85.

Watanabe, M. (ed.). 2017. *The Prefrontal Cortex as an Executive, Emotional, and Social Brain.* Japan: Springer.

Ward-Wimmer, D. 2003. The healing potential of adults at play. In: Charles E. Shaefer (ed), *Play therapy with adults.* New Jersey: John Wiley & Sons.

[i] Embodied learning is an approach to gaining deep structure knowledge and skills through "deliberate use and recognition of multimodal bodymind activities and strategies…" (Munro 2018: 3). A significant amount of scholarly discourse is available on this approach (see for example Bánovčanová & Slavík 2014; Stolz 2015).

[ii] See, for example, the seminal works of Kabat-Zinn (2005) on mindfulness.

[iii] In current research discourse this is referred to as autoethnographic research (see for example Ellis & Bochner 2002; Sparks 2002).

[iv] This meeting took place at Swarthmore in 1998.

[v] See the research done by Kitty Verdolini regarding LK and effective vocal fold activity (for example Peterson, Barkmeier, Verdolini-Marston & Hoffman 1994; Verdolini-Marston, Burke, Lessac, Glaze & Caldwell 1995; Verdolini, Druker, Palmer & Samawi 1998).

[vi] See Gazzaniga's 2005 essay providing an overview of the development of split-brain research. We acknowledge and uphold the interwovenness of the theory on the lateralization of brain functions and Paul McClean's Triune brain theory (Hart 2018) in current neuroscience discourse.

[vii] This perception is now shared by scholars such as Michael MacLachlan (2004).

[viii] Today we embrace this gestalt as a bodymind (Hocking, Haskell, & Linds 2001).

[ix] See Munro (2018: 5-14).

[x] "…words are not concepts, they are 'representation triggers' which present specific structural and functional properties and carry, along with their referential values, a whole fabric of structured relations" (Robert 2008:66). Following Robert it suffices to say that the referentiality and contextuality of language is alive and continuously developing over time, influenced by both cultural and subject formations. Meanings of words, as referential values, shift.

[xi] See Lifter, Foster-Sanda, Arzamarski, Briesch and McClure (2011) for a discussion on the importance of play in early development, Mainemelis and Ronson (2006) for the importance of play for adults in organizational success, and Ward-Wimmer (2003) regarding the healing effects of play on adults.

xii Similar terms are found in other embodied approaches. For example, Hackney (2002) defines dynamic alignment from within the Laban/Bartenieff lexicon.

xiii This progression honours and supports the human developmental movement patterns (see Gallahue, Ozmun & Goodway 2012).

xiv See Titze, (2000) as well as Dargin (2016), for explanations regarding the usage of a straw towards effective vocalization.

xv This is clarified by the "curvo-linear" principle offered in Lessac Kinesensics (Body Wisdom p7).

xvi The 'permission to teach oneself', relates to the prefrontal cortex's executive, emotional and social functions (see Watanabe [2017] for a discussion on the functions of the prefrontal cortex).

xvii The personally unique manifestation and shaping of self relates to the interwoven presence of body plasticity (MacLachlan 2004) and neuroplasticity (Lövdén, Wenger, Mårtensson, Lindenberger, & Bäckmann, 2013), which is continuously informed by the lived experience (Noland 2009).

xviii Here we follow in Lessac's footsteps creating a neologism that demonstrates the monist gestalt that the training promotes.

INTRODUCING BODY WISDOM

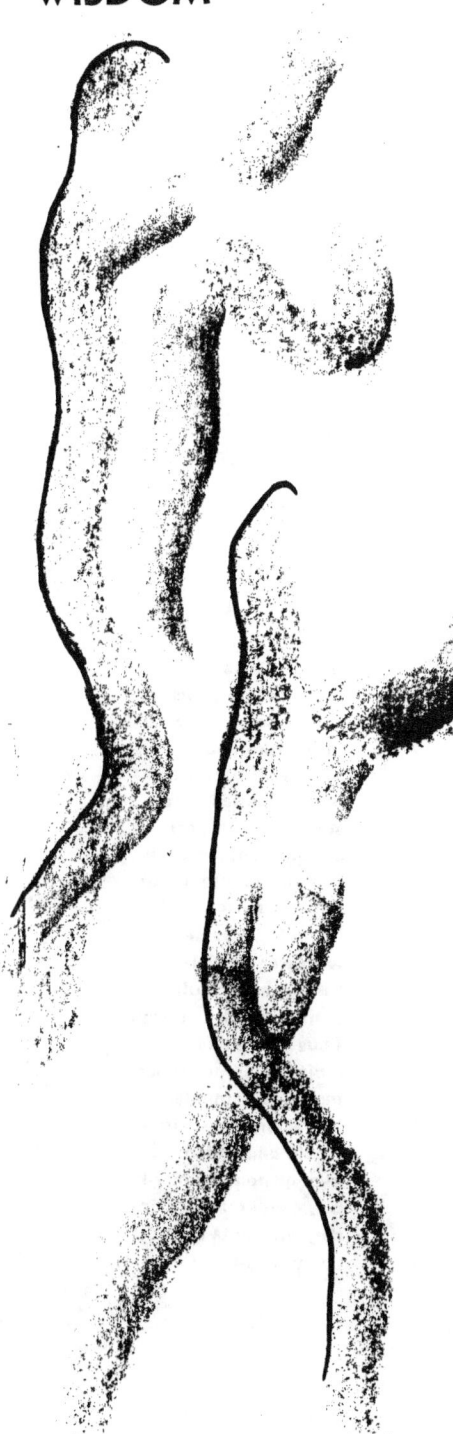

This is a book about dissolving patterns — patterns that work against our natural, instinctive "Body Wisdom," patterns that needlessly put day-to-day (dis)stress and strain on the human organism, patterns that lead to imbalance. *BODY WISDOM* takes us farther along the path first charted with the publication of *The Use and Training of the Human Voice*.

In that work, itself a radical departure from traditional approaches to voice and speech training, I was principally concerned with Vocal Life — seen for the first time as a function of both emotional life and the larger, physical life of the human organism. Here, I am engaged in exploring the language, or more accurately, the many different languages of the body; and discovering how these languages translate and interpret into optimal body functioning.

Since *The Use and Training of the Human Voice* first appeared seventeen years ago, the work has continued, through teaching, therapy, applied research, training workshops, and a series of experimental studies, toward a fuller development of the motor and sensory skills of the entire **human** body. The result of this continuously expanding work is *BODY WISDOM: a new approach to the use and training of the human body* through a new **organic/sensory learning process.**

For many of you who have already applied the experience of our training in voice and speech to your personal and professional lives, *BODY WISDOM* provides not only a companion piece to the first volume, but an umbrella under which verbal and vocal energy can thrive alongside the body's other potent energizers and inter-locking communication systems. For those, from all walks of life, who approach my work for the first time through *BODY WISDOM,* I offer the following introduction to the premises and assumptions of Lessac training.

I believe now, as I did years ago, that with the awareness of certain basic concepts, all human beings can teach themselves to use the "body-whole" constructively, harmoniously, like a finely-tuned instrument — the way nature designed it to be used. Organic defect or accident aside, we all possess the most superb equipment. We are all Stradivari. And we each have the capacity for self-teaching to esthetically realize the full potential of every part of our bodies and of all our body's diversified energy.

We do not need to improve upon our Stradivarius. Rather, we need to teach ourselves how to keep it in tune, **feel** its harmony, consonance,

Introducing
Body
Wisdom

melodies and chords. We need to regard the body as a precious, delicate instrument. And that means using it, not abusing it. Muscles, joints, and nerves are not power tools. They are systems that create motion, as an orchestra creates tone.

The feelings and awareness of sensory experience I want to call forth in you are designed to demonstrate how you can use your body in an optimal way. For the physicist, the optimal principle is a formulation of how nature finds the best way. For us, *BODY WISDOM* is nothing more, but nothing less, than the **optimal use of the human body.** And that is what I want you to teach yourself or rather, recapture for yourself since as children, you and I both possessed this knowledge as instinctive behavior. It was natural. It felt good. But for most of us, it's been deadened or lost and has been replaced by other patterns — anesthetic ones, more rigid ones.

Consider for a moment:

- that one out of three Americans suffers daily from "lower backaches";
- that one in five suffers from such back conditions as scoliosis and lordosis;
- that one in twelve endures chronic belly-aches;
- that one of every three major operations in the U.S. deals with ulcers, gallstones, colitis, ileitis or other similar digestive ailments;
- that head-aches, high back strain, and neck tension are even more common;
- that jaw tension is nearly universal.

NOTE: Certain word hyphenations, such as "indigenous" on page 3, may strike you as somewhat peculiar or ungrammatical. From the standpoint of clear articulation, remedial reading techniques, or esthetic speech qualities, I find it desirable, wherever possible, to start every syllable with a sounded consonant. Thus words like indigenous, remarkable, meditate, reminder, characteristic, unusual would be divided: in-di-ge-nous, re-mar-ka-ble, me-di-tate, re-min-der, cha-rac-te-ris-tic, un-(y)u-su-(w)al.

And then, there are the psycho-physical (dis)stresses of dry throat, nausea, itching, scratching, weariness, paling, helplessness, fear, self-consciousness, discomfiture when sweating, blushing, yawning, sighing, and certain allergies that would benefit from of a sensible diet of Body Wisdom.

That we need a change of diet is clear. That we have been too myopic to recognize and use the proper diet, so close at hand, is also clear. We need to learn how to preserve those natural capacities left behind in childhood that only our consumate athletes, actors, and artists continue to use so instinctively well.

Introducing
Body
Wisdom

You may feel that it is not a simple matter of training to achieve the mastery of a great singer, a great dancer, a great actor, or an Olympic gold medalist. Let us understand each other. I harbor no illusions that everyone will or even could become a Caruso, a Pavlova, an Olivier, or a Jesse Owens. But it is certainly conceivable that some **potential Carusos, Pavlovas, Oliviers, and Owenses** among us are being lost or limited every day, because of conditioned anxieties that block instinctive, organic instructions to the body and place our body's language systems into competitive conflict with one another. As soon as we begin to worry about how we look, how we want to perform, how we need to win, or how we dread losing — all self-images that derive from the outer, not the inner, environment — our body is in conflict with itself, and any greatness that might have been exploited from natural, in-born capacities is instantly aborted.

Let's put it differently. You may or may not ever run Roger Bannister's four-minute mile, or the 3:40 record many milers have since confidently thrust toward. But you **can** learn how to move swiftly and smoothly, using the same "relaxer-energizers" that propel the great runners, without fatigue or undue psycho-physical tension.

You may or may not ever sing like Caruso. But once you investigate the science of vocal art and find that physically, every normal human organism has an optimal vocal range of more than four complete octaves, you'll be much less satisfied with a mere octave and a half. Why not teach yourself to acquire these, rather than waste yourself yearning for them?

Too often, we assume that the use of these natural talents and instinctive skills is simply beyond the reach of average mortals — that these body esthetics, as we perceive them, are somehow gifts from heaven specially sent to the chosen few. This is neither just nor true. What Body Wisdom teaches is the motivation to realistic possibility based on the awareness that one's "art in life" invariably precedes one's "life in art!"

Self-teaching for Body Wisdom is probably the most cost-efficient learning available to us, yielding the maximum return for the minimum investment. Through organic/sensory learning, we can teach ourselves to discover and exploit those human talents and intelligences indige*-nous to the body. In effect, we can teach ourselves by being taught by our bodies. And so doing, **all areas of our brain,** not just the hemispheres we're conditioned to use, becomes active in the process of realizing optimal condition.

*See Marginal note page 2.

*Physical education
    is NOT
    just a
mechanical "conditioning";
    it is
    a coordination
with a state of mind,
with the perceptual
    and emotional
AND artistic process,
with the voice...
    which is a part of
    the body!*

*...effective communication,
psychological health,
    and a
salutary body condition
    are all
    strongly dependent
    upon an
intrinsic interaction
with one another!*

Introducing
Body
Wisdom

Simply put, the self-teaching objectives of Body Wisdom are to train the individual to:

> discover the relationship between body and language in order to explore the "languages of the body";
>
> develop the finest, naturally functioning communicating skills including vocal, verbal, and the body's other physical languages;
>
> coordinate, through organic feeling, all the communicating systems of the body for efficiency and effectiveness;
>
> re-establish the science and art of instinctive body skills and talents;
>
> use these natural skills and instinctive talents with esthetic awareness so that the organic experience is felt, perceived, and responded to; and finally,
>
> apply this esthetic experience to the development of one's full creative potential in the arts, in sports, at work, at home, at play.

*...body wisdom
suggests
we teach
the use of the voice
as a part of
physical fitness...
not only does the voice
need a good body,
but the body
needs
a
good voice!*

As "Body Wisdom" is the universal potential of every human being, indeed the **resource of every human being**, this work is offered to all and accessible to everyone: rich or poor; man or woman; student or teacher; child or adult; university-trained or self-educated. Body Wisdom is a natural human resource, there to be learned from whether the learner went to the best schools or the worst schools; whether widely traveled or sedately sedentary; whether a laborer, an executive, or an athlete, a physicist, a typist, or an actor; whether in business, office work, nursing, industry, government, education, or the arts. And because Body Wisdom is the only constant — the only value-free — body of knowledge, to which all human beings, by being human, can relate, it is intrinsically cross-cultural.

*... our research
and discoveries
about voice
body
language
music
indicates that
there is an instinctive
process in the body that
has intelligence;
that there is an
instinctive
genius
inside our body.
We can see it
in our children
and we must demand it
in ourselves!*

This, then, is a book about the **ecology of the human body**, the ecology of human potential.

This is a book about new languages — new forms of organic communication between ourselves and our bodies; between our voluntary minds and our instincts; between our words and our behavior.

This is a book about the potential health, sanity, balance, focus, esthetics, movement, rhythm of the human body, all inherent within the body environment.

This is a book about being human.

Part One
A HUMAN ECOLOGY

Preface to
PART ONE

On Finding the Way

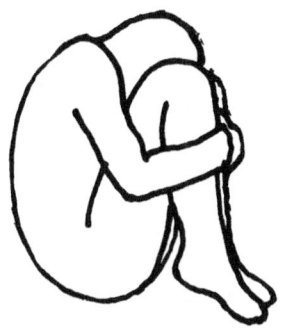

The approach to the use and training of the human body involves a good many principles, premises, and theoretical concepts of current scientific thought. It also incorporates several principles which have been intuitively derived from my experimental work and may be considered "pre-scientific."

At the root of our "feeling process" is an integral view of the human organism, perceived as **naturally** capable of instinctive as well as intellectual life within the single body community. This integral view is reinforced by the recent evidence of "twin-brain" research, which through parallel studies in controlled experiments, has argued persuasively for the "two dominances" within each of us: the intuitive and the logical. The concept of two dominances informs the relationship between body and language, and the very notion of "inner body languages," I first articulated seventeen years ago in *The Use and Training of the Human Voice*. Now, in the present broader work, it becomes the fundamental **gestalt** of my approach to reclaim the natural inheritance of "Body Wisdom;" and underscores the renunciation of the dominance of one side of the body over the other.

Among the integrative concepts indigenous to "Body Wisdom", which will be more fully developed in succeeding chapters, are the following:

- **The "Human Likeness" Principle.** All human organisms, throughout the world, at one and the same time: are the same, vary, and are totally different. Although our dimensions vary and, experientially, each of us is unique, we are all structurally and organically precisely alike.

- **The Human "Musical Instrument" Principle.** The body is a remarkable musical instrument. It is a string instrument, a reed, brass, percussion and sound effect instrument. It can be "played upon" and "play itself."

- **The Principle of "Inner Harmonic Sensing."** Defines the process of a modality of "feeling," through organic sensation and perception, that leads to **kinesthetic understanding and appreciation.** Our term for this kinesthetic understanding, this physical awareness, this body esthetic appreciation, is **"kinesensics."**

Preface
to
Part One

- **The "Perceptive Awareness" Principle.** Perceptual awareness from the outer environment takes place through the five fundamental senses, whereas percep**tive** awareness from the personal inner environment occurs through a synesthesic "harmonic-overtone" sensory system that **feels** the seeing, hearing, touching, and tasting internally and differently, but always with harmony, concord, and order. As soon as perceptual awareness, from the outside, registers in and upon the individual inner environment, it converts to sensation, perception, awareness, and response — and relates directly to the "inner harmonic" senses.

- **The "Habitual Awareness" Principle.** An ongoing, internal sending and receiving system that processes the cues and signals from the performance of any act. The word "habitual" does not here imply a habit-formed awareness. On the contrary, habitual awareness suggests an almost non-voluntary accompaniment of information-gathering intelligence to every conscious and indeed, every subconscious act. It is the state of perception-sensation that accommodates the individual's own response to his own self. Habitual awareness is associated with de-patterned behavior and is inner-directed input **and** output.

- **The "De-Patterning" Principle.** It is possible to establish a foundation of reawakened awareness by which our habit-formed patterns can be de-patterned. That is to say, the awareness will catch those habits in the act; challenge them, redefine them, refamiliarize us with them, make them fluid, and return them to our creative resource(s). Flexibility thus induced, the "habit" is neutralized, negated, and we are then able to respond to internal cues and signals that guard against unbalanced, unnecessary erosion. A habit ceases to be a habit the instant one is aware of it — in use.

- **The "Carefreeness" Principle.** The perception of carefreeness functions as a "safety-cushion," permitting us to sense internal rhythm, or any of our other relaxer-energizer states, as motivation and **reward-satisfaction** in any body act. When we sense "carefree" awareness, we **viscerally** understand how **not** to accommodate tension which results in the absence of tension. It is the positive result of feeling the **something** that took the place of tension. The "Carefreeness Principle" does not involve either "carefulness" (anxiety, apprehension, doubt) or "carelessness" (self-indulgence or complete lack of awareness/perception).

- **The "Balanced Muscle-Tonicity" Principle.** In the performance of any and every act, no matter how vigorous or strenuous, one must experience a **measurable** degree of **active resting** or relaxation; conversely, in every or any experience of body relaxation, one must be able to identify some quality of **dynamic energy.** This suggests an ongoing psycho-physical vitalization of the body wherein all muscles (and nerves) are continuously alive and vibrant — never tight, never dead, always energized.

- **The "Vocal Sound Stream" Principle.** The vocal sound stream differs radically in action, character, and substance from the breath stream. Sound travels at approximately 1200 feet per second; it is a molecular action and resonates any hard substance. Breath travels at approximately 12 feet per second; it is a wind-like sweeping action and disperses particles or sound waves in its path. While science considers the "breath stream" as the "motivator" or "agitator" of voice production, there is no longer certainty on this point. Recent research by French scientists suggests instead that the so-called vocal cords may in fact be stimulated and vibrated by neural impulses, rather than by the breath stream. But even if the breath is indeed the motivator, its relationship to the sound stream at best, is a sequential one working "in relay" with it. As regards voice production and vocal "tone," the contribution of the breath stream terminates at the point that the sound stream initiates its process of conduction, resonance, and wave reflection.

- **The "Curvo-Linear" Principle.** involves three theorems:

    a. that the human organism is to be viewed and experienced as a curvo-linear structure rather than as a linear one — i.e. without "straightness," rigidness," or "fixed stiffness;"

    b. that the body's naturally curved line follows a single, directional blend of the parenthesis-like bow shape, the circle, the wheel, and the sphere;

    c. that the human body evolved from a small, compact spherical ball (or egg shape) — to an expanded, hemispherical shape – to an elongated and extended curve.

The most important curvo-linear area in the human body is the spinal column. Contrary to accepted "fact," the vertebral architecture and postural inter-relationship is such that the spine, naturally and instinctively, follows essentially the shape of a single, parenthesis-like curve rather than a multiple "S" curve. Many of the fundamental objectives and exercises of the later work chapters relate to the Curvo-Linear (C-curve) Principle.

Preface
to
Part One

- **The "Generalization" Principle.** The concept of generalization cuts across energies and body esthetics, and provides a direct follow-through to our concepts of "generalized body balance," "generalized rhythm experience," "generalized concentration," and "generalized attention," all of which pervade *BODY WISDOM*. It also relates to the concept of habitual awareness, which is as easily defined as "generalized awareness" or alertness. I use the term "generalized" in the sense of a holistic, in-depth, cross-quality synthesis that results in an omnipresent, esthetic perceptiveness always in process of movement and change. It is in this sense that we instinctively discover (and can explore) emerging truths regarding the natural extension of body movement to vocal life — of vocal life to posture and breathing — of posture and breathing to balanced vibrant tone — of balanced, vibrant, rich tone to good, communicating inter-involvement — all the way to personal reinforcement and fulfillment through esthetic rhythms, melodies, impulses, images, etc.

- **The "Unique Event" Principle.** When a body activity is experienced so genuinely as to bear no relation to patterned behavior or conditioned repetitiveness, it becomes for us a "unique event." A unique event is, thus, always an "original," fresh experience, never a facsimile of a previous occurrence, even though it may be a prototypical **re-experience** of a "familiar" body event.

Other theoretical constructs independently derived in the laboratories of physicists, physiologists, and biochemists also find application or adaptive use in the investigation of body wisdom. Among these:

- **The Feedback Principle** which we use, as a self-teaching strategy, to communicate to ourselves how we should **feel** when we are doing something **healthy** for the body and therefore, **helpful** and **desirable**.

- **The Distribution Principle** is for us a command principle that helps to distribute the work force, or energy flow, or other physical action over a maximally enlarged area. You don't sing with your throat alone, or lift a weight with your arm alone, or run with your legs alone, or feel enthusiasm with your eyes alone. Even in the event of pain, you can, by involving the "body-whole," transfer its quantity and quality to a point of **disappearance**.

On
Finding
The Way

The Diminishing Fatigue Principle is a corollary of the distribution principle. If a task is shared by as many muscles as possible, if each muscle is minimally stressed, if a minimum of waste products is allowed to accumulate, then fatigue is minimal and each muscle retains a reasonably continuous capacity to function. Energy sites are distributed and "energy flows" are induced and encouraged. Whenever there prevails this absence of local overload, we experience a relaxed energy and relaxation in action.

The "Time-Lag Catch-Up" Principle is really the basis for our pre-scientific principle of "balanced muscle tonicity". As applied to our theory of muscle dynamics, it infers that muscle sensation is altered once a sense of **"loosening"** feeds into the **working, tightened muscle fibre** — and once a "movement-dynamic" feeds into the **resting, relaxed,** muscle. We see finely tuned muscles always vibrating between, as well as during, contraction and extension. They are always "in play" whether relaxed or active. What we adaptively learn from the Time-Lag Catch-Up Principle is that muscles ought never "work" in one direction of maximum stress. But rather, like a vibrating guitar string, while oscillating between opposite states of "maximum stress" they pass through a state of "minimum stress;" thus creating the **feel** of a "third force **optimal stress.**" Muscles in tune with such a dynamic will **play not work**; or better still, they must play **while** they work. The concept uncovered here is a key to the nature of play itself — a constant "looping by-play" between work and relaxation, each one existing integrally within the body of the other. Perhaps this is the secret of never-ending endurance and eagerness-energy of the young child.

The Wave Principle as applied to our understanding of the "body in movement" and "movement within the body," is based on a chain-reacting molecular conductivity. In each molecule, the molecular reaction begins with a state of agitation which is converted to a smooth flow as the stimulus is passed on to the next molecule creating a continuing flow (or wave) of energy.

• **The Kinematic Principle,** applied throughout our work, develops an appreciation of and sensitivity to the fascinating varieties of body movement — i.e. of "the body in motion" as well as "motion in the

Preface
TO
Part One

body." It leads to understanding and perceiving the relative motions, radiations, and "gentle turbulences" functioning within the inner body enviornment: moving muscle, moving energy fields and energy states, moving breath currents, moving brain waves, different moving balances, moving neural impulses, the moving bloodstream, the moving heartbeat, etc.

NOTE: The reader should consider this preface to Part One as a glossary-like introduction to some of the pre-scientific (as well as scientific) principles, concepts, terminology, etc., which I have used in this investigation of body wisdom.

1
MOVING BEYOND WILDNESS

Chapter 1

Moving Beyond Wildness

As we stated in INTRODUCING BODY WISDOM, all human beings have potentially superb equipment, barring illness, defect, or accident. Some human beings manage to realize this potential. Those who do, place themselves on a path to greatness and often become our great athletes, our great talents, our great artists. Unfortunately, the realization of natural human potential is becoming so rare that it is beginning to be perceived as something almost super-human. Natural human potential is an organic combination of physical, emotional, and perceptual relationships. The physical are the most tangible, and once they are understood, the others follow suit.

Life often ends because some vital organ or organs deteriorate prematurely while the rest of the body is still in pretty good shape. Just as vital organs deteriorate, so does human potential.

◄ What Is Natural?

Unhappily, the attrition of Body Wisdom occurs with most people in three ways:

1. we lose relationship and empathy with our body and forget how to communicate with it.

2. the body and the awareness of our body become conditioned to outside constraints, inhibitions, and superimposed "standards."

3. the body, itself, deteriorates much too soon: breathing becomes irregular and inefficient; posture becomes harmfully incorrect; perception becomes restricted and categorized, thereby leading to imitative behavior. Awareness of what is happening to the body is thus inhibited.

These three "destruct patterns" happen together and feed each other, so we never do learn what our body's potential was before it ceased to function!

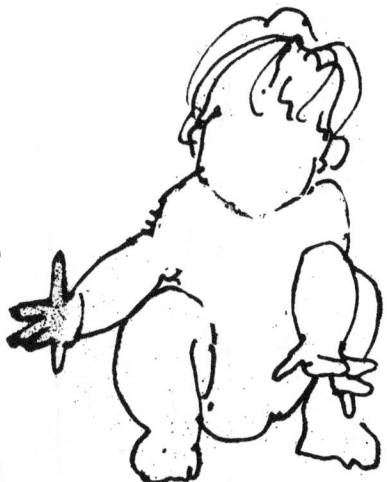

But the capacity to coordinate all of the body's in-born potential remains a natural one. We all once had it. It is still reclaimable. We need to learn how to preserve those natural capacities used so instinctively by the great and natural athletes, singers, actors, artists, scientists, and innovators. But how? Can everyone achieve it? Perhaps not — at least not all of it. However, anyone can achieve significant parts of it, and everyone working to understand and physically feel the "essence" of Body Wisdom will, in time, develop all of it.

A
Human
Ecology

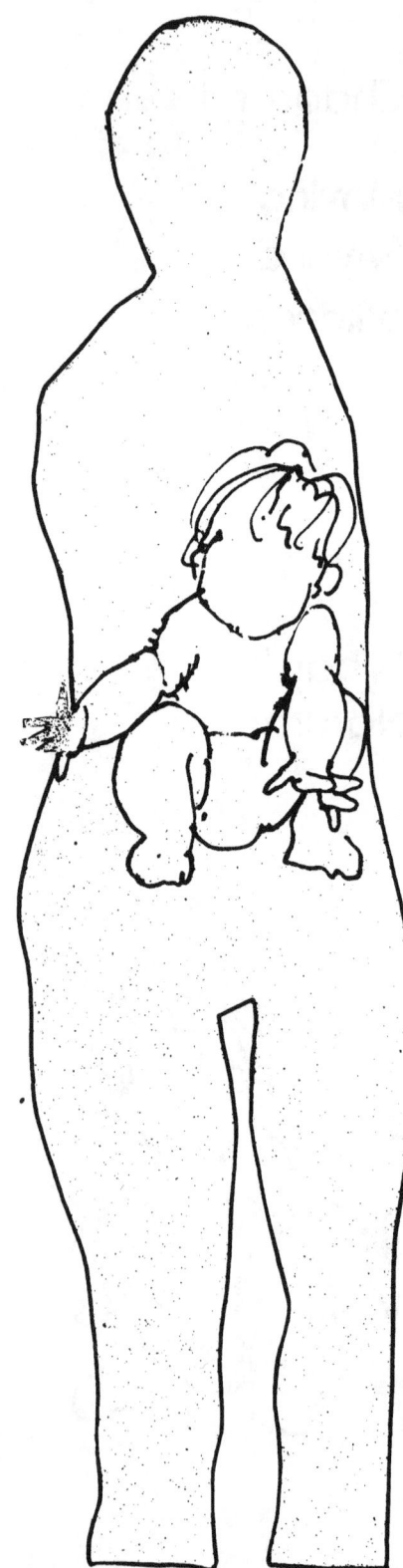

There is an increasing awareness that a certain kind of synchronization and coordination between the body, the mind, and the emotions is a natural inheritance of the young child. It is also an unfortunate fact of modern existence that this natural synchronization is destroyed as the child grows older — as he is conditioned by traditional educational processes and is subject to various imitative forms of how to stand, how to breathe, how to talk, how to read, etc.

What is it about the child that seems so valuable to us? What do children have that we have lost? Or more to the point, what have **we** acquired that the child with its infinite Body Wisdom rejects outright as counter-productive — as an assault upon its natural instincts? Clearly, we do some things better than a child. So what is the "natural" that we must recapture from childhood?

Well, it would be nice to be able to "unlearn" or transform certain kinds of emotional fear. It would be nice to understand how we can deal with fear as an energy state that can be converted to a state of curiosity, enthusiasm, or just plain intensified anticipation.

It would be nice to rid ourselves of useless and debilitating guilt. It would be nice to recapture the spontaneous inventiveness of the child. It would be nice to be able to fall like a child, without falling quite as often as a child.

It would be nice to have a voice, pure and unobstructed, that can sing as well as speak; that can call across great distances without injury or bodily damage. It would be very nice to retain the perpetual ingenuousness and the refreshing ingenuity of the child. All of this would be nice, but we are not children!

It is not easy to enjoy the healthy innocence of the child — to be **childlike** without being **childish**. Our bodies and minds and motivations are different. And they need to be differently synchronized. Besides, truth be told, we do not really trust ourselves to become children, nor do we truly trust the child in the role of guide and mentor — even if the child does seem to have the key to "what is natural."

What we're talking about, here, is the discovery of a process, not merely a vague remembrance of things past. In the most systematic terms, we need to better understand **how it is** that the "pre-conditioned" child uses his natural capacities so well and so spontaneously. True, we once experienced this synchronization. But as children we experienced it without awareness, without understanding and to a large extent, without appreciation.

As adults, we must now relearn this synchronization as a **new learning process**, for it is not a simple inheritance. We can and will relearn how to perceive, recognize, and respond to the primal cues, signals, intelligence, and creativity of the back brain and spine; how to relate to the **intuitive** as well as the so-called **tuitive** or logical hemisphere of the brain. The insight once provided by these areas has been silenced, subdued, and subverted rather than outgrown. We have been categorically conditioned to ignore the cues and signals of our **inner body languages** which, when allowed to atrophy, are easily deposed.

Literally, we need to learn how to speak with ourselves. And that means relearning the languages of the body — how to interpret them, how to communicate with them, how to use them to reclaim the body's natural genius. As we will experience through the later work chapters, this new form of organic communication — in fact, an old intelligence — is rooted in **non-linear language** that "instructs" the body **to do** and **to know what the body is doing** through "feel."

Once reclaimed, the body languages establish a foundation of awareness that softens and melts away habit-conditioned patterns, making them fluid and once again responsive to the day-to-day need for movement and change. Moreover, this foundation yields up the internal cues and signals that serve as empathic guards against unbalanced, unnecessary wear and tear of the body along with its perceptual and emotional systems. In relearning what we once knew, we will teach ourselves how to make the body's natural wisdom an integral and organic part of our active intelligence, our creative skills, our innate talents, our very existence.

Precisely because we are more than ever immersed in chaos, we need to learn how the body **wants** to function, instinctively and naturally, and what are its optimal capacities. At the same time, we need to recognize how present environmental influences destructively condition the individual's inner body environment with the result that our natural capacities and potential are lost to us.

Consider that there are today two separate environments: the inner body environment of each, individual human organism; and the outer collective environment that includes everything outside with everyone else in it. Pitted against each other, both environments are in danger of being destroyed.

...the role of language is not ornamental; it is to teach us to express and speak as we feel and see and hear; we ought not consider a physical, imagistic, emotional, use of language to be "over our heads"!

We traditionally don't feel language in relationship to our body and to our emotions; this is because language is treated as a system of symbols and of "naming", thus having nothing to do with the physical and/or spatial systems!

◀ **The Two Environments**

A
Human
Ecology

We are so conditioned by the outside environment that our very bodily processes have been taught to keep pace with chaos. While keeping pace with chaos might seem to be an achievement, it is in fact a programmed escape – from both environments. Even our intellect has become part of the outer environment, divorced from its birthright in Body Wisdom. Unconsciously caught and unaware of a conflict between the body's native, instinctive response mechanism and the environment's chaotic stimuli from the outside, the problem-solving choices at our disposal only contribute to producing fear, anxiety, conflict, and tension, further advancing the deterioration of the body, its balance and its relationship to feelings and thought.

The outer environment's influences and controls, shaped and shaded as they are by ritual, by convention, by economic considerations, by physical standards, and by imitative **self-images,** are all too casually tolerated as understandable, and therefore acceptable, in the adult world.

Perhaps not so easy to understand or accept are the different clashing effects these influences and controls exert upon the instinctive inclinations and rhythms of the child—of the innocent, naturally inquisitive child. The clash occurs for the "developing, young inner environment" when internal "gut instinct" and intuition collide with externally imposed conditioning and supervision, especially when this conditioning is based upon imitation of vocal and physical behavior which later becomes part of the matured self-image.

The destructive undercurrent of this conflict between the two environments is not always perceived as a clash or felt as non-coordination by the individual. When our entire developmental process is so strongly determined by the external environment, certain standards, certain modes of functioning, certain processes of learning become accepted not only as normal but as the **only** way to do things. The body's natural abilities and capacities become desynchronized early in our development. By the time we reach adulthood, we perceive this as normal; intellectually, we accept it as necessary.

It is neither normal nor necessary. It is a false synchronization resulting from a "least resistance" to outer environment conditioning, and it is a compromised synchronization that in every way is destructive to the achievement of full human capacity. This is unhealthy compromise. How to avoid it?

Moving
Beyond
Wildness

The Two
Environments

One way to begin avoiding it is to recognize that the human body is truly a total community with an ecology all its own. The human organism is a bona fide environment where multifarious activities take place; where there is vital life; where feeling and experiencing processes function; where ongoing regeneration occurs; where germ populations shift and metamorphose; where transformation and conversion of body energy take place; where health-generating and breeder-reactor systems operate; where homeostatic dynamics function; where information, intelligence, and signals are supplied, gathered, and recalled; where different body languages are seeded, grow, and develop if called upon; where all of these wonders and dynamics can mature into a personal culture, into creative and artistic functioning, into living up to the once-cherished "dignity of man." The individual body environment contains its own renaissance, its own humanism, its own unlimited range of realistic possibilities.

Our concept of body ecology and the ecology of human potential requires a process of peaceful co-existence between the two environments; that the small human environment, so potentially fertile, may be sufficiently protected to resist the pulls of the larger, more arid outside environment. Instead of perceiving ourselves totally within the context of our social environment — and deriving our self-image from this unilateral relationship — why can't we begin to understand and re-evaluate our environment **in terms of human potential?** We must reacquire the knowledge to organize and introduce an entirely different set of stimuli, standards, and learning processes that, once again, come **from** the small body environment rather than **to** it. Our task is to discover an inner framework that will instruct us to function satisfactorily within the outer framework, (without being destroyed by it), and eventually to become one with it again.

The healthy body is flexible. If it can accommodate decisions that lead to unhealthy compromise such as accepting the lesser of the two evils, it can also accommodate decisions that lead to healthy compromise of accepting the lesser of the two goods. From the aspect of psychosomatic health, it becomes clear that once attuned to and in tune with the pioneering and radical inner body environment, one can in good conscience make even an unpalatable decision and gain sustenance from having made it. We cannot isolate ourselves from the chaos and insanity of the outer environment forever, nor can we simply withdraw from it.

A
Human
Ecology

We can and must require an environment that permits the development of a **personal culture** within the body. Any collective culture is only the sum total of all the personal cultures within it. Yet personal culture is not and need not be a mirror-image of collective culture. Too many of us are half-people working with only one part of our brain.

The "body-whole," as a psycho-physical instrument, is far more complex than any single one or combination of its experiencing systems, and offers an infinite source for input. When we understand how this "inner input" works and train ourselves to use it, control it, and communicate with it, then will the individual learning process become richer, more intrinsically appropriate and provide more knowledge through self-teaching than through information-processing from the outside world.

In the last analysis, we should recall that all of our education in traditional teaching, training, and learning situations is greatly dependent upon imitation. The way families bring up children — the way institutions educate — the way teachers instruct and train — has to do primarily with learning how to gear one's behavior to imitating (now fashionably called "modeling") the external environment. Essentially, this means the individual, the student, or the child learns to compare, plot, and develop his sense of identity and experience in relation to norms, standards, and even the "natural progressions" of the outside environment.

We learn how outside things work and what they look like. We learn how other people appear, how they talk and walk. We learn how to do and follow what we see and hear. We learn to think in relation to the outside world. **We learn to imitate and we imitate to learn.**

Such learning, dependent upon input from the external environment, is destructive by virtue of the fact that it influences us to accept as right, only one kind of learning that, because of its outer-directedness, obscures our awareness, our attention, and ultimately our ability to learn creatively from **our own internal body environment.**

This does not suggest that our approach to "body wisdom" is to be construed as even a temporary **withdrawal-process** into the individual inner environment. Our path is rather a dynamic process of **perceiving the body's internal movement, stimulation, vitality and gentle turbulence, and of utilizing this intelligence by turning our understanding outward with greater courage and imagination.**

Beyond Wildness

There was a time when the environment, in and of itself, elicited a smooth flowing response from the human organism; a time when the body and mind operated in consonance with one another and in accord with the rhythms of the immediate surroundings; a time when the environment was "wild" and the human animal, in order to survive and survive better, actually had to function better.

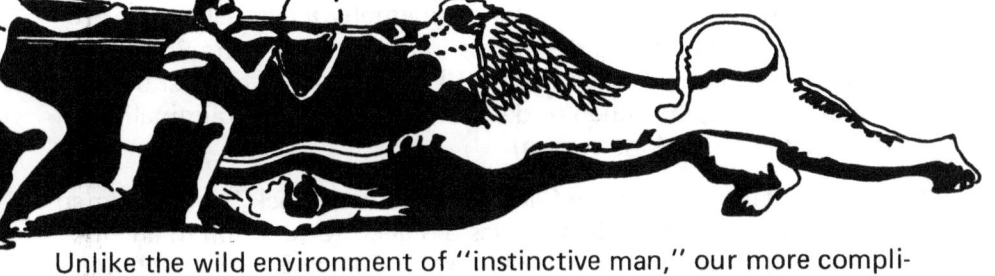

Unlike the wild environment of "instinctive man," our more complicated and socially determined environment no longer **demands** complete health of the human instrument, just various, prescribed forms of "social health." In exchange for the advances of civilization, technology, moral and ethical codes, systems of law and government, social and economic order, and the ascension over all other living beings, we have left behind the instinctive, physically reactive human instrument. It seems a small cost to pay for civilization, and in the past there has always been a balance between what was gained and what was lost.

Indeed, as long as the **psychology of institutions** remains constant, we can continually evolve self-images that make sense. This happens naturally as an adaptive reaction to changing environmental frameworks. But now, those frameworks are shifting. We experience immense changes within the space of a single lifetime. Our entire sense of time has shifted. Body time and social time are out of sync. The natural environment is polluted. Our institutions have become inconsistent. Worse, they are chaotic and contradictory. The "civilized constants" we've become used to are no longer working. Societal frameworks and behavioral standards that allowed us to perceive ourselves within some outer, unchanging context are no longer trusted. Religious and moral constants no longer exist. Political and ideological constants have failed. And even sexual frameworks are in a state of rapid, uncertain transition. The more constants disappear, the more we lose our **own sense of context.**

In other words, the balance is being lost. As a result, we are still deteriorating physically and perceptually, but no longer growing intellectually. We still accept, as normal, poor posture, poor breathing, tension, anxiety; the loss of musicianship in our voices, a lack of perceptual and physical responsiveness; increasingly more frequent psychosomatic illnesses, disease, weakened states of body and mind — only the exchange rate has changed as the justifying norm for these unhealthy compromises has had its bottom drop out.

The chaos and constantly shifting currents of the outer environment have had a jarring effect upon the psycho-physical balance of the human organism. The condition has become so serious, though long in coming, that we've even adopted a common terminology around it. And Alvin Toffler's book, not coincidentally a best-seller, has provided us with a compelling descriptor in the term "Future Shock." We need to protect ourselves against "Future Shock" by first understanding what it is, and then understanding how it is subliminally buffetting the natural instrument.

Properly understood, Future Shock is "Culture Shock" to the human body — at least to the body as it was designed to function in an environment that once was "wild." Because of Future Shock, psychological evolution is no longer a natural process from generation to generation. Consequently, survival in the Age of Future Shock is no longer a question of further "civilization."

What, then, are we looking for? What do we have left to hold onto? Where is the new context, now that the "civilized constants" are no longer working? The fact of the matter is: We (the human organisms) are the only remaining "natural environment" that is reclaimable. This is our context. We may not function, as an adult species, with the health that was implicit in the human instrument when the environment was truly wild, nor would we, if we could, return as knowing, communicating, intellectual beings to that environment.

But we can regain some of the instinctive Body Wisdom that was lost along the way. It is constantly regenerated everytime a child is born and grows naturally until that child is conditioned out of optimal functioning by the imitative standards, now shifting and inconsistent, of the outer environment. It is possible to understand ourselves as natural instinctive environments of our own, and to construct self-images within the context of "kinesensic" awareness. If we reconstruct this awareness as a body of knowledge and allow it to become a complex source of our self-image, we may at least create for ourselves **one** unchanging environment, one constant referent, to which we can organically relate.

To do this means moving not back to wildness, but **beyond wildness.** Wildness is a state of being, involving a sense of self that is simple, impulsive, and instinctive. True wildness — nature's original — does

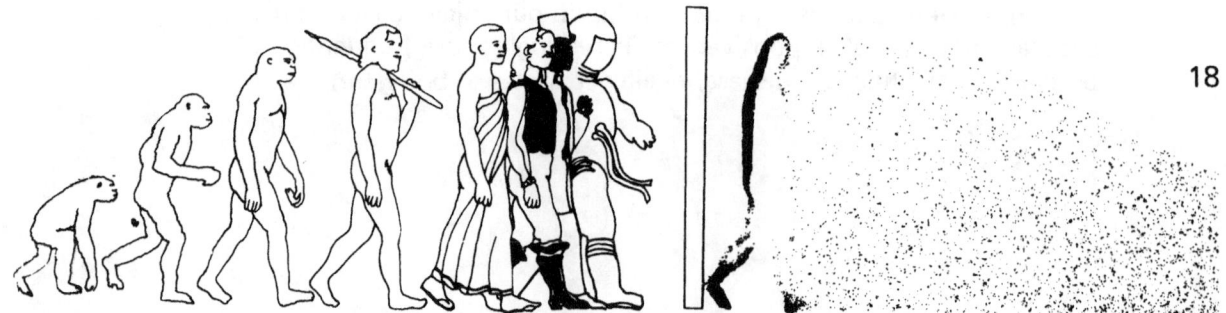

not require any intellectual or derived knowledge, only a naturally responsive physical and sensory instrument. Most importantly, wildness in its pure form is value-free. As such, it does not demand a self-image, merely total body health in order to survive.

Living as we do in an intellectually or symbolically systematized environment, wildness in its original state is an outmoded and obviously inappropriate context — precisely because we all value, and desire more than anything else, a self-image. What we need to reunderstand are the **elements** of true wildness that are still of value to reflective, communicating, social animals who have lost touch with their physical capacities and instinctive body skills.

Look at all of our "return to nature" groups! This contrived search for wildness — (to run naked again, to say what we feel, to feel what we want, to commune with nature and "be natural" again) — within a civilized-socialized environment where the psychology of social institutions has become inconsistent, chaotic, and contradictory, is a searching that leads only to the formation of cults. Thus, the response of a chaotic environment to the yearning to be "natural" — to return to "wildness" — takes the form of programmed escapes from the inhibitions of civilization. Wildness in this pseudo, falsified context is no longer an individual ecology. It is a collective effort requiring formal group support and continuous reinforcement. It is ultimately a contradiction!

We must coordinate into a new understanding of wildness the realization that natural man is now communicating man. We need to move **beyond wildness** — not because nakedness is no longer sufficient (it never was sufficient), but because it has become an acquired taste. It is almost inversely a value of civilization.

"Beyond Wildness" means that we stop equating wildness and nakedness with purity and naturalness. **Wildness is no longer natural.** It, too, has been co-opted by the external environment and converted into an unnatural social value used primarily for escape from that environment. It has become a modish artifact of present-day romanticism and an emblem of misty, value-tinged yearnings.

"Beyond Wildness" means discipline. Wildness was once thought to be the antithesis of discipline and to a large extent, still is. But true wildness lived within the strictest survival discipline of nature. Now our "wildness," or the elements of it we need to reclaim, must live within another discipline. It must live as knowledge within a civilized discipline. And so, in order to regain the Body Wisdom inherent within the human organism without returning to the cave, we must necessarily move **beyond wildness.**

2
A NEW LEARNING PROCESS

Chapter 2
A New Learning Process

The realization of a "civilized discipline," capable of redeveloping body intelligence without retreating from the specific circumstances of contemporary life, demands an entirely new learning process. Self-teaching to Body Wisdom requires that all learning, all self-awareness, be psycho-physical. This means that every act must be felt, perceived, and responded to as organic experience; that we learn from our bodies how to "physicalize" images which then feed back to the body as "organic instructions"; and that our perception of self derives from a new awareness of self as a physically reactive sensory instrument. In short: the new learning process is **organically constitutional** rather than **externally dependent**.

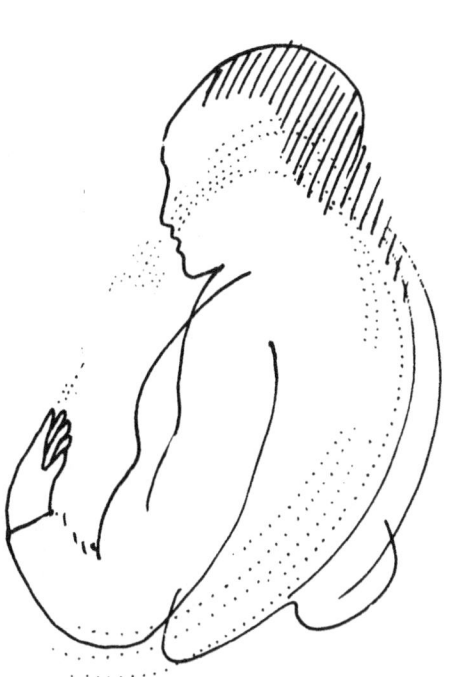

The underlying principle behind this process is that one develops the brain by finding new ways of stimulating the senses, much the way a child is naturally inclined to develop. Through **psychosomatic learning,** we teach ourselves to feel and perceive internal, physical experience and learn experientially that the sensory or **feeling process** is the currency through which we communicate with ourselves, and communicate and relate to others. By "physicalizing" our perception we are tapping into the sources of "instinctual energy" and "objective internalization" that have been heretofore hidden by our conditioned dependence upon input from the external environment, alone.

By "psychosomatic learning", I mean, on the simplest level: the organic awareness of the relationship between our body responses to conscious instructions from the outside and our perception of the physical, gut-level instructions to ourselves from the inside (i.e. from the body organism, itself). Thus, the "feeling process" is the physical continuation of pre-intellectual awareness which perpetuates the awareness itself, on a non-intellectual basis. The more we learn to feel things, the more things we learn to feel.

Organic balance is not something that can be imitated, for imitation itself is both limiting and limited as a learning process. In fact, imitation as a learning process is often destructive to the end result. It can only hope to **reproduce** patterns of behavior on a gross, surface level, while the body wisdom of organic synchronization lies latent and unrevealed beneath the surface.

In other words, conditioned behavior never improves the quality of an act — it can help only in the precise reproduction of the act. **The creative self is not subject to conditioning. To be in good condition does not mean to be conditioned!**

Certain behavior will never adjust to conditioned patterning and
helps form the keystone to Body Wisdom and psychosomatic health.
For instance:

- Prejudice can be conditioned — spontaneous appreciation cannot!

- The manner and pattern of talking and of interrupting can be
  conditioned — creative dialogue cannot!

- A high degree of skill in playing a musical instrument or
  engaging in a sports-art or performing on stage can be conditioned — the interpretation and feeling cannot!

- The five external senses may be subject to degrees of conditioning — the "inner harmonic and overtone sensory system"
  is not subject to that conditioning.

- Learning techniques can be conditioned — the self-teaching
  process cannot!

To register **organic** sensation, perception and response, we cannot
rely very much upon the five outer senses. Outer-directed vision is of
little use to us when trying to understand how the legs want to function. Outside hearing is of no value when trying to understand how
our voice wants to function and how it "feels" internally. The external senses of hearing and vision cannot help us when we want to perceive
our breathing organically and understand how **it** wants to function.

Organic/sensory learning requires a closer, more intimate perceiving
modality. This new perceiving modality is **kine-sensic** — it is a physical
"feeling" modality. Looking, hearing and tasting **inside** our body
environment is the dynamic that permits our emotions to relate to
our physical selves. We are dealing quite simply with a purely psychosomatic learning process. Psychosomatic health is as valid a concept
as psychosomatic disease. And if we are to learn to use our bodies
and our minds and our perceptual apparatus with optimal efficiency,
the greatest ease, and the most esthetic quality, we **must** deal with this
modality. When we have learned the signals and cues of perception,
sensation, and response — what it **feels like** for the body to behave
naturally and optimally — we are then ready to use these feelings as
"organic instructions" to the body.

A New
Learning
Process

Organic Instructions

The concept of the "organic instruction" involves a **conscious** capacity to perceive the body in movement as internal, physicalized experience. It is a first step in the self-teaching process of identifying sensations, acquiring perceptions, responding to awareness, and, through the "inner harmonic senses", training oneself to use these feelings and their images as organic directions to the body.

By contrast, non-organic instructions are commands to the body that are conflicting and confusing. They are commands or instructions that cause the body to behave so competitively that when the words say one thing, the voice says quite another, and the face is at variance with both. They are commands to the body that set the mind and the body into such active opposition that the conflict uses up excessive energy, induces anxiety, and produces friction and damage to the muscles and to the very energy-processing systems of the body.

...the inability to utilize all our communication skills, and the inability to feel at one with the language, is also a cause of neurotic behavior, anxiety, and arrested development... it is not just a symptom!

To the actors a non-organic instruction to the body might be to "throw your voice to the farthest row of the theater!" That is an image and an instruction that demands of the body something it cannot do. The voice cannot be thrown out of the body. The voice can only resonate and vibrate **within** the body. Any attempt of the body to **expel** the voice results in force and violence. The correct, organic instruction in this case would be to "search for the 'bone-conducted feel' of your voice as an 'inside-the-body' experience, and don't treat it as if it were a baseball being thrown through the air!"

Any command to the body to fulfill a specific goal or make a special **effort** — "push yourself to the limit" — "run as hard as you can" — "do twenty-five push-ups" — "press or pull or lift that heavy weight" — may seem like a perfectly reasonable instruction. But in fact, it places the body in unreasonable competition with itself and in conflict with free body rhythm, balance and energy. Thus, it is an externally imposed non-organic instruction that only wears down and destroys the body.

Finding the Familiar Event

When we start our body training in Part Two we will begin by finding the "familiar event." Remember, psychosomatic learning is learning what it **feels** like when we do something right instinctively, hence, what it feels like **to do** it right. So we start by selecting a familiar situation in which we know, from experience, that the body behaves naturally and instinctively well.

This may be an activity you have always performed with ease because of some special talent or skill. Or it may involve a particular act that, from constant doing, functions pleasurably, gracefully, efficiently for **you**. Or it may be an event that, because it invites a natural, pre-conditioned posture, therefore accompanied by correct, comfortable breathing, creates a situation where your body functions smoothly without internal conflict. It may be any of these.

Each of us can find such familiar events, fresh experiences, unique body occurrences; each of us can anticipate those strange yet interesting applications and explore the uncommon carry-overs of healthful body experience. We may have to think and search a bit, perhaps initially with a little coaxing or guidance. But we all have ample resources to draw upon for beginning the new learning process.

Generally speaking, the process will be as follows:

STEP ONE: You will single out one of these natural activities and do it, experiencing the act spontaneously as a fresh event totally opposite from imitation or routine. Because this fresh event is instinctively experienced, giving pleasure and comfort, it can be accepted as a "familiar event."

STEP TWO: As you experience the familiar event instinctively and naturally, with total ease, you will learn to identify its "physical feel" and respond with awareness to this feel as "kine-sensic memory" of a unique event.

STEP THREE: Having isolated these sensations and perceptions as physical sense memories, while experiencing the comfort of the familiar event as a unique event, you will generate the same sensations and perceptions (including the image of that feel) onto a relatively unfamiliar body activity. It will still feel good, but now **strangely** comfortable rather than familiarly so. You'll experience it, not as a repeated action of a prototype, but as a genuinely original, unique experience of another familiar event.

STEP FOUR: You will then be ready to use your awareness and alertness as "image experience"; i.e. to make the image active and learn how to use it as "organic instruction" to the body. The four steps should help you understand the entire experience of the feeling process in any physical act as it directly relates to: **sensation** — **perception** — **awareness** — and **response**.

Consciously or not, we experience different orders of images: inhibitive and non-inhibitive; organic and non-organic; extrinsic and intrinsic. The images that emerge as part of organic feeling become active images for kine-sensic learning; i.e., they first evolve as images of the feel and then convert from **intrinsic effects** of a previous act to **causative factors** directing the body to future acts. (see: Images In Movement, pp. 73, 74)

Image and Action

Thus, an image resulting primarily from association with the initial familiar event will become part of organic physical memory, and then constitute itself as internal, organic motivation for new and future unique events. By appreciating the relationship between image and action as essentially one involving "self-to-self" communication with the body, we teach ourselves to properly channel our mental information into the body and thereby allow the body to behave in a non-conflicting, non-competitive way.

Athletes are beginning to understand this. The great track stars and record-setters now know that the body behaves competitively with itself when it tries to "beat" the four (or by now the three plus) minute mile, which for years remained inviolable. They now know that the real competition is not on the track but inside the runner, between his body and his mind. The mind competes with the body by "informing" the body of the impossibility, or at least monumental difficulty in accomplishing the task.

The new modality of the "feeling process" circumvents the short-circuiting that occurs every time the body and mind are in competitive conflict with one another. This conflict need not necessarily be emotional. At root, it is a conflict between what we intellectually **think** are our goals and what the body actually **needs** in order to live with healthy compromise. The "feeling process" helps to avoid these conflicts as a means of developing new knowledge of the body, and this natural avoidance forms the basis for any relearning of Body Wisdom.

Thus, we look to a learning process that will provide us with a language for self-to-self communication — a language that communicates our thoughts and desires **to** our bodies and receives reinforcement and pleasure and discovery **from** our bodies. Inhibitive instructions, inhibitive language, and inhibitive images are those that are out of context with the "language of understanding" available to the body during a particular period of growth and development.

We are concerned, then, with communication on the one hand and with the way the body understands, on the other. This holds true equally for verbal, vocal, and body language, for all of these languages are physical. All of them respond to psychosomatic intelligence whether such language is communicated on stage, at home, in sports, in the streets, or in the office. Learning Body Wisdom essentially involves **learning the language that the body innately understands.**

This concept of "body training as language training" is further explored in the next chapter, as a consideration of what we call Body Esthetics.

3
BODY ESTHETICS

Chapter 3

Body Esthetics

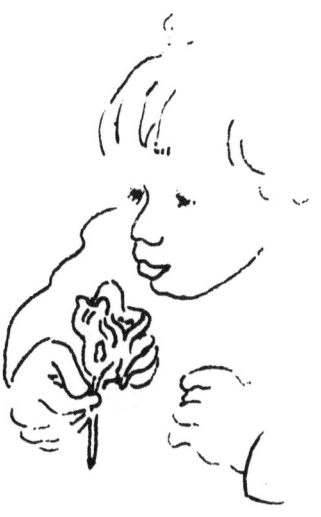

Through the course of civilization, we have so intellectualized the search for **aesthetics** that we have virtually lost touch with **esthesis** — literally, the study of the nature of sensation. Body Wisdom allows us to retrieve the original, archaic sense of the term and construct from it a new aesthetic rooted in optimal condition.

"Body Esthetics" is an intrinsic component of the feeling process. It informs the development of our concepts of sensation, perception, awareness, and response as these relate to psychosomatic learning. And it contains many of the concepts that help us generate those primary (endogenous) images that evolve into organic instructions to the body.

For us:

- Anything that promotes sensitivity and induces awareness of sensation in the body is an **esthetic** . . . a body esthetic; and

- Anything that deadens sensitivity or lessens the awareness or perception of sensation in the organism is an **anesthetic** . . . a body anesthetic.

The evolving images that result from the awareness of a sensation are, in themselves, physical reflections of body esthetics. Thus, they contain a wide variety of physical experiences that can be considered body esthetics. Among these: balance; lightness or weightlessness; curvo-linear and spherical body structure and posture; nimbleness; buoyancy; electricity; flexible strength; body extension; body-internalized rhythm; vocal life; synesthesic activity.* Similarly, the reinforcing psycho-physical experiences of appreciation, satisfaction, enjoyment, are all ingredients of body esthetics that lead to optimal functioning.

Conversely, body anesthetics reflect internal competition in the body as physically manifested in body strain, body heaviness, muscular flabbiness, body "rote" behavior, body exhaustion, a sense of truncated capacity, and other characteristically stressful and harmful conditions.

---

*By synesthesic activity, we mean a sensation felt in one part of the body when another part is stimulated, as when the hearing of certain sounds induces the visualization of certain colors. Through psychosomatic learning, we teach ourselves the **feeling** of seeing sounds, hearing colors, touching smells, etc. This is all synesthesic activity.

Purely intellectual conceptions of "well being" or philosophical appreciation alone of "truth and beauty"— the domain of traditional **aesthetics** — inject values from the outside that more often than not, impose outer-conditioned demands upon the body and thereby feed internal competition within the body. Far from integrating the multiple levels of sensation inherent in the organism, these conditioned aesthetics, filtered through the five outside senses, frequently intrude upon our awareness of self and in fact compartmentalize and therefore emaciate the very essence of sensation. Thus, we grow up to think of various sensing organs or processes primarily in terms of their relationship to the **kinds** of information they transport or transmit. The visual sense becomes a supremely logical, strictly linear kind of input; the auditory sense deposits into our awareness ordered contextual meaning, with practically no registration of subtext; the sense of touch, between live organisms, often conjures up feelings of anxiety rather than of mutual support and trust.

The psycho/physical **esthetic** process, on the other hand, is a continuing exploration of organic/sensory learning in which:

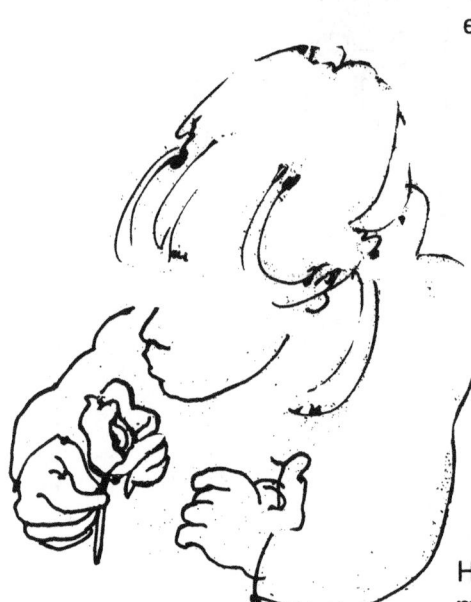

- the body creates the feel, causing an **awareness of sensation;**

- the body receives the feel, creating an **awareness of perception;**

- the body reacts to the feel, receiving an **awareness of response;**

- the body's **awareness of all these feels** reinforces the experience with the final ingredients of satisfaction, enjoyment, and appreciation;

- because it is intrinsic to the feeling process, body esthetics resolves itself into behavior that is, itself, part of the esthetic process.

Henceforth, behavior will here be understood not only as **any body movement**— but also as any movement **within** the body — whether that be the movement of rhythm, of balance, of eager curiosity, of the registration of perception, of imagery, of fantasy, of satisfaction, contentment or appreciation. Behavior must be capable of being sensed, perceived and responded to by our entire perceptual apparatus.

We will be concerned with three qualities of sensory perception and awareness: **incoming** sensation; **resident** sensation; and **output** sensation. Briefly stated:

Body Esthetics

1. **Incoming** sensation originates in the outer environment and is transmitted to our body's inner environment through the five fundamental senses of taste, touch, smell, hearing, and vision. Upon entering the body's inner environment, incoming sensation registers as information and begins to function as resident sensation.

2. **Resident** sensation is the ongoing, internal **feeling awareness** of the body environment. It constitutes the body climate for all **self-to-self response** and creates its own indigenous body input.

3. **Output** sensation begins within the body environment as part of the resident sensation process. Output sensation occurs when input from the body environment is processed by resident sensation and conveyed to the outer environment as **self-to-other communication**.

Hence, the ordering relationship of sensory perception implies that the response to self will always precede and organically prepare for the response to others.

In this context, the "harmonic overtone sensory system" should be understood as the synchronized coordination of input, resident, and output sensation within the body. Whenever the communication of these sensations takes place, body esthetics and the feeling process are working cooperatively or **synergistically**, and we know, through feeling, that we are stimulated, reinforced, and functioning creatively. I find it intriguing to consider the inner, higher senses to be, in effect, the "harmonics" (overtones or partials) of the five, fundamental outer senses. Do we not, after all, accommodate and recognize color, light, design, substance, sound, language, and movement inside as well as outside of us? Are we not, in fact, capable of seeing, hearing, following, and almost "taste-touching" these qualities and actions internally?

It is the "harmonic overtone sensory system" that makes possible the esthetics of organic functioning. It is this coordination of the different dynamics of harmonic perception that allows for tight-rope dancing, bio-feedback, or psychosomatic (visceral) control and adjustments. Clearly, the cerebral thought process is not excluded from the visceral feel process, as we understand it. If we can, indeed, silently see, hear, and follow inner body activities, how far removed is this from "thinking?" If the feeling of what we see, hear, and design inside of us is akin to imaging, reflecting, or integrating, then are we not approaching a fuller, physio-neural awareness of the **feel** of thinking — the **feel** of spirit energy — the **feel** of gut-feeling?

*...body
training
is
language
training!
...it is
a first step
in
bridging
the gap which
separates the
left and right brains!*

*We need to understand
the human body...
as it is physical
as it is thoughtful
as it is impulsive
as it is creative
as it needs
to communicate
as it needs
to feel
as it needs
to express!*

A Human Ecology

> *God spare me from thoughts, that men think in their heads alone*
> *He who sings a lasting song, thinks in the marrow bone!*
>
> — Yeats

...awareness is not to be confused with judgement... it is a sensory reinforcement of the body's perception systems!

The "harmonic overtone sensory system" is fed and synergized by all the experiencing systems of the body: the memory systems, the imaging and associative processes, the nervous systems, the vocal and muscular systems . . . the whole brain! As such, it becomes the prime instrument for reconditioning the body to perform physical action instinctively and naturally.

Within the purview of the "harmonic overtone sensory system," sensory perception can be explored on three, ascending "bio-" levels:

- First and fundamentally, the bio-physical and bio-neural level;

- Second and often correlatively, the bio-psychic level; and

- Ultimately, the distant bio-plasmic level.

...habitual awareness becomes the "fail-safe" servo-mechanism that helps the body stay "on keel"!

...it is the great teacher of of organic balance, rhythm, and humor sensing!

Whereas bio-plasmic and a major part of bio-psychic experience is still uncharted territory for future research, our work — primarily addressed to the **prerequisite** study of bio-physical and bio-neural sensation — establishes important links to certain non-mystical levels of bio-psychic sensation, that deal with the image-supported conversion of body energy states within the individual environment and the transformation of energy fields immediately surrounding the body environment.

By "bio-physical" and "bio-neural," I refer to all the internal experiencing systems physically available to us: **voluntary, semi-voluntary, and in some cases, non-voluntary.** We do not have ready access to all of them, but we know they are there.

Yet even the most accessible, such as voice, muscle movement, etc., we usually misinterpret because we have not learned to register them through the use of our "harmonic overtone sensory system." Organically felt, bio-physical and bio-neural experience includes, among other sensations: inner vibrations/pulsations, flow currents, energy flows, rhythm flows, temperature changes, inner sounds and percussive activity, moving color, designs, shapes, forms, and images, signal and cue warnings, body lightness, and body balance.

...habitual awareness can integrate form content quality and the pleasure principle in a single "gestalt" experience!

A good image to keep in mind is that the feeling process works most sensitively when the body environment is in a state of **gentle, perceptive turbulence.** What a lovely and dynamic image of the body in motion! It is in this gentle and perceptive turbulence that the body absorbs all manner of esthetics with appreciation and, most importantly, with awareness.

Body Training As Language Training

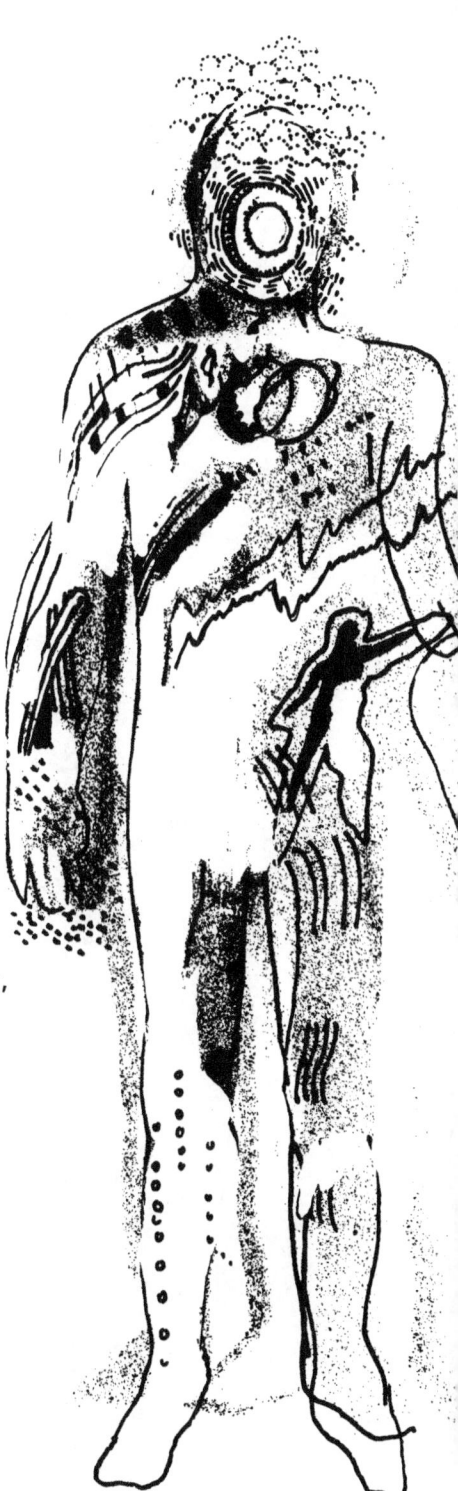

Fundamental to body esthetics, as the study of sensation, is the exploration of language — not just one language, but many. I am concerned with languages of the body that function as bearers of personal intelligence, personal perceptiveness, personal imagination, and personal culture; **sensory languages** within each of us that are both native and foreign, voluntary and non-voluntary. Conversely, any further deforesting of the body's inner languages and dialects will merely add to the considerable rotting of the "body-whole".

Except for poets, the very nature of verbal language is linear and logical — and therefore inappropriate or at least incomplete for organic communication. We need to ask the questions: what kind of body language can we experience when there is absolutely no verbal or vocal code? through what language do we communicate when there is no verbal, but **only** vocal expression as in a cry, a laugh, a sigh, or an exclamation? The retraining of the body to function naturally is, at root, language training.

To function as whole persons means we must function not simply with one forehemisphere of the brain, but with the whole brain! An area of development as seminal as language training (any kind of language), cannot properly be the province of the "mind" alone. Learning a language using only the mind usually results in never enjoying the native accent, the rhythm, the music, the humor, the taste, the sensuousness of the language, its culture, or, people. When we begin to understand the need to find languages within the body that may not be linear, then we begin to understand what we are all about.

In the light of some very hard evidence regarding bio-feedback, (the science, not the cult), psycho-kinetics, and twin-brain research, and of results from our own experiments with the feeling process in therapy, speech, reading readiness, physical education, actor training, and personal development, I am convinced that we possess these languages to help put us in closer touch with our insights, imagination, and instinctive talents. I am convinced that the classification of body activities into voluntary, semi-voluntary, and non-voluntary behavior must give way to a more variable awareness. For what was considered non-voluntary yesterday is seen as semi-voluntary today; what is today considered semi-voluntary could in the very near future become voluntary. A cardinal element is that the body teaches us what there is that is mysterious or undiscovered; that **the perception of the mysterious is the origin of discovery**; and that we are moving toward a training and development that will teach us **how** to discover and explore.

It is basically a matter of evolving, developing, and sensing body languages, body dialects, body styles, body folklore, and body humor. Our task, in this work, is to teach these languages and dialects through the syntax of the feeling process — through self-teaching to feel what the body wants to do and what it is capable of doing. The styles and folklore and humor of the body fall into place as the form and content of Body Esthetics — and through body esthetics, the form and content of body creativity.

Part Two
ENERGY AND RELAXATION

PREFACE TO PART TWO

Unifying the Two Opposites

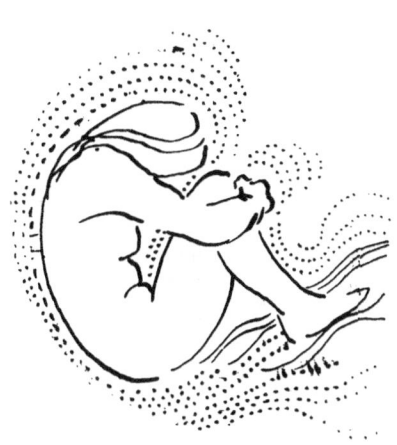

All energy is a form of intelligence and can be decoded into body language. To understand how the "pre-conditioned" body once functioned and can again function instinctively well, we begin this first of two work sections by investigating the body's diversified **energy states** and appropriating, for self-teaching, its energy-giving behavior. Through a sequence of guided exercises or "experiments," we will be exploring the body's different "energy feels" and learning to identify their special character: from the vibrant, potent energy state to that of gentle "idling"; from being able to viscerally "taste" an absence of (dis-)stress to actually feeling the presence of **dynamic relaxation**.

Once experienced kine-sensically, these different energy states can be categorized, recognized for their synergistic inter-relationships, and perceived as "unique/familiar events." We will then be ready to objectively observe how our body behaves within each of these categories. Seeing this first in ourselves will allow us to see it in others.

Thus, we'll be able to watch a dancer, gymnast, actor, basketball player, skier, or percussionist in active rest or restful action and say: "There, you see! There's the 'floating buoyancy' esthetic! There's the 'electric radiancy alert' dynamic! There's the flexible 'body strength potency!' There's the 'shake-vibrating relaxer-energizer'; the emotional inter-involvement'; the 'reserve safety-cushion regulator'; the 'inner rhythm dynamic' ". In PART TWO, we will be examining and experiencing all of these energy feels, all of the **non-derived** or **intrinsic energy states** that fuel and feed the body's activities.

Central to the focus of PART TWO and basic to all the work chapters is the principle of **Energy and Relaxation** — seen as a new, "third force unity of opposites." We all understand the terms "relaxation" and "energy" as routinely applied to stress technology. But because these concepts are commonly misunderstood to be two separate entities, we understand far less their self-application for Body Wisdom.

Energy is usually associated with **action**; relaxation with **inaction**. At best, they are regarded as a duality, capable of some sort of integration or mixed combination. In truth, they are complementary opposites that incline toward synergy or cross-quality synthesis; complementary opposites such as male and female, higher and lower, stillness and movement.

When we investigate the use of body energy in terms of its "resting" or "equilibrating" component and the use of relaxation in terms of its "active" or "dynamic" component, we approach optimal functioning. As we experience **relaxation** through its intrinsic dynamic properties and perceive the use of **energy** through its intrinsic resting properties, our harmonic overtone sensory system teaches us why these opposites (or seeming dualities) should never be disengaged; how each draws substance from the other and is contained within the other; how together, they become **relaxer-energizers** for the body.

By building an organic bridge between active rest and restful action, this third force unity of opposites gives rise to our principles of relaxed energy and energetic relaxation, or to resting up and resting down simultaneously; it is precisely this bridge between 'active rest' and 'restful action' that leaves an only barely noticeable difference between voice, speech, and body training. This holistic, cross-quality approach or "generalization of energies" carries over, throughout BODY WISDOM, to the related concepts of generalized body balance, generalized concentration and attention, generalized body awareness, and generalized rhythm experience.

We accord special treatment in PART TWO to rhythm — **organically felt rhythm** — as a significant intelligence and distinct, non-verbal "body dialect." Our concern is with the perception of rhythm as internal energy-dynamics and the tapping of the rhythm complex for generating organic instructions.

Watching the artist-athletes at the Olympic Games, anyone trained in kine-sensics could see how they coordinate rhythm with movement, inner music with outer melody. Whether in pole vault, high jump, track, swimming, skiing, or gymnastics, you could objectively observe the way their eyes and faces were genuinely, joyously involved with their body's self-to-self communication. When you see and read all of this in their optimal performance, you know that something additional is happening. You know, from kinesensic awareness, that there is a set of esthetics fomenting their performance that not only informs, but is, in the final analysis essential to the physical skills involved. And you leave the Olympic Games confirmed in the knowledge that with Body Wisdom, you needn't be an Olympics athlete to experience the skills and inner rhythms of body esthetics!

From this point forward, the general principles of the feeling process, set forth in PART ONE, become part of a **practical program** of self-teaching experiments. No longer a passive auditor, you are now an active partner in the work/play of Body Wisdom. So scratch that itch, close the door to the next room, find a more comfortable chair, or lie down if you prefer. But prepare yourself to experience, rather than merely read, what follows.

From here on, don't take anything I say for granted. Test it, reject it, accept it! Catch the purpose of each experiment! Then put the book down, try the exercises, experience each body esthetic with increasing awareness, and return to the text for the next step.

4
THE BODY ENERGIZERS

Chapter 4

The Body Energizers

Kinesensic training begins with the discovery that the individual inner environment can organically experience at least seven potent "body energizers." Those of you familiar with *The Use and Training of the Human Voice* have already experienced three of these organic energizers: the three **derived energy states** of "structural, tonal, and consonant action." For those new to kinesensics, an appended brief summary of these vocal or verbal energies, learned either by example, inclination, or specific instruction, is provided at the conclusion of this chapter along with a listing of benefits and exercise classifications.

Our primary concern here is with the four **non-derived, primitive energy states** intrinsic to the body environment and fundamental to the total use and training of the human body: **Buoyancy, Radiancy, Potency,** and **Inter-Involvement.** As you will learn for yourself, each of these non-derived energy states has its own characteristics, its own quality of sustained, physical reach-extension, its own particular **feel**.

IN BUOYANCY, the body feels as if it were oxygen-charged. Through an "elastic-legato" physical reach and a sustained extension flow, buoyancy supports a floating, volatile, lighter-than-air body in three, distinct variations:

- **rising buoyancy:** or the feel of floating up like the expanding dough of a yeast bread;

- **floating buoyancy:** or just level floating like a feather wafting in windless air; and

- **settling-down buoyancy:** or floating down and when reaching the surface, feeling as weightless as an air-filled balloon.

IN RADIANCY, the body feels as if it were impulse-charged. Radiancy involves an eager, electric-like physical reach and a spirited sustained extension that supports an agile, darting, "Chaplinesque" body. Radiancy energy induces the feeling of spontaneity.

IN POTENCY or MUSCLE-YAWN, the body feels like it is chemically charged. The sustained extension of potency is a power-potential reach, its flexible, muscular strength supporting a powerful, yawn-stretching body.

IN INTER-INVOLVEMENT, the body feels as if it were emotionally charged. Here, the physical reach (sustained extension) is motivational or "self-to-other," supporting a body fed by its instinctive needs and emotions rather than by muscle awareness.

Energy
and
Relaxation

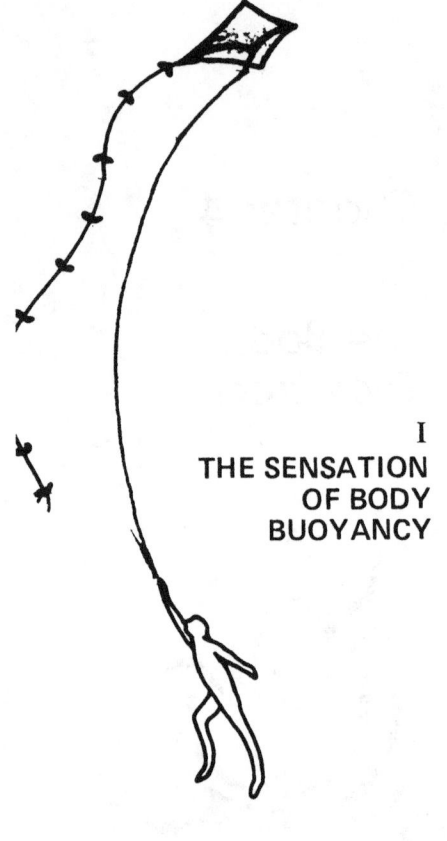

Organically felt, these four non-derived energy states can rightfully be considered body dialects with intonations, inflections, and accents all their own. Used individually or in varying combinations, they add dynamic and esthetic styling to the syntax of our personal culture and physical development.

**I
THE SENSATION
OF BODY
BUOYANCY**

In a phrase, buoyancy feels like "dynamic relaxation." It infuses into relaxation an active feel totally opposed to that "sinking feeling" or body-heavy sensation or limp-floppy relaxation we all know so well. Body buoyancy is a relaxed energy state that when kinesensically experienced, yields up a new perception of body movement, of movement that feels virtually weightless.

To experience buoyancy, we must be aware of an external, energy-support field surrounding the body. This may be an actual support field such as a body of water. Or it may be a field of magnetic or wind currents, a self-suggested field where an image is energized, or even a physically generated support field, such as one produced by breath-energy.

As regards the breath-buoyancy relationship, you will find in the following experiments that whether in water or air:

- a fully inhaled breath promotes the sensation of rising buoyancy;

- a half-exhaled breath maintains even-floating buoyancy;

- a fully-exhaled breath induces settling-down buoyancy.

Let's begin!

**Buoyancy
Experiment One:**

**Recognizing The Feel
of Weightlessness**

(A) • Guided by the illustration, press the back of one hand, from the wrist joint to the first knuckles, firmly against a flat wall for approximately four seconds.

- Now step lightly away from the wall and allow your hand and arm, as a unit, to float up by itself.

- Do the same with the other hand and arm.

- Repeat the exercise with both hands and arms pressing firmly against the door frame, then floating up as you step away.

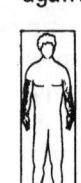
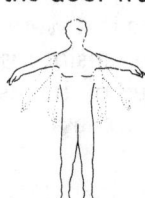
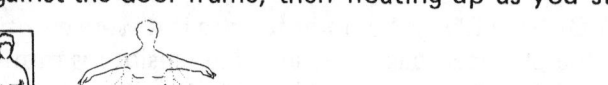

Body
Energizers
(Buoyancy)

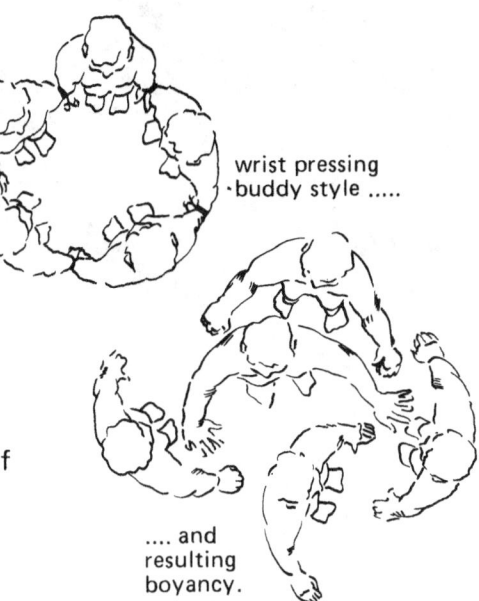

wrist pressing -buddy style .....

.... and resulting boyancy.

You have experienced what amounts to weightlessness. This is the feel of rising buoyancy.

(B) • Select a covered, hard surface, i.e. a blanketed or carpeted floor, and lie down on your back.

• Think of the weightless, rising quality of buoyancy you have just felt and inhale a full breath. Note that before inhalation, even **thinking** buoyancy did not completely dispel the **feeling** of weight in the arm and hand. But after full inhalation, the arm and hand buoyed itself up with no apparent difficulty.

• Now try it with just the fingers.

• Now with just the hand.

• Now with the entire arm.

• Do it with the other arm.

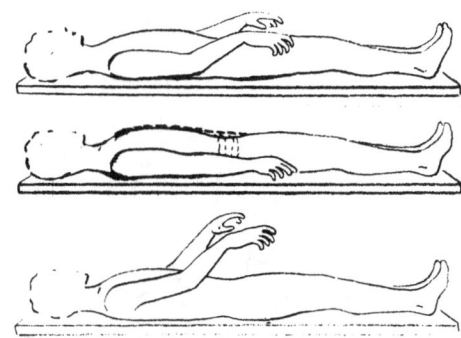

• Now with both arms simultaneously. Notice how the arms float downward when you exhale half your breath and then float easily at the halfway mark.

• Exhale all your breath. Note the settling-down buoyancy or flotation of the arm and hand.

• Now inhale again and notice the rising buoyancy of the arm and hand. These breath-induced buoyancies appear to be **semi-voluntary** events.

(C) • Imagine yourself floating on water.

• Let the "image energy" become so pervasive that you begin to sense a "floating, wafting feeling" — a feel of gentle, inner turbulence in both the movement and the relaxation. If your arms and legs feel weightless, then you are beginning to experience body buoyancy — but subjectively, at least insofar as your muscles are concerned.

A More Objectively Structured Exploration: First Water, Then Air!

The direct affinity between buoyancy and the body's breathing process should now be apparent to you. That affinity persists whether in water or air. But you will find that, in water, breathing buoyancy deals with the **actual sensation**, whereas in air it calls forth the **muscle recall/sense memory** of rising, floating, and settling-down buoyancy.

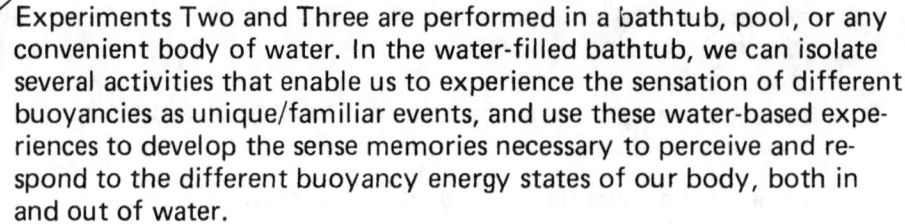

Energy
and
Relaxation

Experiments Two and Three are performed in a bathtub, pool, or any convenient body of water. In the water-filled bathtub, we can isolate several activities that enable us to experience the sensation of different buoyancies as unique/familiar events, and use these water-based experiences to develop the sense memories necessary to perceive and respond to the different buoyancy energy states of our body, both in and out of water.

The sensations of body weightlessness, of lightness of body contact, of legato, wave-like, inner body rhythms are most objectively sensed and perceived in water. In water, the body experiences movement and relaxation simultaneously and spontaneously, moving and resting in a state of equilibrium that yields ultimate understanding of "restful energy" and "energetic rest." Thus, the water that provides the circumstances in which the body functions organically and reacts to its environment in a natural manner, can become a familiar event for objectively experiencing the sensations of body buoyancy.

Experiment Two:

Water Buoyancy Energy

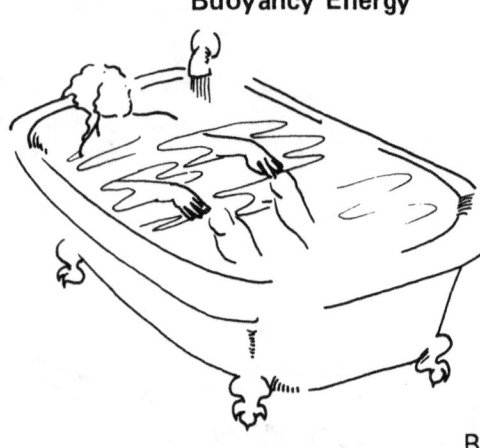

A • Lie in a bathtub that is nearly filled with comfortably warm water. Lie on your back, relaxed and flexible, with head resting on the rim of the tub as in the illustration.

• As you notice your arms and hands floating up almost above the surface of the water, you'll feel your arms responding to the sensation of buoyancy. The movement of the arm in the water will seem weightless, yet with a momentum and direction to it.

• Repeat this movement again and again, until you become familiar with the feel.

• Try it with either arm, then with both arms together.

• To what extent can you feel a similar sensory experience with your legs and feet — first one, then the other, then both?

B • Consciously take and hold a full breath. Note how the body as a whole now experiences the sensation of dynamic rising buoyancy, and holds that position just as long as you hold your breath.

• Exhale about half your breath and register the sensation of the body buoyantly floating beneath the water's surface. This floating buoyancy is maintained as long as your body sustains half the inhalation.

Body
Energizers
(Buoyancy)

- Now exhale all your breath and feel your body float gently all the way down as you experience settling-down buoyancy.

- Review the illustrations and recognize how each of these buoyancy activities appears to exemplify "resting up" and "resting down" at the same time.

C • Again take a full breath and note, as in illustrations, that nearly your whole body buoyantly floats to the water's surface, resting up and resting down at the same time.

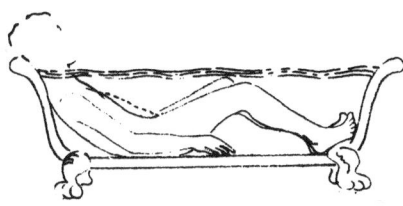

- Again exhale all your breath and feel the entire body floating weightlessly down to the bottom of the tub, in settling-down buoyancy. Respond pleasantly with natural vulnerability, so that you do not inhibit the movement and note that here too, at the bottom of the tub, you are resting down and up at the same time.

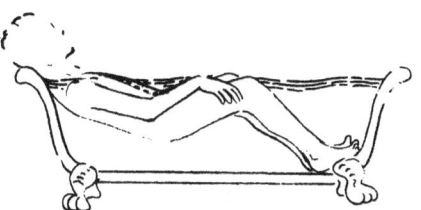

D • Study the illustrations. Then, with your head and feet resting on the rim of the tub, breathe in fully and watch your body rise buoyantly to the surface.

- Sense-record the feel of weightlessness under your head and feet, as well as the smooth movement, floating rhythm, and salutary dynamic relaxation that accompanies the act.

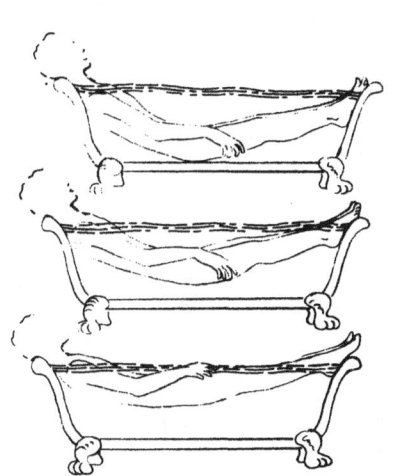

What you are exploring and discovering here is the feel of vanishing pressure at a given contact point, (in this case at the head and feet). This "Contact Vanishing Point" results from pure movement devoid of muscle strain and body weight; it is a "zero-pressure" experience intimately connected with body balance and truly relaxed activity.

E • Still in the water, place your index finger to the floor of the bathtub and take a breath. Notice how your body rises while you remain balanced on one finger.

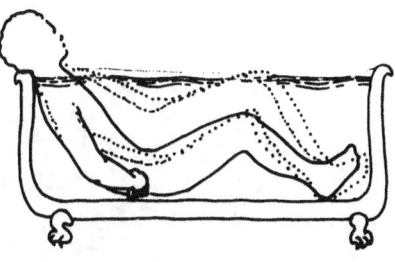

- Exhale and your body buoyantly settles down, while you are still balanced on one finger.

- Repeat the exercise, only this time using one toe rather than your index finger, with your head continuing to rest on the rim of the tub.

Energy
and
Relaxation

Now that you know the feels of weightlessness, relaxation, balance, and rhythm in water and have appropriated these as familiar events, you will want to re-experience these same sensations out of water. And you can! But first, while still in the water, we must learn how to **convert** the actual sensation of water buoyancy into the sense memory of those buoyancy energy states — that we may re-experience them in air by recalling how they felt in water.

In other words, the physical feels that you instinctively experienced during the familiar event of the first experiment, and perceived as natural to the body during the new familiar events of the second experiment, will for the first time be freshly experienced as they are carried over into a set of non-familiar events. Those activities of buoyancy that were part of involuntary and semi-voluntary behavior will now become part of **conscious voluntary control**, through concrete feedback from the body to the brain of sensory messages relayed during the spontaneous experience of water buoyancy. This will become immediately clear with the experiments that follow. Still in the warm-water bathtub:

- "inhale your body" to a state of rising buoyancy. As you do so, self-suggest that: "Once I have completely exhaled, **my body will maintain its upward floating position.**" So exhale, and,

- your body will still feel weightless and equilibrated. It will still be floating on the surface, only with this difference: you are now using your body's "recall" of the sensation of rising buoyancy as an organic instruction to the body, to respond **as if** it were still filled with air! What was before a non-voluntary body movement has become, under your control, an intentional, voluntary act. Your own organic instructions to your own body's inner environment have taken over the responsibility previously lodged in the outside, surrounding energy-field — the actual body of water.

- now conduct the experiment in reverse: inhale, hold your breath, and **instruct** your body to **feel** itself settling down buoyantly, without heaviness or forced pressure.

- as you work **against** the breath flow, observe your arm, your hand, your torso freshly experience the feeling of a familiar event within the frame of a new, strange set of behavioral circumstances.

39

Body
Energizers
(Buoyancy)

So far, in your water experiments you have learned:

1 the feel of body wafting and floating in response to water flows and currents, as well as to moving breath streams;

2 the sensation of the body resting with optimal relaxation — your hands resting more comfortably on the surface of the water than on a table or someone's shoulder outside the water, your sitting position in the bathtub with feet upraised (see illustration) much lighter, more vitally relaxed and "gravity-free" feeling than sitting on a stool or chair out of the water;

...gravity
(or gravitation)
is best managed
by levity
(or levitation)!

3 the experience of effortless balance on one toe or one finger, within the water-energy field — constituting a sense memory, or **direct image**, for future organic instruction to the body;

4 the feel of eurhythmic*, legato, slow-motion movement in water — the floating buoyancy sensation that will be applied, out of water, to fluid, loose-jointed, flowing body activity in standing, walking, rolling, running, climbing, dancing with free-form expressiveness, etc.

5 the awareness of self-teaching through a new kind of sensory intelligence which previously appeared to be involuntary or semi-voluntary and can now be used as conscious, voluntary organic instruction to the body.

In this experiment, we pretend still to be in water but using the prior water-energy experience as a kinesensic guide, we now recreate these sensations out of water.

Experiment Four:

**Out of the *WATER*
And Into The *AIR***

A • Lie down on your back, well rested and flexed, on a mat or comfortable rug.

• Pretend you are lying in a brim-full warm-water bath.

• Concentrate on all the sensations you felt and perceptions you experienced while in the water. Don't focus on the "doing." Just feel what you felt.

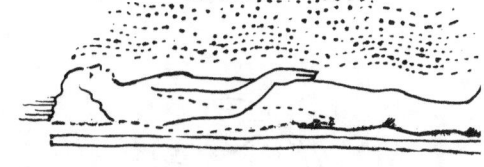

• Using your breath energy, try to re-experience all the sensations of lightness, balance, weightlessness, and floating movement associated with water buoyancy. Recall the feel of arm floating, as in previous illustrations. Remember how it felt when the

*good and beautiful movement.

arm and hand floated up in similar fashion, but without help from the water or wrist pressure against the wall.

- Now inhale a full breath and as you do, activate the "image-feel" of the arm floating up as it did in the bath.

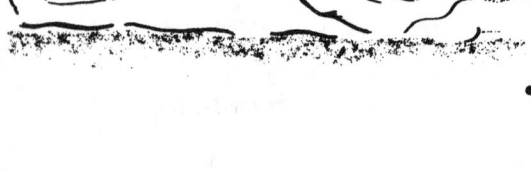

- Notice how your arms and hands float up a foot or more above the ground in rising buoyancy. Stay there for awhile in floating buoyancy.

- Then exhale gently and note how easily they float downward again in settling-down buoyancy.

- Just as in water, if you take a full breath, your arms and hands are almost involuntarily drawn upward, except now, you have willed the act through breath energy and direct image. Likewise, as you partially exhale, they will float easily halfway down and remain there with little or no fatigue. Upon complete exhalation, the arms and hands will rest gently and so lightly on the ground as to hardly sense its support.

B
- On the floor, repeat several of the buoyancy activities first explored in the bathtub: sitting postures, leg lifts, wafting and waving, Contact Vanishing Point, etc. To start you off, repeat the actions involving:

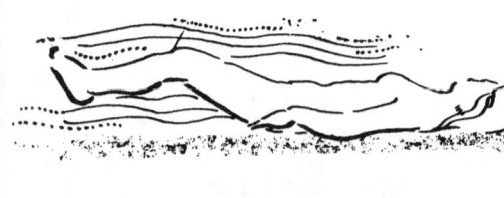

  ○ feet and legs, singly and together, as in the illustration, with feet straight up (not flopping sideways);

  ○ raising the torso while resting on the pelvis, as if approaching a "sit-up,"

  ○ balancing on the pelvic bone with feet and torso off the ground,

  ○ raising the torso with knees bent and feet off the floor in a balanced, compact sitting position,

  ○ wafting and waving, as though you were being gently moved in all directions by the currents and flow of the water.

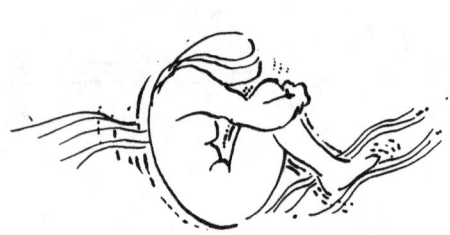

- As you perform each exercise, check whether the quality of buoyancy differs as your "image-instruction" takes you in and out of the water. Is it the same? Does the energy state you experience on the floor bring you full circle back to the feel of water buoyancy?

Body
Energizers
(Buoyancy)

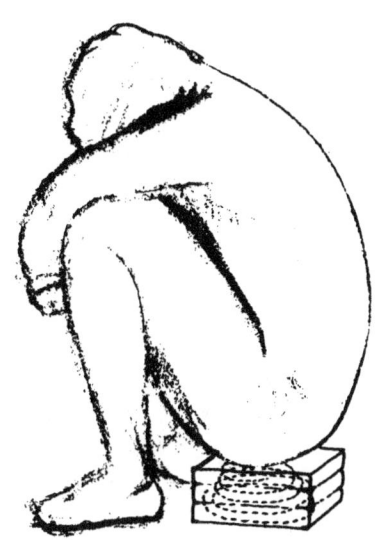

- Try sitting on an object no more than four to six inches high. Hardly sense the body contact. Pretend you are sitting in water. Can you recreate the feel of lightness of contact upon the hard surface? Pretend you are sitting on a large but delicate watch-spring. Can you feel the lightness of almost zero-pressure on its springy surface?

- As you move through these various exercises and positions, insert different breathing variations (full breath, half-exhalation, full exhalation) and register the varying sensations. What moves? What expands? What extends and "reaches?" What is the progression of movement? What is the rhythm of the motion?

- Consider the breathing action in these postures as a major part of the familiar event. Develop an awareness of this organic experience for future adaptation to other body postures where you will be off the floor. You'll discover, as you progress, a number of strong image and muscle memory instructions that influence muscle-sharing and which create a sharper, discriminatory climate for perception and awareness. You are beginning, here, to teach yourself the concept of "balanced muscle tonicity."

Experiment Five:

**In The Air -
Off Your Back -
On Your Feet**

In this experiment, continue with the "water image." Only now, you will be standing and your whole body will be unceasingly stimulated and motivated by the image of the water's gentle turbulence. Keeping that image in mind will help your body to feel gravity-free and to function as a "center of gravity" as it is wafted and waved in dynamic equilibrium.

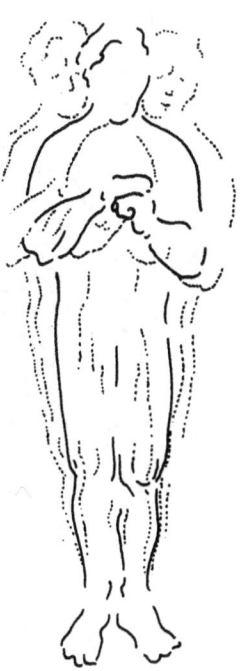

- Standing, with eyes open, waft and wave your body sideways, all the time maintaining balance, (see illustration).

- Repeat, wafting and waving forward and backward...now diagonally...then in circles, both clockwise and counter-clockwise, (see illustration).

- Coordinate this wafting and waving with breathing-energy and feel the resultant body extension and expansion. Feel the body respond to the sensation of either floating or rising buoyancy.

- Avoid a rag-doll floppiness anywhere in the body, but especially in the head, neck, and shoulders.

Energy
and
Relaxation

- When, on occasion, you find yourself wafting beyond a comfortable balance, simply let your feet shift gently and floatingly to an adjoining spot on the floor.

- Continue wafting without thinking about losing balance. In other words, enjoy **finding** additional balance without fear of falling. How? By turning the falling movement into a new improvisation of body expressiveness, a new step, or new discovery of balanced movement, a new challenge to achieve weightlessness.

- Exhale your breath slowly and feel the body float and waft downward toward a settling-down buoyancy. Check with illustrations. If it feels right, you're doing it right. Your knees will be loose and flexed; your back will form a "C" curve or bow-shaped bend very much like that of a fine skier moving down a gentle slope on the start of a cross-country ski hike.

- Repeat the exhalation but stop at the halfway mark. Note how your body pauses as it wafts and waves and balances in floating buoyancy, just as it did in the water.

- Continue exhaling until the body has settled all the way down, wafting and waving in balance almost to a sitting position — like the skier gathering speed just before a jump.

- Now inhale and feel your body respond, as it floats gently but unhesitatingly upward with rising buoyancy to standing posture.

- Still standing, with feet remaining in place and the "simulated" body of water still acting as your surrounding energy field, imagine the water's turbulence and its swirling, exciting changes of current. Feel these molding, sculpting, urging your body into spontaneous, free-form, rhythmic, asymmetrical, slow-motion movements of body expressiveness.

- Settle down buoyantly to supine position and do the floating sit-up as illustrated. Experience the sit-up as a body-reaching, body-extending dreamy-legato that is sustained throughout the extension. This buoyant reaching and extending appears to move right through the breathing network, forming a kinesthetic continuum and follow-through of the breath energy, itself. As you evolve the sit-up, reach buoyantly with one arm, then with the other, then with both. Add the reaching, floating head; the reaching neck; the reaching shoulder; the reaching back, until the whole body responds in a unity of energy to floating buoyancy and your floating sit-up becomes one with the buoyancy reach.

further described on p.113

43

Body
Energizers
(Buoyancy)

- You'll feel your breath energy internally distributed throughout the body and at the same time, it will feel as if the breath energy were being transmitted out of the body through the fingers, toes, ears, nose, elbows, shoulders, head, knees, and neck as well as through the surface pores. When this transmission of breath energy to outside space occurs, the reaching of any part of the body, now felt as an integral extension of the breath flow itself, forms a communicating link to the environmental space immediately surrounding the body.

- The benefits of this body reaching and extending are many. It forms one of the first interesting experiences in the discovery of plastique movement and genuinely original, personal body dancing. It reveals internal plastic rhythm dynamics that accompany the different reaches of body and breath energy. As the body reaches and extends in floating buoyancy, there is a discernible carry-over of the feel of peacefulness, of contemplative calm, of weightlessness, and of absolutely effortless "doing." It becomes an extremely effective way to reclaim body balance and balanced muscle tonicity.

...peace of mind and tense muscles are always mutually exclusive!

Still standing but with eyes closed, the waft or wave experiences, sensations, and perceptions of body buoyancy are uniquely different. In this experiment, you need no longer entertain the water image. You are now in your own inner space, consciously and intentionally, imaging various atmospheric conditions such as stronger winds for body-waving and body-rocking, gentler breezes for body-wafting, quiet air for body-floating and body-soaring.

In this as in the previous experiments, you must respond with the same effortless, light buoyancy and weightlessness. No new demand for conscious use of muscles, joints, hinges, or bones will be made, but you will find revealed to your sensory and perceptual awareness a new battery of fascinating images that can be "hired" for organic instruction.

- With eyes comfortably but fully closed, waft and wave from side to side.

- Continue wafting and waving, with eyes still closed, but now move forward and backward...then diagonally...then conically...

- Waft and wave downward, eyes closed, floating down to a sitting position; then waft back up to upright posture. Your eyelids should be inquisitively relaxed.

Experiment Six:

**Wafting Rhythmically
With Eyes Closed
In Almost
'Motionless Movement'**

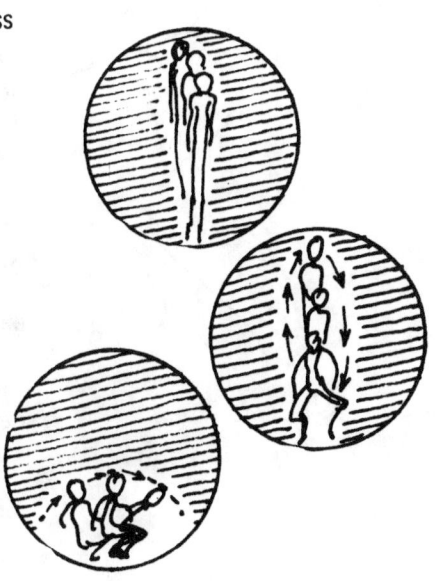

Energy
and
Relaxation

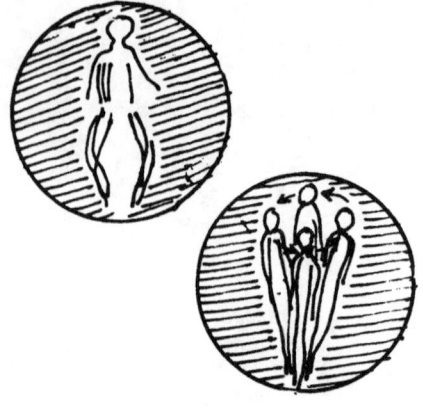

- Move **slowly** as deliberately as you can, but do not halt the motion.

- Register your sensations of wafting and waving with eyes closed: your feelings during the movement; your evolving images as you waft and wave in different directions; your perception, awareness, and response to all of these.

Three fundamental components specifically relate to this experiment and generally serve to develop your awareness and sense-memory feedback: breath, space, and creative calm.

BREATH! While wafting and waving, always try for quiet, smooth breathing; breathing gently and quietly through the nose while the tongue softly blankets the velvety lining of your hard palate and your lips stay gently apart. Inhaling and exhaling should feel like a gentle, satisfying sigh, a soft sigh reflecting the feeling of appreciation, contentment, even wistfulness.

When you breathe in, you feel yourself fueling and feeding and vitalizing the body. As you sense yourself distributing breath energy throughout the body, trace the movement of distribution to parts and limbs, outer surfaces and pores, through veins and arteries. As you track the energy distribution through the feeling process, you'll sense in the movement a feel of inner rhythm and body potential.

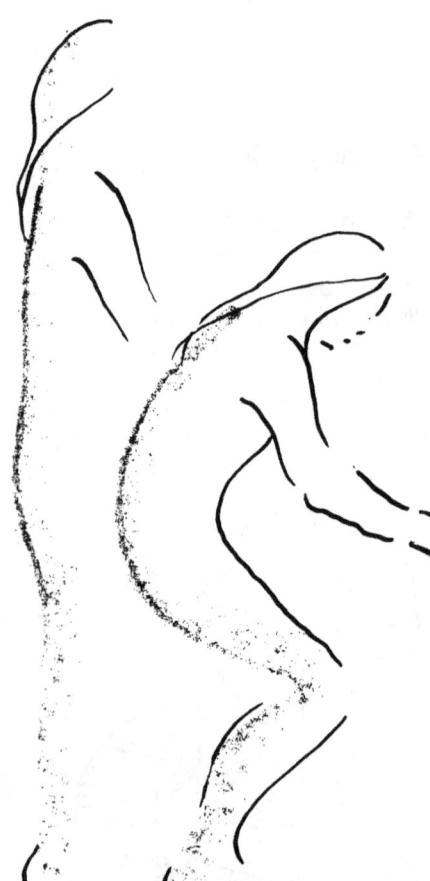

The slower and farther you waft and wave in any direction, the slower, longer, quieter, and gentler will be the "inspired inhalation;" i.e. an inhalation that literally "inspires" the body, both viscerally and esthetically. As you coordinate body-wafting with inhaled inspiring, you'll begin to experience a more sophisticated awareness of the rhythm-feel of breath energy.

SPACE! As you work with the inner rhythms of wafting, waving, and breathing, you will sense the feeling of increased spatial expanse within the body environment. With your eyes closed, you feel this body extension and expansion — imaging yourself as a "vital vehicle" soaring or floating freely through internal space, cruising in any direction, at any speed, at any height or depth through vast internal expanse. It is the feeling that the slower and gentler you waft, the slower and quieter you breathe and the faster your body vehicle seems to travel through a vastly more prodigious inner space.

The key image is that of "listening within" our body organism. We seem to be using our five outer senses inwardly, but in a new and different frequency, in a new and unfamiliar environment. It is this "feeling within" our still strange, inner body environment that allows us to discover the sensation and perception of every nuance and shade, every shape and substance of our harmonic overtone sensory system.

CREATIVE CALM! Whether you are being wafted by actual or imaged support fields, or you maneuver the wafting consciously, the significant fact is that the experience occurs within a body climate of almost perfect equilibrium. The movement-dynamics of the breath/buoyancy energy state — whether felt through the esthetics of balance, rhythm, languorous plastique motion, or any combination of these — become a veritable study of both "stillness in motion" and the "movement of stillness."

The images that derive from breath-floating buoyancy and support this activity may be peaceful and benign, but they are simultaneously active and curiously vital; they appear to stimulate and sensitize a progressively new approach to meditation discipline. The feel of these diverse images and sensations, that induce wide-ranging body expressiveness, are all perceived as part of psycho-physical body esthetics.

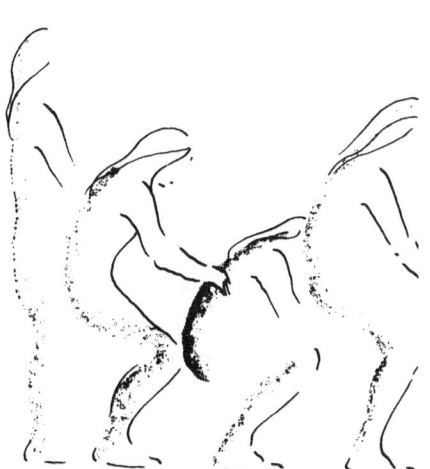

Buoyancy Summary

In summarizing the buoyancy activities exemplified in Experiments #1 through #6, let me underscore those essential, carry-over experiences that recur throughout the remaining work chapters:

1. the sensations and perceptions of **breathing-body-buoyancy**, our first, primitive body energy state, as a physical expression of "live weight" vs. "dead weight;"

2. **buoyant wafting and waving out of water, with eyes closed,** as a regenerator of instinctive balance; of the feel of the body traveling through inner space; of "moving meditation" or contemplative calm; of weightlessness and plastique body expressiveness;

3. **buoyant wafting and waving out of water, with eyes open,** as a causal factor in sensory awareness; conscious body skill and control; buoyant muscle elasticity and body expansion; incipient, mimetic movement that introduces the feel of a personal art of mime; and rhythmic, slow motion composition that evolves into a personal and original Tai-Chi;

4. the **floating sit-up** organically experienced in harmonious balance as part of muscle-free, buoyant body reach;

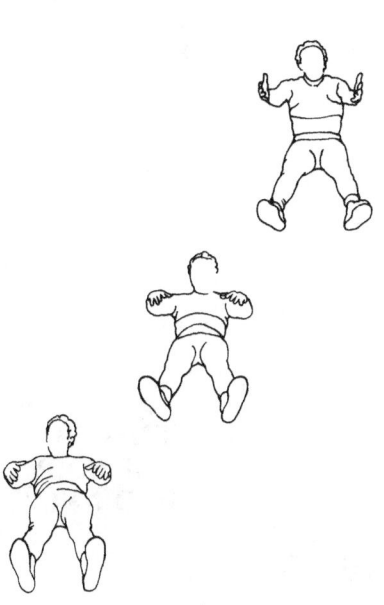

5   the quality of **body reaching** (extending and bending) as a function of the buoyancy-breathing energy state;

6   **plastique movement,** or plastic body molding, expressing a sculptural inter-relationship between the body in spontaneous, balanced motion and the surrounding space;

7   avoiding the **fear of falling** through body sensations that accompany the events of rising, floating, and settling-down buoyancy and which induce the feel of weightlessness — constituting at least partial discovery of the feeling of fear diffusion;

8   images generated by the breathing-buoyancy energy state that can eventually be "hired" as images for organic instruction, including:

  ◦ floating, balanced body reaching;

  ◦ feeling the vanishing of weight at any given, body contact point;

  ◦ zero pressure or zero stress as an effect of body weightlessness in equilibrium;

  ◦ body images suggesting the potent power of breath, the sensory feel of fluid internal body exercise, the awareness of breath power as potential inner eurhythmics;

9   the use of **body esthetics,** a concomitant of the feeling process, as the only effective antidote to the anesthetics of pain, discomfort, pressure, and a lack of creative awareness;

10 the decoding of **buoyancy-feel** as a "regional dialect" of one's individual body language and personal culture.

II THE SENSATION OF BODY RADIANCY

The feeling of "radiancy," like buoyancy, is one of the physical idioms of body language. The "radiancy energy state" provokes and stimulates at least three body dialects:

- sophisticated muscle-shaking and a radiating feel of body-vibrato;

- electric body-spark, or flick, that promotes agility and physical dexterity; and

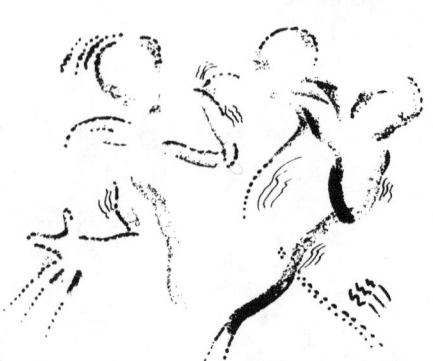

Body
Energizers
(Radiancy)

- a visible sense of eagerness, alertness, or anticipation which induces the sensation of spontaneity.

As a vital nervous energy release, body radiancy is a freely expressive, exciting, tingling, always trigger-ready awareness.

As a vital muscle energy release, it represents the personification of deftness, nimbleness, and agility.

As anticipation energy release, it is like the carefree but meaningful vitality of all child-like "work-play" behavior; the unrestrained eagerness and excited curiosity of the child waiting for its "surprise" to unfold; the child's wide-eyed rapture at a magic show or circus; the child's ingenuous inquisitiveness of whatever is happening **now**, etc., of its exploring; etc.

The precocious kitten with its unpredictable moves and its fascinating, electric eyes — prancing, playing, leaping, turning, rolling, sudden stopping — is all radiancy energy! The artful, ever-alert body behavior of Charlie Chaplin or Laurel and Hardy in the old silent movies is radiancy at work! The deer on sudden guard at the first scent of intruders — the great "lighter-than-air" tap dancing of immortal Bill Robinson — the night-watch always loose in order to be always on guard — the track-runner just before the Go signal — the symphony musicians on sudden "nerve-tingly" anticipation of their maestro's first downbeat — all of these images obtain to radiancy energy.

Radiancy energy release, especially with the young child, always starts in the eyes and is often accompanied by an equally eager hand dexterity and finger-dancing. It is reflected in the wide-eyed look of impish delight, the leprechaun look of sudden surprise or amusement, the astonished and breathlessly eager look when captivated by the storyteller, the circus clown, or the magician. Try it!

- Open **your** eyes with impish delight.

- Dart your eyes in different directions and at different people or objects with the feeling of eagerness and pleasure that will induce "that wide-eyed look" all the way to your ears and through the back of your head.

- Infuse your entire face with these quick, dart-like movements and assume the face of a kitten...a rabbit...a pixy, etc.

- Continue the deft, nimble, amusing, elf-like expressions and movements of the eyes and carry them over, as a flowing cur-

Experiment One:

Radiancy In The Eyes

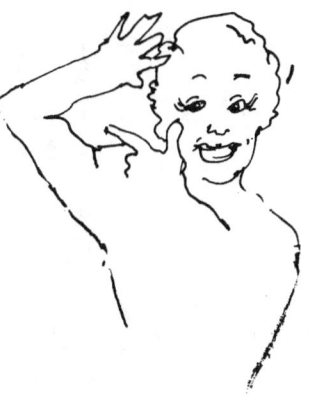

rent, to the fingers, the finger-tips, the hands and arms — maintaining that pleasure-fun principle of being fully **childlike** but never childish. This is a transferral that has infused the art of several of our greatest actors and modern choreographers.

Experiment Two:

Radiancy Energy State

The radiancy of anticipation energy could be regarded as a **heightened boyancy feel,** the boyancy energy state agitated by tingling nerve impulses.

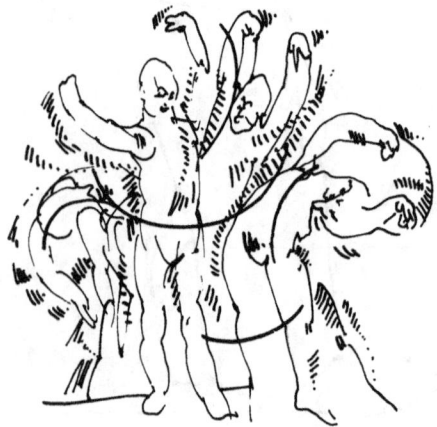

- Sculpt the space around you with a peaceful, calm breathing-buoyancy floating action.

- Suddenly punctuate that calm floatation with darting, staccato-like gestures, similar to the flickering antics of excited puppets.

- Register the new sensation and perception. It is as if you were to leave or disengage the calm trust of weightless balance and legato extension to spontaneously join the alert, trigger-like, kinetic vitality of nervous energy. It is the image of calm contemplation unexpectedly overtaken by the lambent eyes of a child's radiant face, or the flicking tongues of flame darting to and fro within the glow and blaze of the fireplace.

Experiment Three:

Radiancy Images

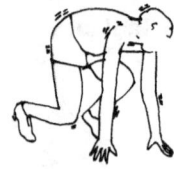

A • The Sprinter Image:

- Imagine yourself a sprinter and put yourself into "get-ready" position. You are full of anticipation as your attention is captured by the imminent "go" command. But the real experiment in feeling radiancy energy is at the get-set signal. As the starter calls it out, your body fibers galvanize and without any apparent movement, you trigger-set to GO!

- Try this several times, in each instance feeling your body "light up" and elastically expand with the electricity of anticipation energy. Feel it as "muscle-release" energy.

B • The Stalking Hunter Image:

- Imagine yourself a hunter about to snare your quarry.

- Improvise a stalking, stealthy, almost motionless advance, like a cat silently moving forward but so low that its belly nearly touches the ground.

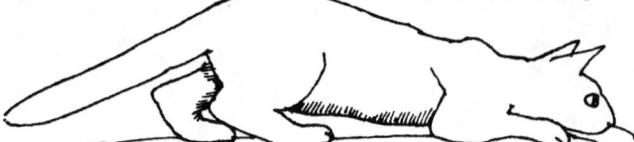

Body
Energizers
(Radiancy)

- Then, like the cat, playfully and lambently flick out at your target.

- Sense-record the feel of anticipation, vibration, and muscle-release as you again experience this electricity-like, nerve-energy state.

The other character of radiancy energy is the shimmering, vibratory, radiating feel. This is the stimulation that agitates a flicker-like tremble; a spark that combusts into small, shooting flames; a darting staccato that becomes a restless, vibrating **agitato**.

Experiment Four:

Vibratory Trembling, Shaking, and The Coil-Spring Sit-Up

- Imagine an event, surprise, or experience so pleasurable that it starts you literally trembling with excitement. Note how differently you perceive the tremble when it is associated with something pleasurable rather than something frightening. **Feel the difference** and add it to your sense memory bank.

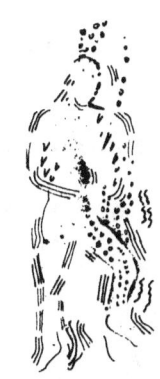

- Now try to refine this body shaking to a kind so subtle and sophisticated that all you respond to is the rhythm and the underlying pulsation of the quiver. Register the feel of this sensation as a quiver-vibrato, a kind of vibrant, internal "gut message." This feeling is, in fact, a stimulant to the body in dynamic live weight, eliminating the dead weight of floppy, hanging-loose, body heaviness. Body quivering with radiancy energy is, in this sense, another body energizer.

- Repeat the sit-up exercise, but this time think of it as a "nervous energy sit-up." Or as a "coil-spring sit-up" — a sit-up that expresses a quick, yet quiet excitement in body reaching especially revealed in the eyes and face. As you coil-spring sit up, your arms, hands and fingertips should reach out with their own sparkle of effervescence, and the lightness you feel is that of a body suddenly released. It is the lightness of the deer or kitten, the flicking tongue of the cat rhythmically lapping up its milk. Your body is now nimbly relaxed and as you stand up, you'll feel a sensation of "dancing relaxation." That is the lingering effect of radiancy energy!

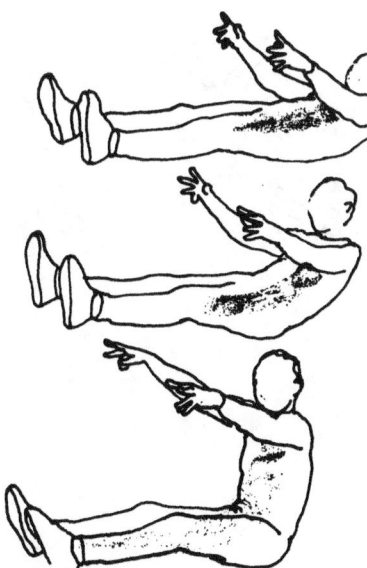

Remember that with radiancy, one can speak as trippingly with the eyes, toes, and fingers as with the tongue. Radiancy affords a special quality of motivation to muscle expansion and muscle reaching. You now know how to induce into your muscles and joints the sense of radiating vibrato that is at the core of radiancy nerve energy.

further described on p.114

As you incorporate these experiments and adapt them to everyday life, you will notice a qualitative change in your increasingly balanced muscle tonicity. Nothing will seem heavy, forced, or tight — only light, tingly, agile, and deft! You'll experience a greater vitality and kinetic energy in performing daily tasks.

Note: Please keep in mind that all the experiments presented in this chapter are designed to offer you experimental opportunity to explore and discover ABOUT the body energy states. Specific exercise training is covered in the work chapters of Part Three.

III THE SENSATION OF BODY POTENCY or MUSCLE - YAWN ENERGY

Before discussing this concept, let us move directly into

Experiment One:

Power Potential Potency

- As you have often seen a cat or dog do, and as indicated in the illustration, get your body into a natural body-yawn stretch as though trying to stretch the sleep out of your body.

- Next, breathe in and at the top of the breath, close your fists around an imaginary lead pipe.

- Picture yourself, on your mental screen, in super-charged body yawn stretch and grip — and **feel** yourself bending that pipe.

- Then, take a jar with a cover too tightly fastened to unscrew by sheer muscle force or a bottle too tightly corked to pull out by hand.

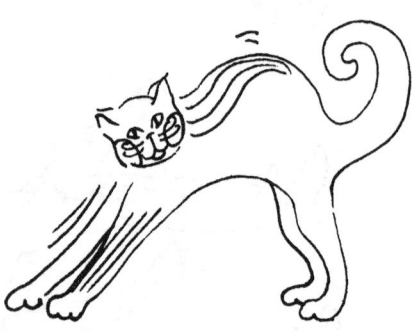

- Recalling the feel of the body-yawn stretch you just experienced in bending the imaginary pipe, apply it to unscrewing the jar or uncorking the bottle. Breathe in and at the top of the breath, close your fists around the jar cap or cork and accompany the full yawn-stretch with the vocal expression, "Oh, it feels so-so-o g-oo-ood!"

Performed without struggle, irritation, or outside assistance, chances are you will loosen the jar-cover or slide out the cork, slowly but smoothly. And in the process, you will appreciate how much more creatively powerful is the body's strength potential in a body-yawn stretch, than in an act that tightens the muscles to strain or force.

Body
Energizers
(Potency)

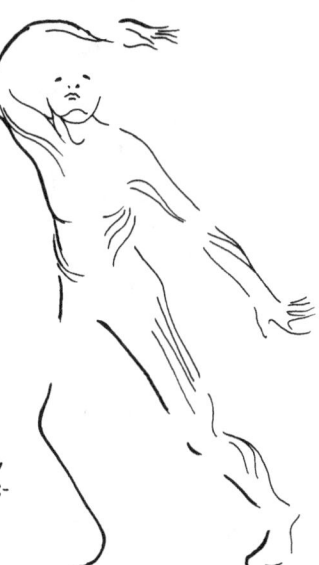

I consider this phenomenon a form of chemical energy that generates an invariably maximal physical action. If, as suggested by the illustration, you have experimented honestly using genuine body-yawn freedom, then you will have experienced a far greater, hidden reserve of physical strength or power potential than you knew you had. Potency always carries the feel of a high-voltage, muscle-yawn stretch that vitalizes the body with a sense of fierce and deep intensity (often supported by "gut-felt," expressive vocal accompaniment), a feeling, precisely, of unlimited potency. Interesting enough, it is an energy activity that relaxes as it empowers, both actions functioning simultaneously at optimal efficiency.

Experiment Two:

Body-Yawn Push-Ups and Chin-Ups

A •   Lying on your stomach, start stretching as though just waking in the morning. Enjoy the full-bodied quality of the stretch and allow it to feel good.

• Next, place your hands in push-up position (finger knuckles to the floor as illustrated) and as you move into a body-yawn, stretch yourself into a push-up — first from the knees, then from the toes.

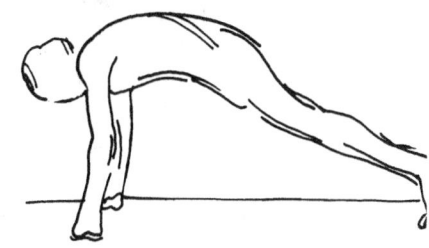

• Do as many of these as you like, but with each one imagine yourself stretching the body out of sleep and tell yourself, "Oh, what a **beautiful** morning!" Do your body-yawn push-ups with personal involvement while genuinely enjoying the stretching.

• A few hours later, do the same push-up series in the usual muscle-forced way. Compare the number of repetitions and the ease or dis-ease with which they were done, relative to the previous yawn-stretch series. Then immediately after, repeat the push-ups with body yawn and check to feel which are more comfortable and more pleasurable.

B • Do the same with a series of chin-ups, as illustrated. Find a ledge or bar or sturdy branch and try to pull yourself up by brute force.

• Then, perform the same chin-up allowing the body-yawn stretch, with full breath held at the top, to pull you up.

• Compare the feel and endurance ability of both kinds of chin-ups.

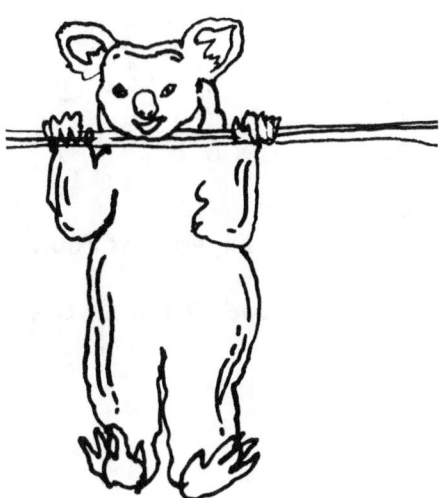

Energy
and
Relaxation

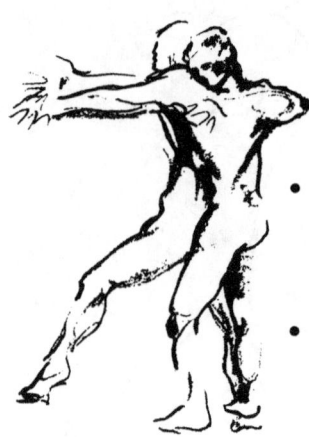

- Remember: You must be genuinely involved with a good, salutary body-yawn stretch. Remember, too, that the body can yawn-stretch itself with or without the regular throat yawn. In this experiment, the yawn-stretch is muscular, not respirative.
- For those of you who have trouble getting started with the chin-up, notice how the body-yawn stretch **prepares** the body for the act and feels good in the process.

Experiment Three: A

Buddy Work

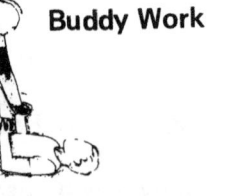

- Perform this experiment with a friend. As indicated in the illustration, lie on your back, elbows on the ground, ready to hold up your buddy who in push-up style, will attempt to keep you pinned down while you try to push him/her all the way up to arm's length using sheer muscle power.
- Repeating the exercise, substitute the body yawn-stretch for muscle power. Once again, accompany the stretch with the genuinely felt vocal expression, "Oh, it **feels** so-o-o g-oo-ood" — recalling the first stretch of the morning.
- You will discover the dramatic and remarkable experience that what was strenuous and difficult with muscle power becomes an exciting, exhilarating and adventurous energy exploration with body-yawn stretch.

B
- Again working with a buddy, extend your arm towards an object or person in body-yawn stretch as part of a **motivated** reaching action.
- During that motivated reach, your buddy will try to flex (not break) your arm at the elbow.

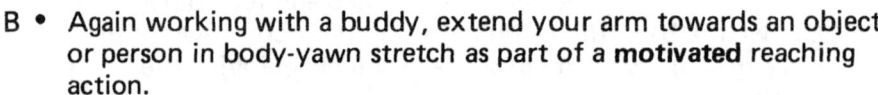

- If your arm is truly muscle-yawning and genuinely reaching **through** the object or person rather than merely to it, your friend will have a pretty difficult time bending your arm, (see illustration).
- The surprising experience is that you will achieve the same result with the floating-buoyancy energy state as you did with the muscle-yawn stretch.

Experiment Four:

Body-Yawn Sit-Ups

- Do the sit-up but this time, in coordination with a body-yawn stretch: first with fingers and hands; then progressively, with arms, shoulders, neck, head and back, pelvis, thighs, legs and

Body
Energizers
(Potency)

feet. Do it, as illustrated, in a flexible, wiry, spring-like yet yawn-stretch manner.

- This will work only if you avoid the traditional sit-up and become genuinely involved in **feeling** the potency of muscle-yawn energy which draws you up, almost without your knowing it.

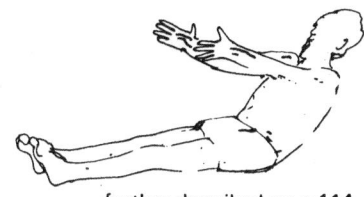

further described on p.114

Body-yawn energy, when turned off, resolves the follow-through action into a stimulating floating-buoyancy energy state.

Experiment Five:

From Body-Yawn To Floating Buoyancy

- Repeat the first buoyancy experiment involving the back of the wrist pressing against the flat wall. Only this time, while pressing your wrist, be sure to feel the urge of the body-yawn stretch through the entire arm and shoulder. When you step away from the wall, giving your arm free space to move, observe the phenomenon of floating buoyancy coming directly out of the potent body-yawn energy state. Clearly then, if in any physical action you turn off (or dilute) the stretch power of the body-yawn feel, you will be left with the floating power of body buoyancy.

- Body-yawn stretch your back and arms, as illustrated, and during the action simply turn off the muscle-yawn stretch. The immediate result is that the energy flow circles back to the sensation of water buoyancy, yielding up an incredible feeling of relaxation. It feels as if the yawn is expired by the muscles while they are, simultaneously, inspired by the buoyancy energy. The body yawn is expended, but leaves in its wake the quieter, gentler, breath-buoyancy feel as a follow-through energy state. Not a drop of body-yawn fuel is left in the tank, yet the gliding, cruising, flying capacity appears to float on and on, indefinitely.

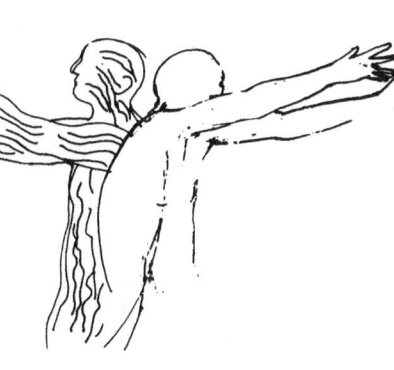

- Now try space-sculpting with body-yawn energy. An interesting transformation occurs. While you experience the same free-form plastique body movement, it is now fed with the ardent intensity of the body-yawn reach and stretch, instead of the legato floating-reach of buoyancy, or the sparkling vibratory-reach of radiancy.

- Finally, repeat the body-yawn sit-up and alternate it with the characteristics of the buoyancy sit-up, then the radiancy sit-up. In each case, experience the new sensations, new qualities of resilient power, speed, agility, flexibility, durability, and strength; in each case perceive the new idioms of relaxation, rhythm, and balance.

Energy
and
Relaxation

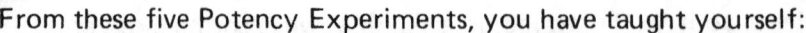

From these five Potency Experiments, you have taught yourself:

1   the FEEL of the most intense body strength without force or strain;

2   the FEEL of the most dynamic body extension;

3   the FEEL of the most energetic relaxation;

4   the FEEL of experiencing breathing-buoyancy energy as a natural continuation of ardent, intense body-yawn energy; and

5   the FEEL of never over-exploiting the body's musculature, which offers you a "reserve cushion" so that even more extension or vigorous activity can be anticipated and explored without fear of strain or body stress.

IV THE SENSATION OF INTER-INVOLVEMENT

To the extent we are personally involved, to that extent do we lessen technical work, whether in professional performance or in the initial step of training. Even the purest technique is poor technique when inner personal involvement is lacking. But to be self-involved with the perception of your own body energy states is not quite the same thing as the sensation of inter-involvement!

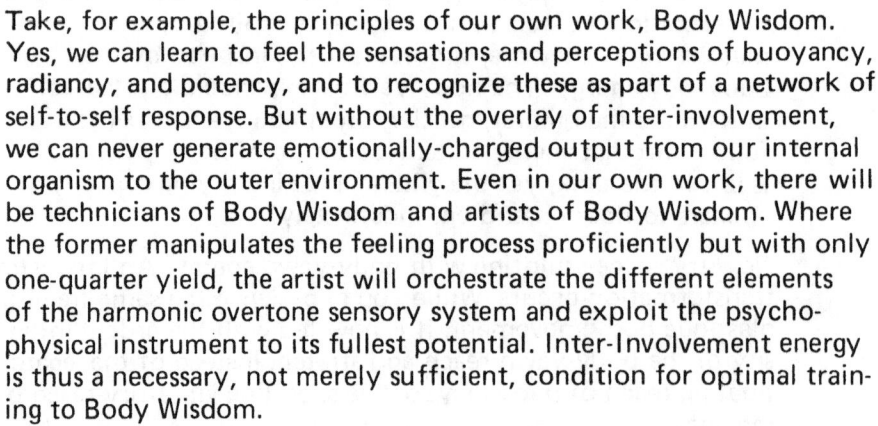

Take, for example, the principles of our own work, Body Wisdom. Yes, we can learn to feel the sensations and perceptions of buoyancy, radiancy, and potency, and to recognize these as part of a network of self-to-self response. But without the overlay of inter-involvement, we can never generate emotionally-charged output from our internal organism to the outer environment. Even in our own work, there will be technicians of Body Wisdom and artists of Body Wisdom. Where the former manipulates the feeling process proficiently but with only one-quarter yield, the artist will orchestrate the different elements of the harmonic overtone sensory system and exploit the psycho-physical instrument to its fullest potential. Inter-Involvement energy is thus a necessary, not merely sufficient, condition for optimal training to Body Wisdom.

Inter-Involvement energy serves as an instrument for committed communication. It is a personally motivated relating to others directed by our emotional experiencing system. Through inter-involvement energy, the internalized **feeling** of self-to-self response is transmitted to the larger, outside environment. This can best be demonstrated through the following experiment:

Body
Energizers
(Inter-Involvement)

- Let us do the sit-up once more. We have already "floated up," "radiated up," and "yawn-stretched up" in preceding sit-up exercises. Now let's do an "emo-tivated" sit-up, one that is emotionally charged — that functions as vital communication and communicating vitality at the same time.

- Lie on your back and starting with your eyes, infuse every body fibre with climactic, emotional body reaching. Whether you select a searching, inspirational, or intensely critical motivation, the emotional reach will involve not only the eyes, the face, the arms, hands, and fingers, but as well the nuances, shadings, intonations, and inflections of the entire body that are being fed by the instinctive needs and emotions rather than by muscle awareness. Here is total reaching, nourished by a magnetic force diametrically opposed to sheer brawn.

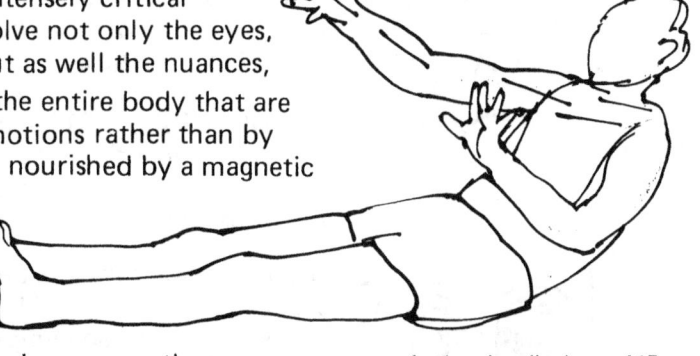

- Now repeat the sit-up using first breathing-buoyancy, then radiancy energy, then body-yawn stretch. Underscore each body energizing sit-up with inter-involvement and sense the extra ease and enjoyment in performing the sit-up with emo-tivated weightlessness, emo-tivated agility, and emo-tivated power potential.

further described on p.115

- Note the common denominator: Your involvement energy is so dominant it removes all concentration from muscle responsibility. In **Inter-Involvement,** the muscles are pre-empted and the emotional experiencing system, in synergic cooperation with the body's communicating systems, appears to take charge with such vigor that it bypasses the muscular system and all consciousness of kinesthetic exertion.

   SO FAR:

1. You are learning about an inner awareness of different levels, degrees, qualities, and rhythms of four intrinsic, body energy states — and how these inter-relate, synthesize, and balance one another. In other words, we have come full circle back to the concept of the cross-quality "generalization of energies."

2. You are learning that it is possible and reasonable to tune into a body energy state at any time, whether your body is totally relaxed in a resting condition or vigorously active — and that all four of our balanced, primitive energy states are therapeutic, relaxing agents for the body.

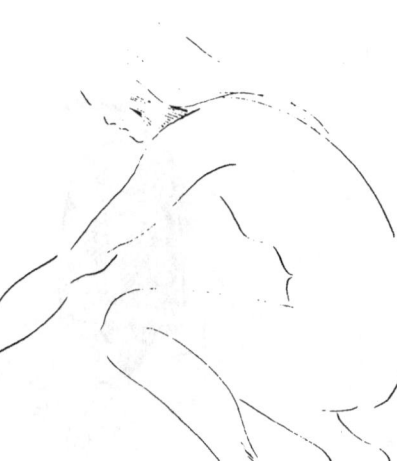

3. You are aware that all of these energy experiences provide definitive feelings of pleasure, comfort, health, body improvement, and psycho-physical tension-relief. That is to say, they provide a strategy for, and make available, an infinite variety of "body esthetics" to your internal experiencing systems.

APPENDIX: The Three "VOCAL LIFE" Body Energy States

For the benefit of newcomers, entering our work for the first time through *BODY WISDOM*, there follows a brief, outlined introduction to the three vocal or verbal **derived energy states** that were fully treated in *The Use and Training of the Human Voice.* *

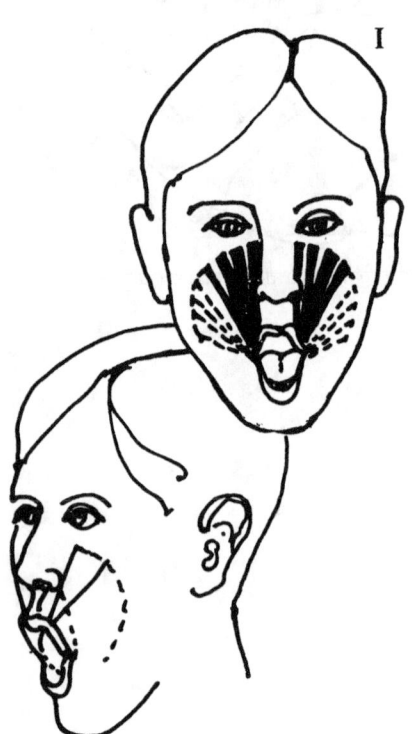

I **STRUCTURAL ACTION: A kinesthetic energy state** related to facial posture (proper formation of the "cervical spine" and head posture carried over to optimal facial form and alignment) revealing the existence, nature, and functioning of an unconditioned reflex of the jaw.

Benefits: Achieves most efficient and effective size-shape of the vocal sound box that self-regulates color, body, resonance, strength, esthetics of vocal tone for any voice and speech situation. Contributes to protection and maintenance of dental health. Provides continuing tension relief for the entire mandibular, neck, throat areas, with attendant relief in face, chin, head, and shoulders as well. Also produces good muscle tone in face, throat, and shoulder areas.

Applications and Results: An organic physio-sensory formation and awareness of perfect vowel production and natural, kinesthetic pronunciation process.

Exercise Classifications: Structural Stretch; Instinctively induced Rounded Lips for Rounder Vowels; Relaxing the Jaw; Enlivening a previously crowded Tongue; Stretch and Relaxation; Phonetics by Feeling; Structural Vowels; A Simpler Phonetics; Woo-Woe-Waw-Wow Exercise; Word List and Drill for Structural Perception; Word Lists and Sentences; Reading Selections; Personal Projects and Improvisation in Communication through Structural Action. (See pp. 56-78 in *The Use and Training of the Human Voice*).

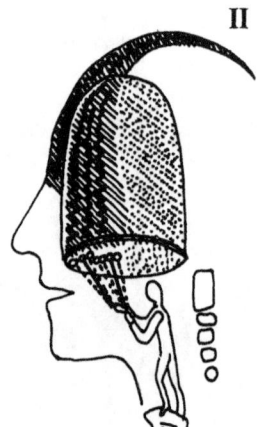

II **TONAL ACTION: A vibrative energy state** relating to phonation, voice production, tonal resonance, color quality, vocal expressiveness, and the emotional experiencing system.

Benefits: Tonal action is a natural relaxing agent; it is at the same time integrally joined, in a one-to-one relationship, with the emotional experiencing system.

Applications and Results: Develops internal vibratory therapy **and** body exercise. Constitutes protective device against strain and throatiness. Relieves tension and provides "built-in vibratory beam" to give

Vocal Life
Energy States

directional guidance to your speech. Attacks and helps cure bad vocal habits such as throatiness, nasality, denasality, and breathiness. Tonal Action is a defending force against pain, anger, strain, distress, pressures; it is an intrinsic "feeling modality" that can be used as a revolutionary approach in training the deaf and hearing-impaired to develop rich, resonant, normal speaking and singing voices.

Exercise Classifications: Ybuzz Exercises and Word Lists, Muscle Shaking, Ybuzz Sentences, Ybuzz Improvisation, The Plus Ybuzz, Plus Ybuzz and Carry-Over Exercises including Ybuzz Communication, Reading Selections, and Improvisation in Communication through the Ybuzz Focus. Also, Call Exercises #1 - #19. See Tonal Action I – "The Ybuzz," pages 79-94, and Tonal Action II – "The Call," pages 110-128 in *The Use and Training of the Human Voice*.

CONSONANT ACTION: A musical instrument energy experience related to rhythm and music in speech, intelligibility, and articulatory skills.

Benefits: The recognition of consonant music and rhythm as major and dominating components of speech. The development and awareness of the "consonant orchestra."

Applications and Results: A clinical aid in speech and voice therapy in areas such as stuttering, cleft palate, hysterical aphonia, deafness and hearing impairments, etc. Restores clarity, musicality, and natural rhythm to poorly conditioned, sloppy speech — eliminating enervation, carelessness, and poor diction. Consonant action functions as a natural and significant relaxing agent. Fully developed, it adds meaning, emphasis, and emotional content to your speech.

Exercise Classifications: The Consonant Orchestra Tuning Exercises including: the N violin, the M viola, the V cello, the F sound effect, the Z bass fiddle, the S sound effect, the B tympani drumbeat, the P bassdrum drumbeat, the D tympani drumbeat, the T snare drum drumbeat, the G tympani drumbeat, the K tom-tom drumbeat, the TH clarinet, the TH sound effect, the SH sound effect, the ZH bassoon, the L saxophone, the NG oboe, the DG chinese cymbal, the CH crash cymbal, the DZ tambourine, the TS after-beat cymbal, the H sound effect, the W flute, the Y french horn, the R trombone, the DL and TL woodblocks, etc. See pages 129-178 in *The Use and Training of the Human Voice*. (See Chapter XI, pp. 144 - 147).

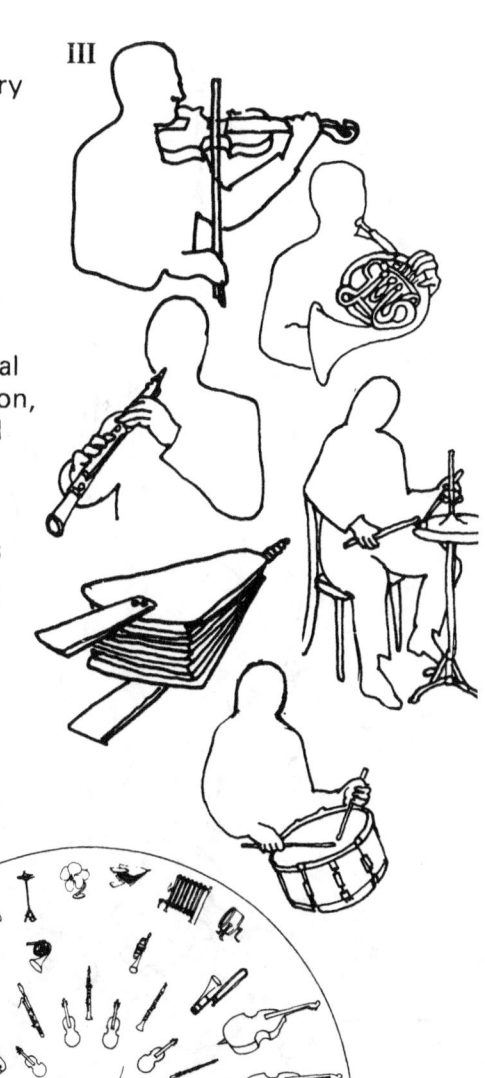

III

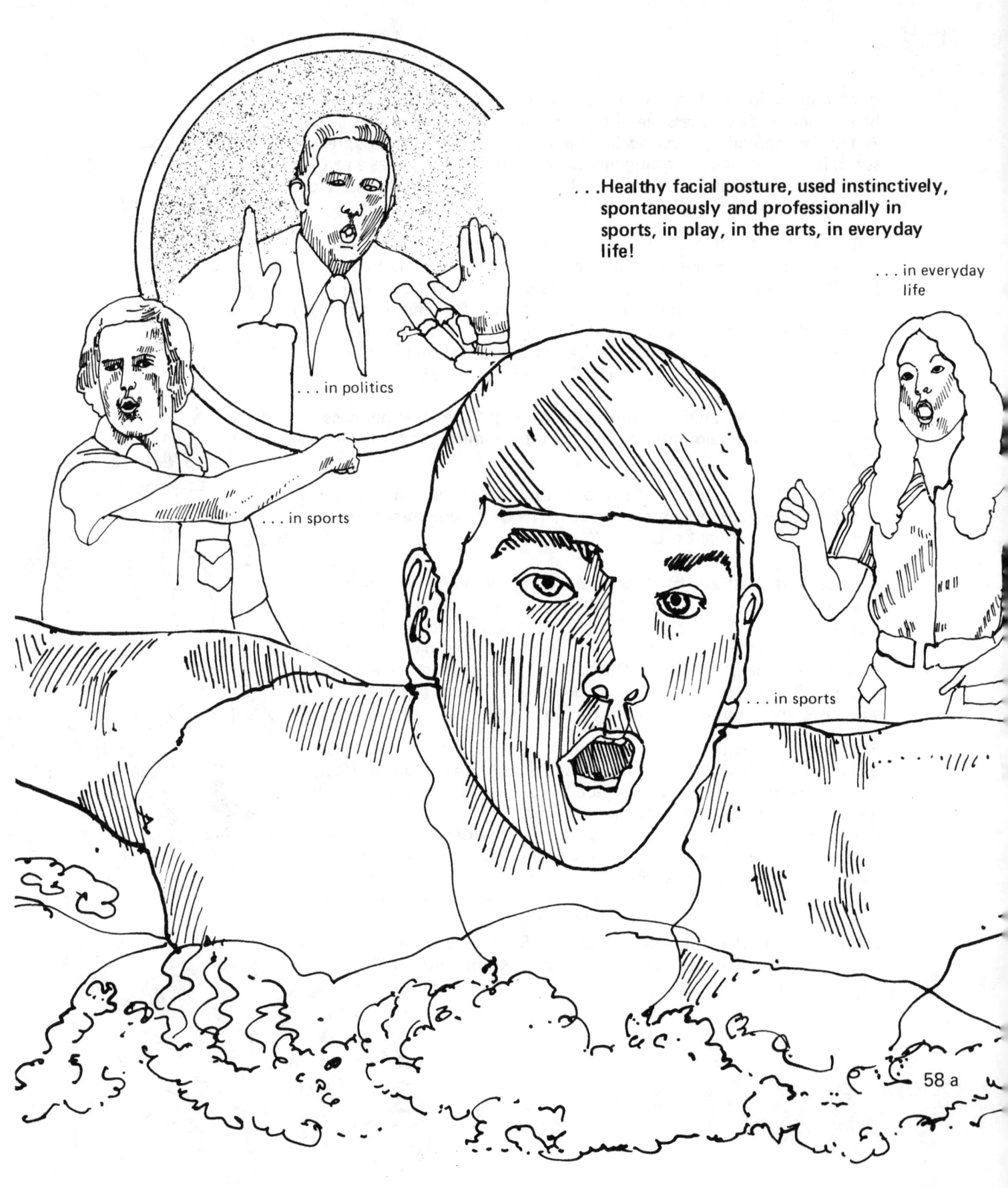

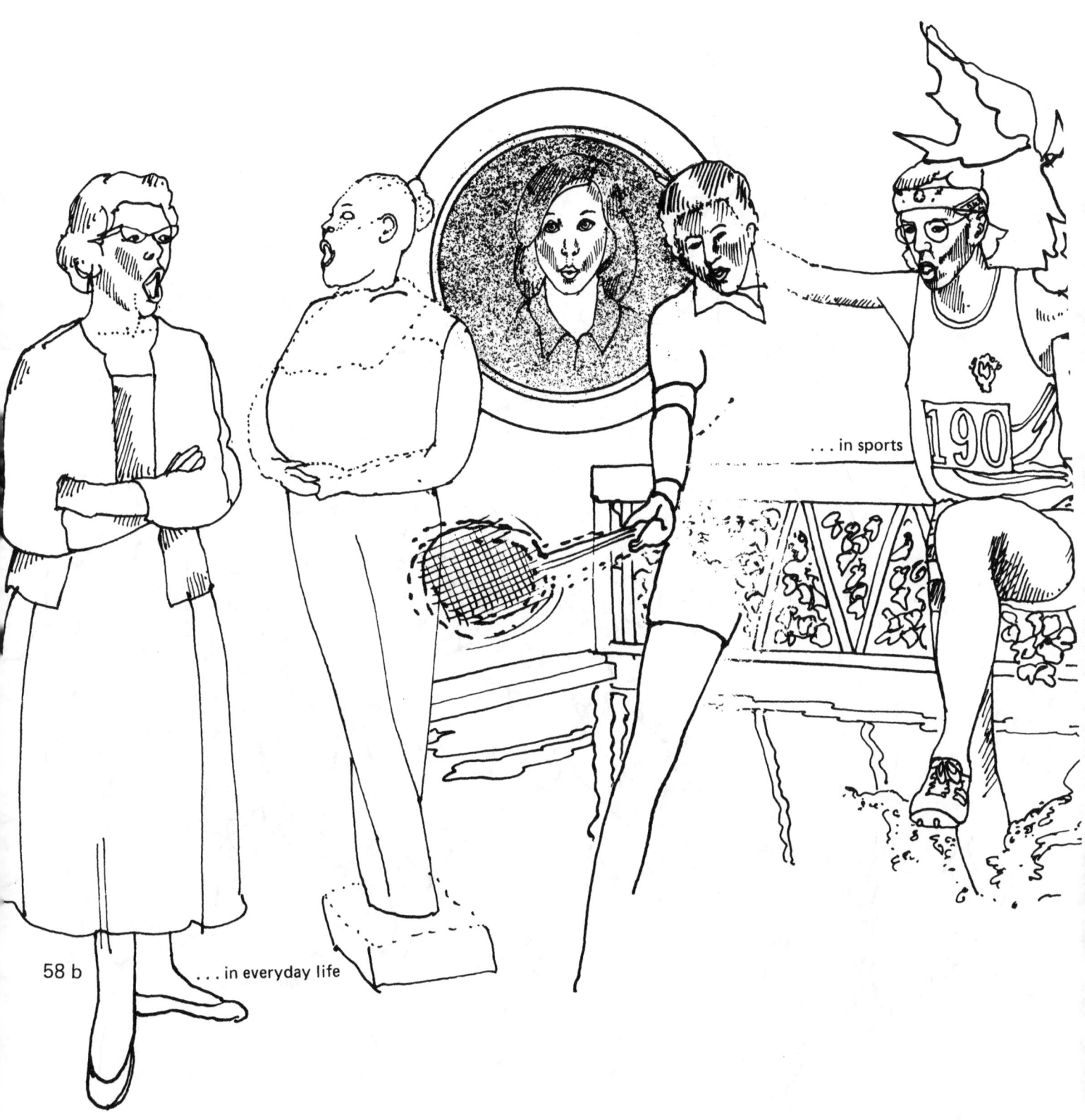

58 b ...in everyday life ...in sports

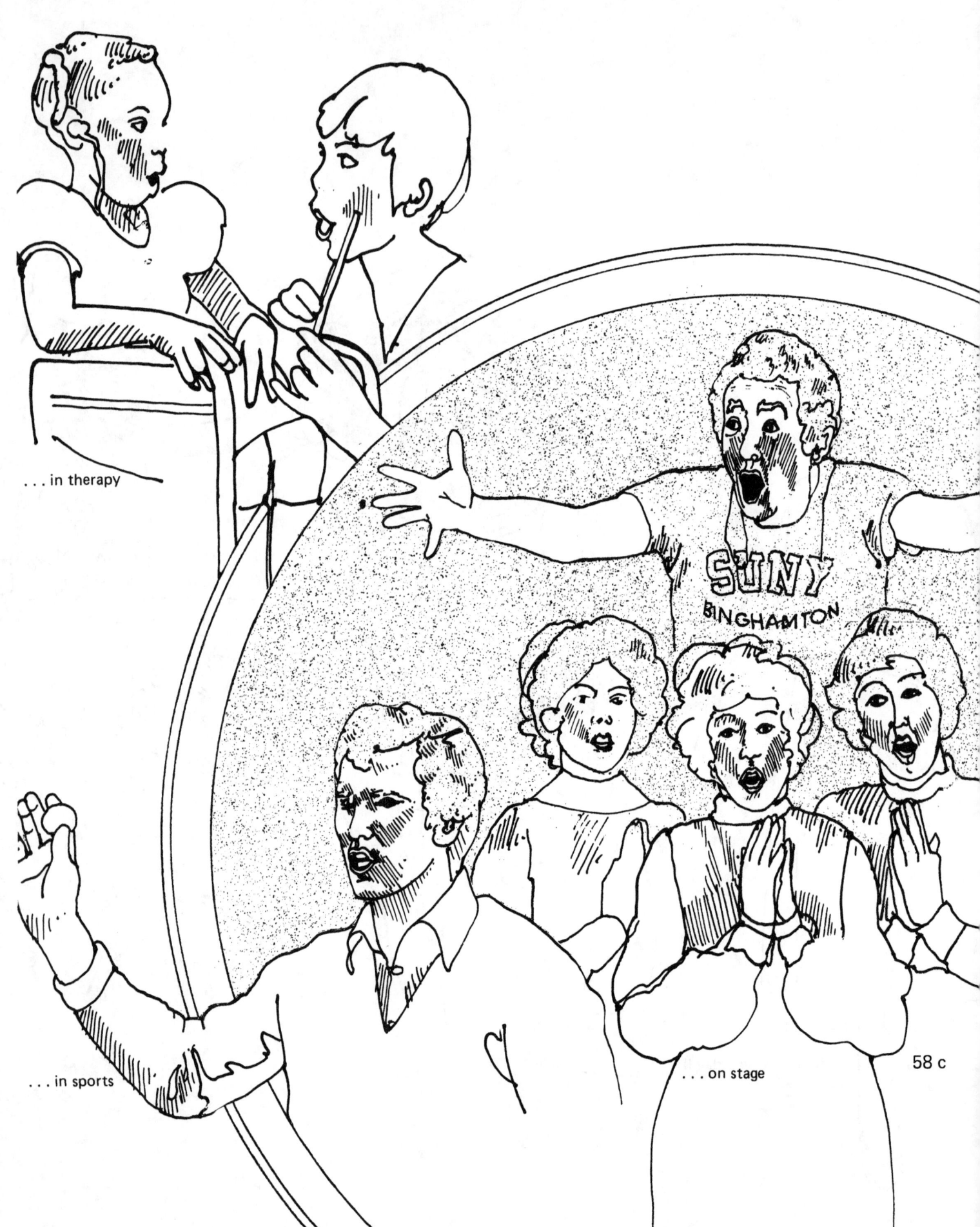

...in therapy

...in sports

...on stage

58 c

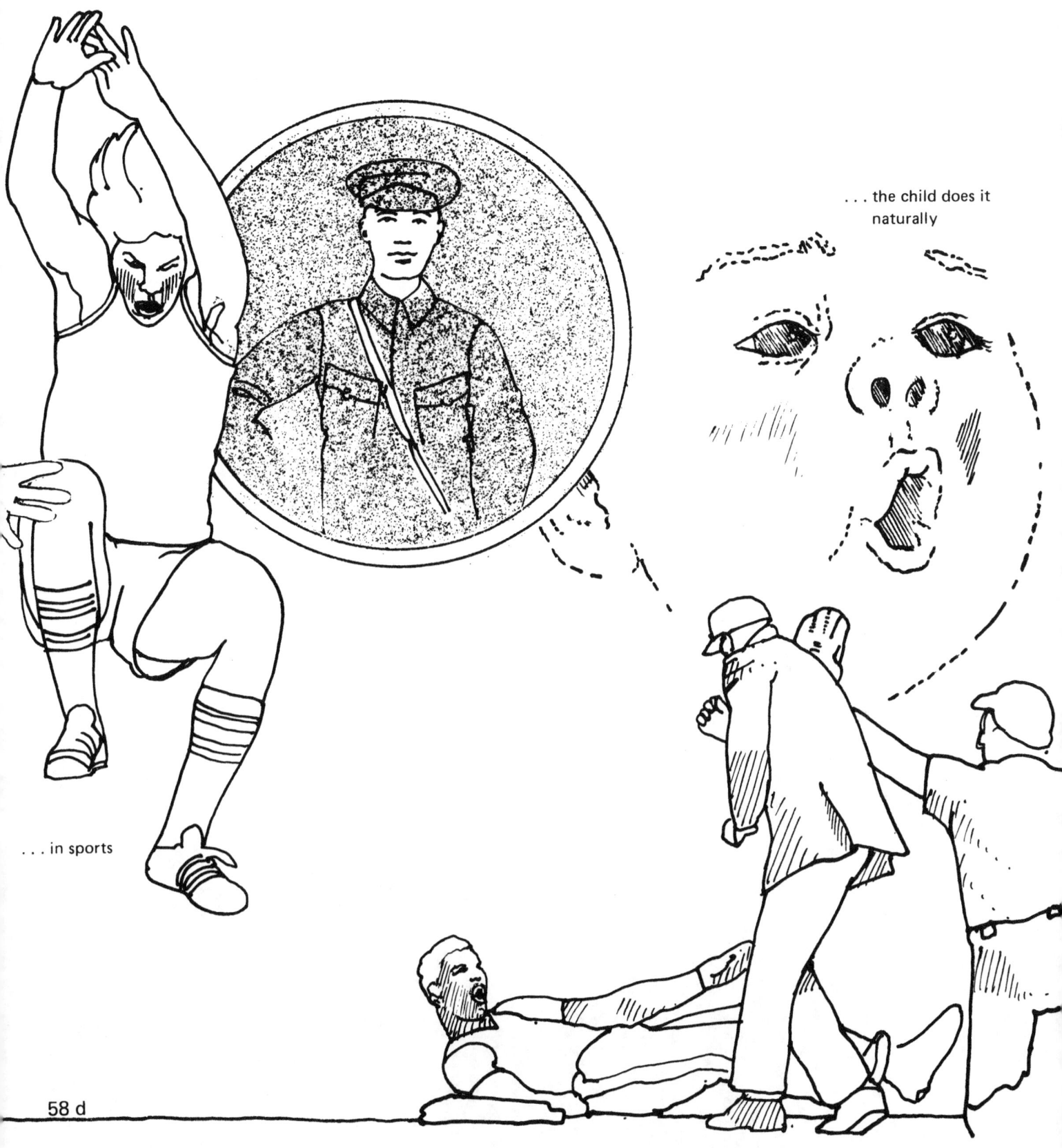

... in sports

... the child does it naturally

... in sports

58 d

5
RELAXER-ENERGIZERS

Body Wisdom husbands a great store of natural relaxer-energizers to which the body instinctively resorts, usually on a non-voluntary or semi-voluntary basis. Our task is to convert this intuitive storehouse into a reservoir of voluntary events accompanied by conscious awareness.

We began PART TWO with the corrective that energy and relaxation are not so much a duality as complementary opposites which incline toward synergy or third-force unity. Venturing a definition of relaxer-energizers, we can now affirm that: any body activity that will free muscles, relieve tension, maintain body awareness, support personal pleasure and salutary feeling, and sustain body inquisitiveness and vitality can be considered a **relaxer-energizer**.

Therefore, in self-use, a relaxer-energizer infers two qualities, both of which qualify as body esthetics:

- The act must embody both relaxer and vitalizer agents. Since both components make you "feel good," the exact proportion of one to the other becomes irrelevant.

- In performing the act, the existence and functioning of both relaxer and vitalizer agents will be **consciously** perceived, the **awareness** compounding the pleasure and reinforcement of the act.

Only natural, instinctive body functioning can serve as a relaxer-energizer. Patterned or habit-conditioned behavior will rarely, if ever, qualify.

Natural relaxer-energizers must be, and always are salutary esthetic experiences. Yet they can rather easily be transformed into anesthetic desensitizers through the imposition of conditioned functioning, vanity, ego conflicts, or patterned behavior. Fortunately, the reverse is also true.

The experiments of the last chapter have shown you how and why active rest and restful action promote the experience of esthetic balance and rhythm — how, together, they contribute to your feeling good. But if, during a physical effort, your body sends out the message: "Don't bother me now with the idea of resting;" or if, during rest, your body signals: "Please don't disturb me with the concept of movement, let me rest" — then your inner experiencing systems will be in competitive conflict with each other, leaving the body susceptible to psychosomatic deterioration.

Chapter 5

Relaxer - Energizers

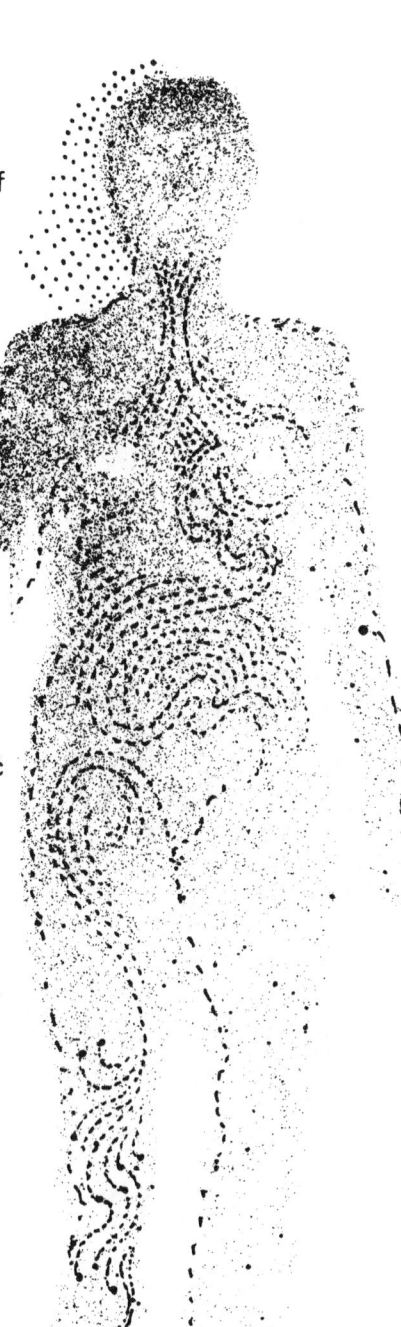

Energy
and
Relaxation

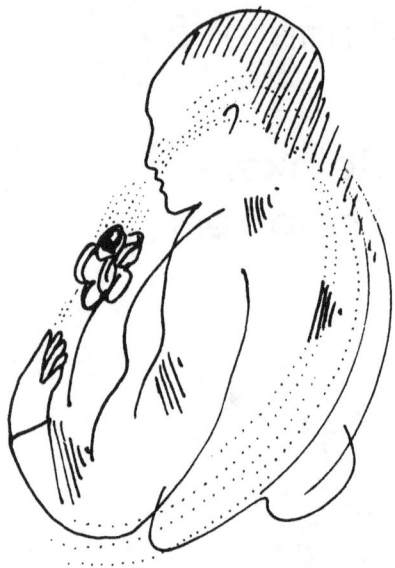

For example: the act of breathing on the instructions, "stand up straight, shoulders back, chest out, chin in", may not seem harmful or painful. Yet, the body cannot respond to such instructions with psychosomatic health, (no matter how fresh or clean the air), because poor posture always adversely affects one's breathing. Conversely, poor breathing always induces poor posture. However, when one breathes that fresh, clean air in a natural and spontaneous manner as one impulsively smells a favorite flower, then breathing becomes instinctive and deconditioned. That kind of breathing is a smelling in of the air with a gentle sigh of contentment as part of an inspired, awareful act that just **feels SO good!**

In this breathing-sighing-scenting activity, the body is intuitively doing everything right, and thereby offers up one of its natural relaxer-energizers for self-use. By instinctively inhaling the fresh spring air — the invigorating, cold clean air, the aroma of delicious, exotic foods, the scent of delicate perfume — and consciously enjoying it, we can transform patterned, harmful breathing into a natural relaxer-energizer that feeds and fuels the body and rewards it at the same time.

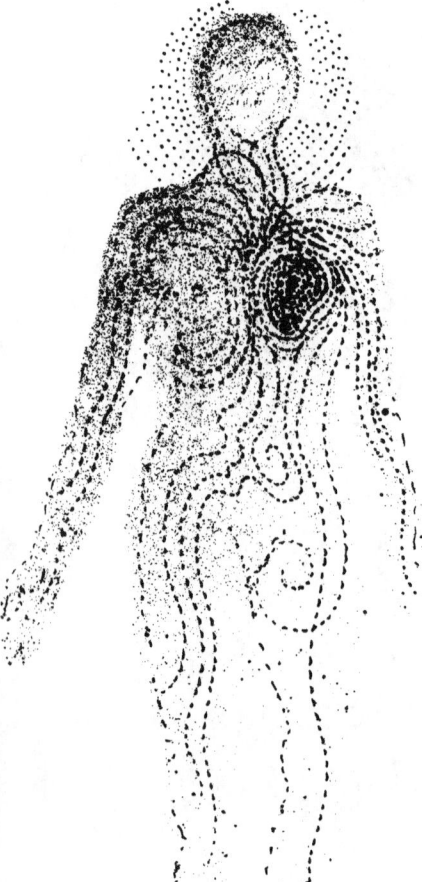

To take another illustration: Although swallowing is as natural and primal to Man as sucking, attempting to swallow when the throat is dry will prove neither relaxing nor energizing. But using your tongue to stimulate the salivary glands, and then swallowing, converts the act into a full-bodied relaxer-energizer that restores natural functioning and makes you feel good. Test this for yourself.

Relaxer-energizers are neither talents, skills, nor techniques and cannot be practiced as such. When a "sigh" is fabricated, it is no longer a sigh! If the sigh is contrived by technical manipulation, it is no longer natural or effortless and it will therefore, not relax **or** energize the body. But when our awareness is tuned into experience and sensation of natural events, when we teach ourselves the "feel" and perceptions of the esthetic, rhythmic, and rewarding body dynamics during these acts, at that moment our relaxer-energizers become part of kinesensic intelligence.

Relaxer-energizers are there for the having — if we will only engage them, enjoy them, and use them. It's exactly this level of body awareness that makes the feeling process so readily accessible. All relaxer-energizers are either natural or derived "familiar/unique events" which function instinctively as body esthetics.

Relaxer
Energizers

Investigate for your personal exploration, the dozen or so body activities that I consider natural, organic relaxer-energizers. No doubt there are a good many more, but those indicated suffice to initiate your relaxer-energizer experimenting and self-teaching.

A guiding principle: As you discover and explore, try to recognize that the more unrestrained, the more "child-like" your response, the more easily you'll achieve the best results.

BREATHING:

Breathing and posture constitute a most important set of inter-dependent dualities. If you stand properly, you will breathe well. If you breathe correctly, your posture will be good (i.e. salutary). During sleeping hours, our bodies may not be inhaling very deeply. But because our sleeping postures are normally unvictimized by outside conditioning, the body does breathe instinctively and consistently well.

On the other hand, during waking hours, while we do periodically and sporadically breathe deeply, two significant factors contribute to the pollution of our respiratory systems:

- Our universally poor and harmful postures in standing, walking, sitting, running, etc; and

- Extremely shallow inhaling, often to the point of not breathing at all. Aside from moments of fear, guilt, anxiety, and apprehension which affect our breathing rhythms, we tend unconsciously to suspend breathing while **doing** things — particularly while listening, concentrating, reading or conversing. This is probably one reason for the yawn which, among other functions, enforces deep breathing by body demand.

Normal, everyday breathing, in terms of sensation, perception, and awareness, does not necessarily fulfill the objective requirements of a relaxer-energizer. However, with the awareness of the respiratory process turned into an instinctive, optimal breathing experience, natural inhalation and exhalation become one of the body's major relaxer-energizers.

Some Cues and Signals: *

Breathing becomes instinctive

- Whenever the body position utilizes a single **convex back** (dorsal) **curve** or bend as in the actions of sitting, squatting, leaning, wafting, dancing, golfing, conducting, skiing, sculpting, crouching, etc.

- In any **spherical** body rolling, rocking, tumbling, or balance action.

- Whenever inhaling occurs through the **natural**, self-absorbing actions of smelling, sighing, yawning, or laughing.

SWALLOWING:

Much of the muscle tension that usually lodges in the jaw, neck, shoulders, and head can be relieved by converting conditioned swallowing into a pleasurable, conscious oral activity — especially when combined with a viable head and neck posture.

- With space between the teeth, lips parted or in gentle surface-to-surface touch, engage your tongue in a smooth, supple-like swirling in all directions; as though tasting the soft, slippery lining of the mouth embracing cheeks, gums, roof, floor, and the inside of the lips. This gentle swirling stimulates your salivary glands.

- Now collect the supply of saliva and let it trickle unhurriedly toward the throat, helping it along with a soft, slow, awareful swallow.

- Notice how the lubricated throat passage relaxes the entire area, massaging the internal throat and loosening the neck muscles. If you're a teeth gritter or grinder, as so many of us are, notice how this kind of activity relieves that tendency. You have just turned swallowing into a **relaxer-energizer**.

---

*Chapter XI: THE BODY AS A CRESCENT-Standing Up — provides a special detailed section on the breathing process.

Relaxer
Energizers

Using the illustrations as guides, expand your repertoire of "body-yawn" explorations to include the following:

YAWNING:

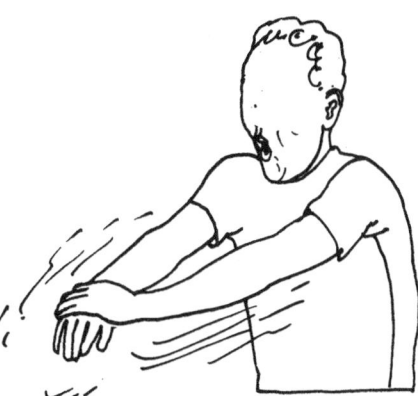

The Forward or Hard-Palate Facial Yawn Energy

As indicated by the illustration, this is a forward facial-stretching posture.

- Begin by sustaining the "aw" vowel sound, as in the word "bore" or "crawl."

- As you sustain the easy, comfortably pitched vowel, allow the **vocal sound** of the yawn to resound through the hard palate in the roof of your mouth.

The Backward or Soft-Palate Facial Yawn Energy

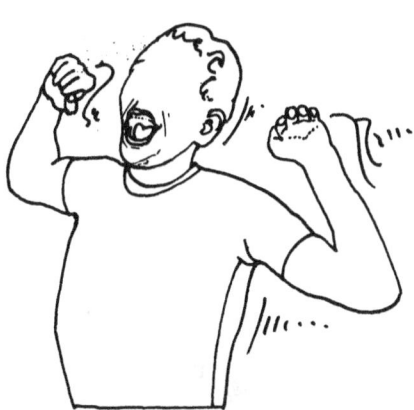

As indicated in the illustration, this is an upward facial-stretching posture.

- Generate the vocal sound of an "a" vowel (as in "gal" or "task") in the highly arched soft palate in the back of your mouth on an easy, yet high pitched, tone.

- Now steer the sound so that it is caught up into the bone of the nose and forehead, while sustaining the same vowel sound.

- Feel the muscles stretching the cheeks and mouth upward and outward into a comfortable facial yawn stretch.

- Compare your sensation-image of this soft-palate stretch with that suggested by the illustration.

The Muscle Yawn-Stretch Energy of the Whole Body

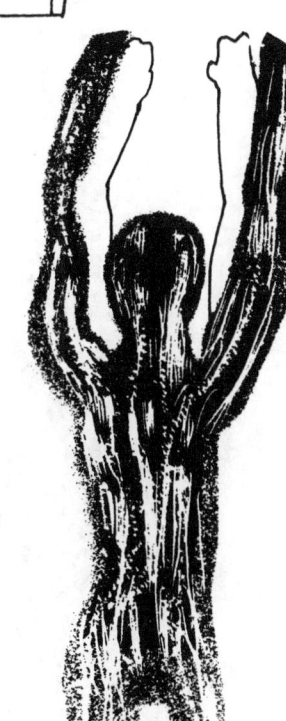

You already know this exercise from our exploration of the potency energy state. To review:

- Stretch the entire body as you would when getting up from a full night's sleep, as though your body just had to uncramp itself before starting another day.

- Note that as you stretch, the body feels like it wants to test its stretching capacity to the fullest.

- Move with this feel, sensing both the relaxation and the stimulation in the stretch itself.

- Notice how the relaxer and the energizer effects stay with you beyond the stretch.

DO IT... DON'T PRACTICE IT!

HUMMING:
Here again, the relaxation and the stimulation are in the doing. Just hum for pleasure and have fun tasting the sensation of the sound.

- One generally hums on an "M," so start that way.

- Then hum on all the sustainable, voiced consonants: "N;" "N" combined with "M;" "N" combined with "NG," with "L."

- Now try "Y" (as in "beyond"); "V;" "Z;" "ZH" (as in leisure); "W;" "R;" and finally "TH" (as in breathe).

- Don't just hum; hum melodies. Invent tunes. Respond to your images as you hum along. Feel them as though they were pictures or metaphors for orchestral music whose instrumental sounds appeal to you.

SIGHING:
No heaving of chest, no baring of breast, no self-pitying sigh will induce relaxation and stimulation. Instead, begin to feel the relaxer-energizer in gentle sighs of satisfaction and thoughtful sighs of contemplation or anticipation.

SHAKING:
Several body shakes, each with its own character, quality, and strength, function as tension-reducing relaxer-energizers. Among these:

- the vigorous, large muscle shake;

- the quieter, controlled smaller muscle shake (or major key rhythmics);

- the subtle, delicate quiver shake (or minor key rhythmics);

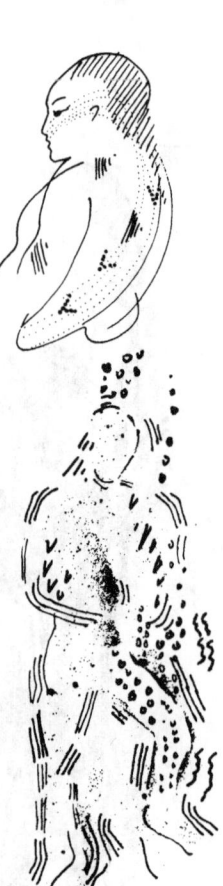

Relaxer
Energizers

- the varying, vibrative shakes such as shivering, fluttering, quivering, and flickering . . . the uncontrolled, trembling shakes of the infirm and the aged . . . the character shakes of nervousness, stress, anxiety, and eager exhilaration or anticipation;

- the reciprocal shakes in certain parts of the body that are induced by specific, voluntary shakes in other parts of the body.

All of these shakes can be converted into relaxer-energizer behavior.

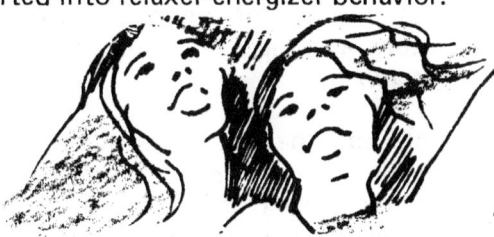

SMILING: Just do it! Let it be in response to a thought, to something, to someone. Or to something you see, hear, touch, taste, or smell. Better yet, smile in response to something you feel. Let it start in, and with, your eyes. Allow it to subtly reveal your sense of humor or permit the smile to begin the process of developing one **for** you.

SINGING: No nonsense about having a poor voice, no "ear," or no ability to carry a tune! Simply sing, as carefreely and unselfconsciously as you do in the shower. Only now sing at least three or four times a day — in the shower, throughout the apartment, outdoors, or in the car. Remember: singing is not the same as humming on consonants. We sing on vowels. Sing quietly, strongly, happily, sadly, angrily — with any emotional involvement that feels natural. Just make sure that it is **your** singing and not an imitation of your favorite crooner or song stylist. Don't worry about remembering the lyrics or melodies of particular songs. This is not a rehearsal for opening night. Your own melodies on LA, DO, RE, or toot-toot-ta-toot, if you prefer, are far better if you feel good physically doing them. And as you sing, become aware of the pleasurable sensations this activity produces in your head and throughout the body.

LAUGHING: Of course, if you don't smile very much, you'll hardly be inclined to laugh. The only difference between smiling and laughing is that while the former is usually a silent activity, the latter is generally vocal. If you feel timid about drawing attention to yourself with hearty, contagious laughter, or with "belly-laughing," then tune into the music and lovely sensations of chortles, giggles, chuckles, or soft melodic laughter.

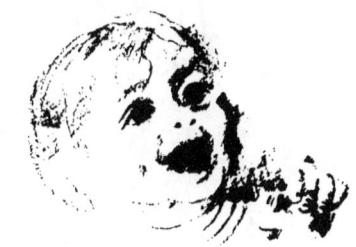

Try to combine your laughter with your singing, as they share much in common. The important thing is to begin experiencing these natural relaxer-energizers every day, and several times a day.

THE ELONGATED SPINE: The longer the spine, the healthier the spine. The longest and healthiest spine is a "single-curved" spine or the closest thing to it. The convex spine influences an expanding and extending back that is salutary for the organism. Its shape and structure favor a more natural alignment and more instinctively correct inclination of movement.

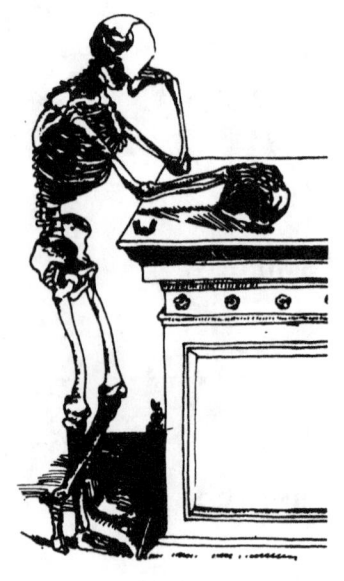

Note, too, that in some postures the convex curve can be completed into an arc of a circle. In some, it can be opened to a "C" curve (as in running or dancing) and in some, the two ends of the "bend" can be extended into an upright, bow-shaped crescent (as in walking and standing).

Emulate the golfer, skier, orchestra conductor, or dancer. As you elongate the spine into a single curve, **feel** the extension and expansion flowing radially from the lower-spine energy center into the pelvis and back thigh muscles. Experience the sensation of an antigravity current flowing through the upper-spine energy center into your shoulders, neck, and head. This becomes a remarkable relaxer-energizer, or better still, energizer-relaxer.

DANCING: Again, no excuses about lack of rhythm or not knowing how!

- Begin exploring by mixing equal parts of relaxer-energizers consisting of: breathing, humming, shaking, smiling, and elongated spinal activity.

- Shake well and don't let it settle; vibrate, and you're dancing!

As your varying "esthetic shakes" work into a sense of rhythm, you will, at the same time, really begin sensing a personal dance experience.

RHYTHM: One of the most sophisticated body relaxer-energizers, rhythm is fundamental to all body movement. It functions as a self-regulating device and provides the esthetic experience of body symmetry, balance, and expression. Because of its importance and special place among relaxer-energizers, rhythm is accorded special treatment in the next chapter.

RHYTHM 6

Chapter 6

Rhythm

Rhythm, in terms of our work, may be specifically defined as: the "organic appreciation of motion in the body." As such, it becomes one of the kinesensic manifestations that inevitably energizes (and relaxes) the body by its gentle turbulence.

Rhythm may not be an energy in itself, but it is clearly related — for us, it is viscerally connected — to the body energy states discussed in the two preceding chapters. Certainly, we can all agree that "rhythm feel" is analogous to experiencing intelligence through one of the body's communicating languages. Rhythm speaks to us through our body and, at the same time, speaks to our body through us. Therefore, we need to expand the definition of rhythm to include its various levels of perception.

A significant intelligence

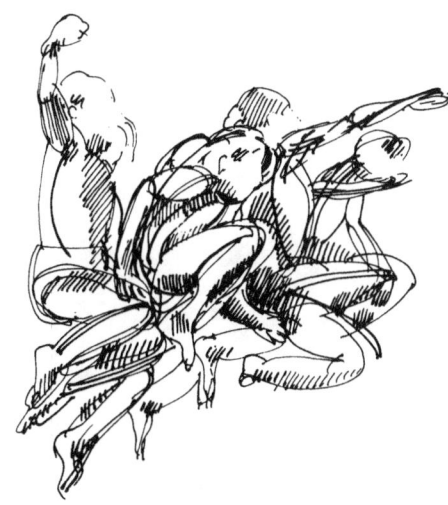

Perceivable rhythms range from basic, verbally defined tempos- meters- beats, to cyclical body clocks, to organically felt rhythms that are internally perceived as harmonic-sensory experience. Rhythm can be found, experienced, and appreciated in a dance, a poem, a sport, the smile of a friend, the laughter of a child, the traffic of the city, the crying of a new-born infant, etc. In previous chapters, we have experienced rhythm in restful action and active rest; in buoyancy, radiancy, potency, shaking, breathing, et al. Our perception of rhythm in each of these instinctive body activities now permits us to integrate the manifold movement dynamics of the body-whole.

Rhythm, seen in this wider context, becomes a perceptual vehicle with applicable relationship to fear-diffusion, pain-therapy, alleviation of anxiety, self-regulating safety cushions, and various energy conversions. Let us examine two such applications where **rhythm** functioning as **organic instruction** changes the quality and perception of a physical sensation. In both instances, a transformation process occurs, effecting the psycho-physical perception of those physiological and psychosomatic body movements directly involved in the behaviors of fear, hysteria, and/or pain.

Organic instruction

Under severe pain, an individual is normally involved in a body activity we commonly call "writhing." Writhing is characterized by an unusual accompanying rhythm that is **always part of an extension stretch-release and curvo-linear body-reach.** These descriptive categories are by now familiar to you from our exploration of the four non-derived energy states.

Writhing

Writhing, then, seems to be the body's way of loosening impingements and melting away fixations in order to alleviate pain, and bring a degree of comfort to the injured area. It is critical that we recognize writhing as a **positive** and creative body activity. Instead, we usually associate it with discomfort, fear, and a sense of helplessness; i.e. with a negative and destructive experience produced by a conditioned association that in fact only creates a climate of competition within the body.

If our associations were based not upon outer conditioning but instead upon direct sensory experience, we could choose to experience writhing as **an esthetic expression of the body's instinctive response to pain.** That this is uncommon makes it no less accessible. When we concentrate on the **rhythm-dynamic** of writhing and on the rewarding satisfaction of experiencing its physical yawn-stretch qualities, we learn to appreciate the positive aspects of writhing.

Through this conversion process, we actually assist the pain in re-expressing itself. By changing the perception of writhing from discomfort and anxiety to a comfortable awareness of salutary body therapy, we can begin to enjoy the movement of writhing as an aesthetic (as well as esthetic) rhythm, the opposite of what we originally perceived. In so doing, we will have taught ourselves a most effective method for diffusing fear, and for reinterpreting anxiety into **usable energy** and non-destructive emotion.

This process involves a very real transformation of psychic energy which produces a change of perception and a therapy, in and of itself. The process can also work in reverse, becoming an equally effective strategy for self-control and perceptual relaxation.

The Bug-Blade-Bead Association

As a second example of rhythm functioning as organic instruction, take the sunbather's mounting discomfiture and annoyance as he violently reacts to what he thinks is the persistent creeping of a bug over his body. Suddenly, he **transforms** this tension and irritation into gentle pleasure and even thrill, when he realizes the sensations were caused not by a bug at all, but by a sun-fed bead of perspiration or by a blade of grass gracefully caressing his body. The situation is self-evident.

By **voluntarily** studying and re-experiencing the good feeling of the wafting blade of grass or the rolling beads of perspiration, a transformation process ensues. Through the effected change in perception, the sunbather can now comfortably and consciously accommodate to the bug itself. Or the actor can use the bug image as conveniently and creatively as he could the blade of grass, or bead of perspiration, even though he may perceive a different rhythm as he moves from a "bug" to a "bead of perspiration."

Rhythm:
An Organic
Instruction

Hence the active search for rhythm in an emotion, in anxiety, nervousness, or pain, becomes more than merely a method to distract attention from the unpleasant. Stage fright and nervousness can shift into constructive excitement when the performer or athlete or teacher learns how to:

- tune in feelingly to rhythms of nervous energy;

- perceive that energy as an esthetic force; and

- image it within the energy state of anticipation, eagerness, curiosity and, quite literally, a sensing of humor!

Furthermore, when positive, beneficial dynamics of organic body esthetics are applied to negative dynamics of pain, fear, stage fright, or personal imbalance, our converted and transformed discoveries and explorations are likely to become manifest as **talent**!

As you learn to perceive and identify the rhythms inside your body, your perceptions and response-mechanisms will grow to appreciate rhythms in the external environment as well. Feeling rhythm in music, for example, is one sub-area; rhythm in dancing, painting, sculpting, building, designing, acting, walking, climbing, track-running, ice-skating, skiing, gymnastics, singing, etc., are others. To perceive such qualities in the context of rhythm is to perceive them in the context of all other movements and kinetic forces in the body. As such, they participate in the larger composite of overall "aesthetics."

As stated at the outset of PART TWO, our concern is with the perception of rhythm as internal energy-dynamics, and the use of rhythm as part of the "organic instruction" process. To perceive rhythm as a quality and to use that quality as organic instruction is a way of understanding internal rhythm as a causative component of instinctive body behavior.

The example of writhing is instructive in this regard. But it extends into a larger reality: that **underlying** most states of pain, nervousness, anxiety, and irritation is a basic body rhythm. In learning to perceive and appreciate the subtextual rhythms of pain or anxiety, we teach ourselves doubly well to deal with the normal rhythms of conscious behavior. And in turn, we learn how our body copes and how to help the body cope by reinforcing its internal rhythms. We begin to reconnect our imagination with the body and with our body's imaginative intelligence for learning, self-teaching, and perceiving rhythms as organic phenomena.

Experienced internally as movement and image-maker, the rhythm energy state ceases to harbor negative or conditioned values. It can then probe our semi-voluntary and even non-voluntary body dynamics while simultaneously entering the higher harmonics of awareness, reinforcement, reward, and pleasure as both impetus and inspiration.

Summing up, no one can teach you what an organic feeling of rhythm is. You simply have to experience it with awareness. By becoming aware of internal rhythm as a vehicle within the individual body environment, driving on both conscious and subconscious levels, you will teach **yourself** to **feel** its special character as a relaxer-energizer; to **perceive** it as a significant intelligence of the body; and to **utilize** it as an organic instruction for optimal functioning and psychosomatic health. (See also Balance and Rhythm, pp. 75, 76; refer to Index for further treatment of Rhythm dynamics.)

Part Three
ENERGY AND RELAXATION IN MOVEMENT

PREFACE TO PART THREE

Play, Images, Balance-Rhythm Evolving Body Curve

PART THREE calls for skillful and creative application of energy and relaxation **in movement**, within a progressive program of self-teaching experiments that, in effect, reconstitute the evolutionary development of the human body and turn it into a plan for reconditioning the body to maximal efficiency. Working with the **body sphere in movement** (chapters 7 through 12) from a fetal-like "small ball" position through expanding orb, crescent curves, circles, wheels and loops, we evolve into those "personal space spheres" (chapter 13) which we will come to perceive as natural extensions of the body's basic structure, organic energy states, and "outer senses," and ultimately, as the body's breeding ground for manifold "self-images." (chapter 14)

As a bridge between PART TWO, which concluded with the notion of rhythm as a major dialect within the body's complex language system, and the upcoming work chapters of PART THREE, I would like to devote this connecting preface to a consideration of "balance and rhythm" as an organic duality in movement, and briefly explore the nature of "play" and "image" as these participate in the overall duality of energy and relaxation in movement.

What Is Play?

- Play is the "work" of babies, children, and kittens.
- Play is the "work" of athletes, musicians, actors, dancers, circus clowns, and story tellers.
- Play is also the "creative labor" of innovators, inventors, architects, sculptors, and others who make of their work something imaginative, creative, and healthful.

In point of fact, "play" is the "work" that takes place in any **labor of love!**

Having, literally, a personal tap on this sense of play regears the body to function differently. If we can combine this tap with four or five principles that reveal the way muscles **should** work, we will have succeeded in discovering a systematic means for exploring the relationship between work and play, truly understanding what is meant by the expression, "the child at play."

... when rhythm is "felt" or perceived even sub-consciously, the sense of strain, or "hard" work disappears!

As stated earlier, we all marvel at the incredible natural endurance, endless eager enthusiasm, remarkable body talents, and fascinating qualities of relaxation demonstrated by children throughout their play. What we forget is that, as adults, we can also naturally and instinctively enjoy these qualities and capacities if only we would

Preface
to
Part Three

tune in more intuitively to our own work as a labor of love. Our outer-environment conditioning has not yet eroded the inner climate beyond reclaim; it is a climate that still retains the energy-spark in which such esthetic strategy can once again take root and grow healthier than ever.

But for most of us, play has taken on other codes of meaning that bear no resemblance to the inflection of feeling experienced through natural growth by the child, or even the kitten, at play. Some adults engage in "play" on doctor's orders; others out of family duty. For some, "play" represents the programmed pursuit of prescribed fun, or often, proscribed indulgence. For others, a dose of play is taken as stimulant or tranquilizer, as enforced exercise or soporific duller of the senses. But fewer and fewer of us, in adult life, feel they can experience either play or work within the sense of a "labor of love." How can Body Wisdom help? How can it initiate a personal turn-around against the storms of future shock? How can we, as individuals, discover another **beginning process** through Body Wisdom that can fortify us for current struggles and our future evolvement within the outside environment? One modest approach is to reflect on the child and pre-occupy ourselves with the many ways its inherent Body Wisdom works.

If we would constantly remind ourselves how full of curves the child and the kitten both are, how they both always move **through** curves — if we would marvel less and remember more how they instinctively use all our relaxer-energizers as natural food, fuel, and fulfillment — and how they naturally activate, through movement, all the body energies and esthetic qualities we've been discussing, then we could relearn as adults what we once knew as children and were taught to forget. In other words, the sense memory of these once familiar events could become the image ingredient for redeveloping a positive relationship to our own familiar event behavior, a **semi-direct image** that we could reactivate as organic instruction to our own body.

Clearly, we cannot play **at** being a very young child in order to relearn the natural play **of** the child. That would be sheer imitation and pretense. But we can learn how to recapture the child's organic instructions to himself during the act of play.

Without knowing it, the child's instructions to himself are always organic because they are invariably instinctive. The child's very freedom and carefreeness is essentially a "focus," rather than a lack of it. This is an important perception. It is the child's carefreeness that allows him, whether subliminally or consciously, to concentrate on the total action. And that essentially is what our work in Body

Play, Images
Balance-Rhythm
Evolving
Body Curve

Wisdom is all about: relearning the experience of carefreeness, and with it "painfreeness" and "harmfreeness," so that as adults we can function as matured evolvements of the natural, instinctive child.

To do this, we must come to grips with the organic duality of movement in the body and the body in motion. Through the harmonic overtone sensory system, images within the body must be considered part of this duality. For the feeling process, images are both input and output of resident sensation within the body; registering as sensation, perception, awareness, and response. Images describe, suggest, guide, invent, and potentially instruct the body to function organically without internal competition. Let's take a look at various orders of images available to the body for organic instruction.

*...harmonic sensing
is a
bio-psychic system
of
intelligence gathering!*

- **Direct Images:**

Certain images are so directly related to body functioning and body experience that they already constitute perfect organic instructions to the body. When, for example, you suggest to your body that it experience a "stretch" instead of a "push" or a "pull," the response and result is immediate. In yawn-stretching, we do something that we and our body already know very well. For self-teaching, the only difference in the use of the muscle-yawn stretch is applying our **perceptual experience** of it to a brand new task.

Images In Movement

The direct image is always an organic instruction that supports the body-whole at the same time as it supports a specific, physical act. Importantly, there is no shift in personal identity when you deal with direct, organic images. The direct image always constitutes a familiar event.

- **Semi-Direct Images:**

This is the order of image at work in our sense memory of what it felt like to be in a body of water, as in the buoyancy experiments of PART TWO. When you **suggest to yourself** that "you are in a body of water," recalling how it felt, you are using a semi-direct image. You imagine the physical feel of rising, floating, or settling-down buoyantly in water, and then project **conscious sensation and perception** of these body energy states upon the imagined physical feel.

Like direct images, these secondary images are based on experience you know very well. Only **now**, as semi-direct images, they are always applied to another task in a situation where the original experience, no longer present, has been replaced by the **sense memory** of that experience.

Preface
to
Part Three

- **Indirect Images:**

    Indirect images usually involve a shifting of identity. That is, you imagine you are a plant or an animal, having to transplant yourself into another identity, in order to creatively construct images you want to use for any given behavior in any given situation.

    An indirect image may become direct, and thus akin to organic instruction, if while you support the image it becomes associated with any of the body's energy states or esthetics. For example, imagine that you are a plant (indirect image). As a plant, imagine that you are being wafted by the breeze (semi-direct image that sense recalls the feel of being wafted but now applied to a new task). Still supporting the image, you begin physically to experience the buoyancy energy of wafting. As soon as this occurs, the image becomes direct and relates to organic feeling.

- **Inspirational Images:**

    These are not images summoned up to create a feeling, but images we come upon by serendipity and support with feeling. They provoke, motivate, and inspire inter-involvement energetics. They belong to the imaging realm of inspirational flight, fancy, and fantasy, but are not, necessarily, related to organic instruction.

    In a curious way, after teaching ourselves the "feel," "taste," and "music" of body and vocal energy states, we may no longer require the original images for organic instruction. When this occurs, these images take flight, turning into inspirational, free-wheeling explorations. They are no longer organic, but, now purely inspirational images.

- **Hiring An Image**

    Recall that, in transforming the perception of writhing from discomfort and anxiety to a comfortable awareness of salutary body therapy, or the perception of the bug crawling over a sun bather's body into the pleasing feel of a sun-fed bead of perspiration, we "hired an image." Any conversion or transformation process will, especially in therapeutic circumstances, hire an image to do the job.

    Thus, to control a cough or ease its intensity, you can hire the image/feel of a frog-like, easy clearing of the throat. To reduce a severe emotional reaction to a body limp, you would hire and work on the image/feel of rhythm and balance in the limp action; thereby introducing to the limp a smoothness and grace of movement that could even improve the physical condition. If you are exhausted beyond measure, bring in the image/feel of music, melody, or dance

Play, Images
Balance-Rhythm
Evolving
Body Curve

and work with it to diminish and often liquidate body fatigue. What you're **playing** with here are the two ends of the movement spectrum — balance and rhythm — each functioning as a body esthetic.

Balance and Rhythm

Balance and rhythm, complementing energy and relaxation, and play and work, constitute another third-force organic duality. It makes sense to us to talk about the rhythm in balance as well as the balance in rhythm. As two ends of the movement spectrum, balance is associated with a recognizable **dynamic stillness** while rhythm is associated with a recognizable **dynamic movement**. Yet, rhythm and balance are intrinsic to each other. They operate in a symbiotic duality of movement. We must have the body in movement before we can "feel" balance; and we must have the body in a state of balance before we can experience rhythm.

From whichever point of the movement spectrum balance is viewed, it needs to be seen primarily as a direct image and recognized as a composite category unto itself, functioning as hub or fulcrum. It is interesting to note that the "balance experience" feels the same whether its equilibrium is **in moving stillness** or is **stillness in movement**, retaining throughout its character as energy and esthetic. In kinesensics, we perceive these characteristics embracing not only rising, floating, and settling-down buoyancy but also the equilibrium concept of "pedestal balance," "pinpoint balance," and "moving or traveling balance."

Body balance, by implication, always brings together two opposing directions without losing its own indigenous sensation of movement. In the case of "relaxed-energy" and "energetic-relaxation", a double duality is brought together into a single dynamic esthetic and primary image. Also, in "resting up" energetically and "resting down" weightlessly, the body is organically instructed, through a direct image, to experience body balance. However, body balance can also be applied, in broader context, as either a semi-direct, indirect, or inspirational image.

Recall the involuntary "arm raising" after pressing the wrist against the wall, immediately followed by reproducing the same act without wrist-pressing. Or remember the carry-over of arm-raising, after inhalation, in the bathtub to the same act out of the water. In both instances, semi-direct organic images were active in instructing the body to the feel of body balance.

Preface
to
Part Three

If, as you perform your push-ups, chin-ups, sit-ups, and leg-lifts, you shift your identity into the image of a stalking panther, you will be hiring an indirect image to experience the body balance of "resting and working" at the same time. Another indirect image for instructing the body to feel itself in a state of balance would picture some muscle fibers shortening and contracting, while other muscle fibers are lengthening and relaxing in the very **same** muscle during a physical act. The indirect image, generating an organic instruction, will actually produce the feel of "balanced muscle tonicity."

Motivating body balance through an inspirational image might involve the following construct: Imagine that your nervous system has been converted into an electrical wiring system, that your veins and arteries have become waterways, airways, and thruways, and when the switch is pulled, all the electric, oxygen, and heartbeat juices stream into the network with such a confluence that you feel suddenly "lit up," "light-weight," "gently vitalized," and "potently strong" all at the same time. The feel of total balance follows upon the flight of free-wheeling fancy.

The Evolving Body Curve

Once we learn how to feel these multi-faceted sensations and perceptions of body balance, we begin to apprehend the **evolving body curve** in movement. Put another way, we begin to perceive that the balance of standing has a great deal to do with the psychology of moving. Body Wisdom is based on movement, balance, and body curves, not on rigid, sharp-edged straight lines that have to be constantly propped up lest they fall down.

We have no interest in teaching you specifically, or prescriptively, how to stand or sit or breathe or sing or run. But we are concerned that you acquire a new sensory awareness of the causative relationships between movement, standing, good vocal tone, healthful breathing, running, et al. Think of it this way: **If posture derives from movement as much as movement from posture, and if neither posture nor movement is rigid, then the connecting lines between the two must be spherical and curvo-linear.**

One thing is clear. When the body is perceived as a body-whole, not metaphorically but psycho-physically, when everything is taken together and all is seen to function at optimum, then certain causative truths emerge. Because body movement must be curved and esthetically smooth, body movement naturally extends into good, rounded, balanced posture. The natural extension of balanced posture is good breathing. The natural extension of good breathing and balanced posture is good, balanced vocal tone. The natural extension

Play, Images
Balance-Rhythm
Evolving
Body Curve

of good vocal tone is effective communication and inter-involvement. And the natural extension of effective communication and inter-involvement is nicely balanced rhythms, music, impulses, and creative dialogue. In the final analysis, we sense the body and the individual as a totality of kinetic, rather than static, activity. Our self-image and everything we perceive around us derives from this perception of movement; and all of our organic instructions become essentially instructions for movement!

Let's take the inter-connecting links of the causative chain a step further. If I perceive the duality of balance and rhythm in the light of other organic dualities (energy and relaxation, resting up and resting down, play and work), and understand how they inter-relate, constituting between them a whole series of auxiliary images, I can find body balance by thinking buoyancy; buoyancy by thinking gravity-free energy flow or resting up and resting down simultaneously; the physical urge of anti-gravity energy flow by thinking body-yawn potency, and so on. What occurs in the process, not so much as a side benefit but as a necessary consequence, is that my focus on failure is removed from the task. In other words, by introducing a system of inter-related organic instructions, by providing an integrative way of perceiving the overall movement of the body, we elude the tendency to break down individual tasks into directional specifics that invariably include a built-in fear component.

In exploring balance and rhythm through the contiguous continuity of breathing, posture, and the **C-curve** of the back, we are simultaneously exploring the "fear of falling." In fact, we perceive the body in movement in a way that **allows** for falling as a variable choice — the way the skilled skier falls, without fear, to avoid injury; the way the accomplished actor falls in a stage battle without seeming artful or contrived; the way the prima ballerina falls with design into the poignant movement of the dying swan. Only if I **wish** to remain in the "anesthetic" realm of fear, falling, tension, and pain will I inevitably and helplessly concentrate on the **goal** of fear, falling, tension, and pain. But should I **choose** to fall as part of a process or strategy, I will do anything but concentrate on the goal of falling.

Through an inverse dynamic that most of us experience frequently, we succeed in accomplishing the exact opposite of what we intend. Concentrate on the goal of not falling from a high place, and with enough concentration, you'll probably fall. Concentrate on stage on the goal of not being nervous, and you're guaranteed to be a nervous wreck. If I religiously pursue body balance by putting all of my conscious attention to the task of balance, I'll more than likely fall precisely because the concentration on balance is so great, that

Preface
to
Part Three

"losing it" (the fear of falling) becomes the viable and dominant image. In order to relearn the carefreeness of the natural, instinctive child, we must find for every task the relevant aspect **not** to pay attention to! I have always advised athletes that if they want to win in an important sports event, they must never concentrate on winning — but should instead tune in, psycho-physically, on the esthetic dynamics occurring **inside** their bodies. Similarly, I have always told my actors, dancers, and singers that if they are required to laugh, cry, yawn, fall, cough or feel pain on stage, the creative approach is to avoid these goals, concentrating instead on how to **keep from laughing, crying, intentionally falling, etc.; thus exciting the "feel" and perception of the inter-related process that provokes these emotional behaviors in an instinctively natural experience.** The reason why many of our instructions to the body to cry, laugh, cough, or intentionally fall, get hopelessly jammed up is that we are plagued with so many entangled, competitive instructions related to these emotions and goals.

If you share this view, and can internalize it, then the work chapters that follow will really become play. You'll appreciate why we avoid the anesthetic instructions of "push" and "force" at all points, and instead require only the other esthetic feel activities. And you'll find yourself performing all kinds of physical tasks without fear, but rather with awareness and body-responsiveness that, once again, feels natural.

We are now ready to take the fundamental concepts, skills, and talents we need to know, and learn how to sense, perceive, and respond to them through six stages of movement: from the perception of the body as a small ball to the perception of the body evolving into a small sphere, an expanded sphere, a crescent lying down, a crescent standing up, leading finally to the perception of the body in the upright.

7
GETTING THE BODY INTO A COMPACT BALL

Ready? Let's begin with the

Five Floating Squats

These positions follow directly the experience of "equilibrium and floating" you discovered in the wafting and waving experiments of Chapter 4 ("Body Energizers"). They apply several concepts with which you are already familiar: multi-directional and curvo-linear movements; the three different buoyancies; vibrative wafting and waving; gravity-free "live weight" vs. floppy, hanging "dead weight;" and lightness of touch-feel or vanishing contact pressure.

Recall how the variable (multi-directional and curvo-linear) movements, from upright to sitting position and back again, produced that floating, melting sensation without your slightest physical awareness that muscles were at work. With this in mind, picture your squat position (see illustration) as the sitting position, only now your seat floats down toward gentle contact with the ground. You may know this posture under a different name — the "deep knee-bend." For us, the deep bending of the knee is less the point than the weightless buoyancy experienced during the downward and upward gliding action, and the lightness of touch-feel (vanishing contact pressure) between the feet surfaces and the ground.

If you **send** your body weight into the ground, you will, in effect, be sinking it into the ground and you'll feel every pound as floppy dead weight. If instead, you **settle down buoyantly**, your body will perceive itself floating to the ground while still feeling the "vibrato" of the wafting and waving movement. Throughout the action, your body will feel like gravity-free live weight, in other words, "weightless."

Chapter 7

Getting the Body into a Compact Ball

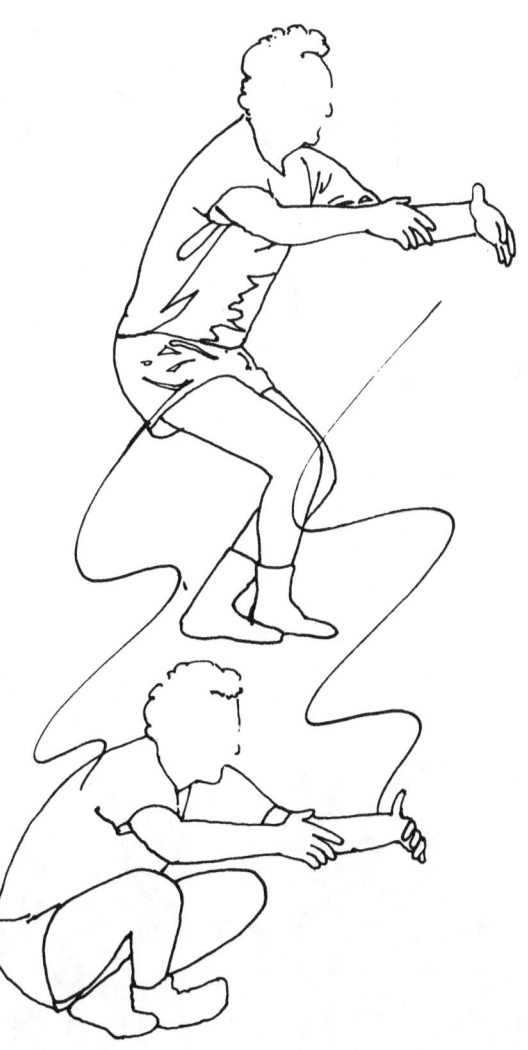

Energy and
Relaxation
in Movement

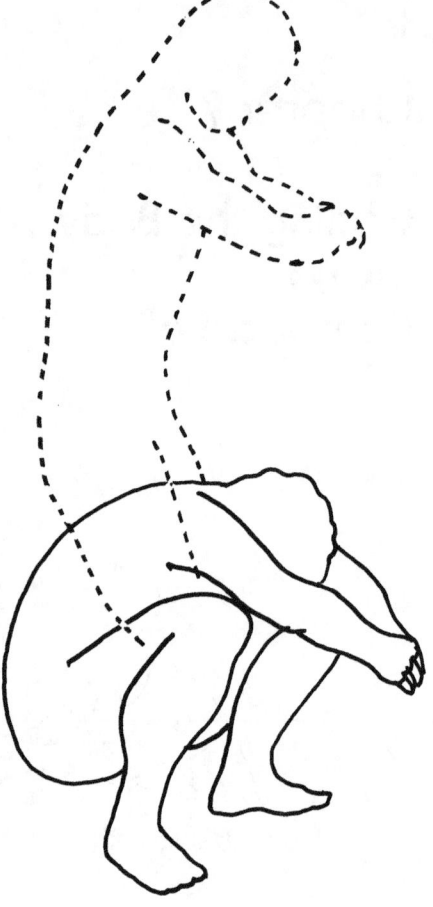

So, as you perform the five floating squats:

° avoid doing stressful deep knee-bends that send your weight into the ground;

° avoid a "pulling tight" at the knee joints;

° avoid a "pressured pushing" or "heavy sinking" into sitting position; and

° avoid all the accompanying images of these body anesthetics.

° use instead the images of the floating squat, with its almost antigravitational urge and lambent buoyancy that never ceases its waft and wave body vibrato.

Follow these cues, and you should experience a body sense of practically total effort-free muscle functioning. A vital relaxing plus a body lightness will result from the maximal distribution of muscle-cell activity, and both will combine to help avoid pressure or strain in and around the knee-joint area.

The illustrations reveal our five squat postures:

1. the **flat-sole** (1st position) **squat,** heels on ground with toes apart;

2. the **toe-stretch squat,** on the balls of the feet cushioned by a pad;

3. the **flat-sole** (2nd position) **squat,** heels and soles on ground with toes pointing straight ahead in American Indian style;

4. the **criss-cross squat,** with alternating crossing of the legs; and

5. the **two-bladed squat,** performed on the outer edges of the feet.

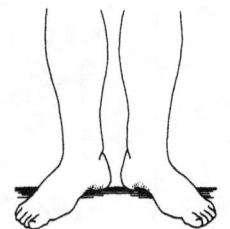 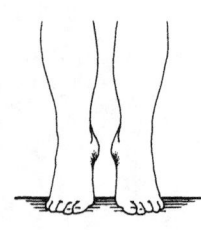 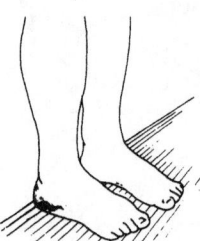 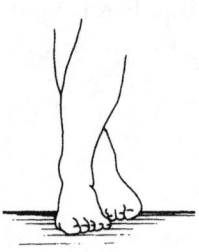 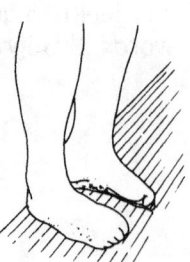

The Five Squats

- At first, practice the floating squats in the order indicated above. Later you may make your own selection.

- In some of the squats you may sense a strange balance experience as you waft and vibrate downward to a near-touching position with the floor. Don't be disconcerted if your body does not always manage to maintain steady or complete balance. As soon as you begin to waver, turn the wavering into **waving**, and let yourself waft into a new balance in the most immediately proximal position. See illustrations in Chapter 4.

- Note from the side-view illustrations that the natural squat movement is a downward-sitting **spherical** action — not a "leaning forward" sitting motion. Remember that we are preparing the body for exercise within the structural form of a small compact ball.

- Do the exercise series as described below, in **all** the squat positions.

- With each squat, waft-wave-vibrate yourself down until you feel the floor imperceptibly rising to gently, subtly touch your "sitting bones."

- Reinforce your wafting and waving by recognizing the oscillating and vibrating motion as one of the body dynamics that loosens and lightens rather than tenses and tightens. Adopt it also as a safety device against losing body balance, as discussed above, being always vibrantly aware that it contributes to the discovery of new, balanced positions resulting from body shifts. This will assist you in dispelling any "fear of falling." By going with the motion and rhythm of the movement, rather than against it, you diminish the probability and eliminate the action of falling since the follow-through movements will merge coincidentally into newly explored, initiating movement.

Some General Instructions and Observations:

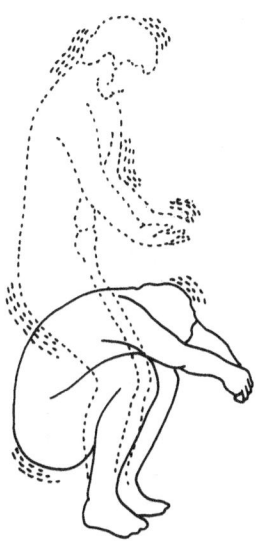

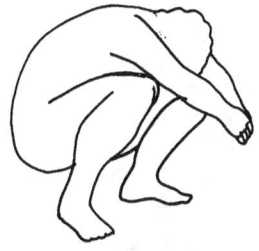

Check references to wafting and waving in Chapter 5

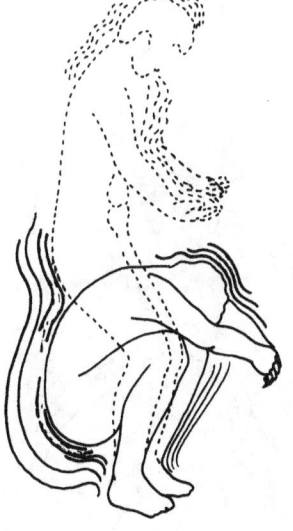

Energy and
Relaxation
in Movement

Exercises for the Five Squat Positions

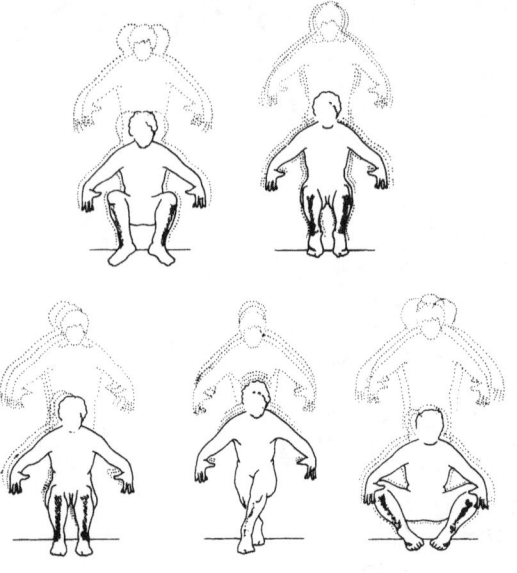

Series One:

- In relaxed, buoyant upright posture, waft and wave in each squat position. First do it multi-directionally in each squat position; then from left to right and reverse...diagonally...clockwise...counter-clockwise...crescent-like...settling down and rising up. (see Illustrations)

- Coordinated with breathing energy, waft down and up a dozen times but do it weightlessly, gracefully, and buoyantly.

- Observe and respond to the lightest possible touch contact of your feet to the ground — of an anti-gravitational urge in your back — of your breathing energy consolidating body balance and alleviating body weight.

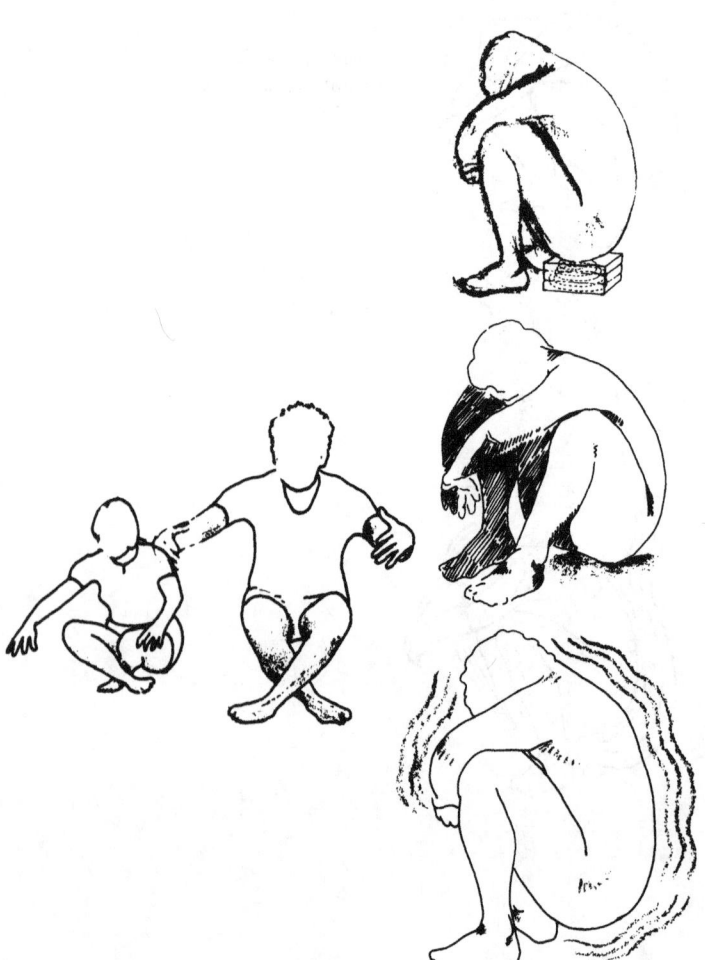

Series Two:

- In each squat, melt yourself closest to the ground and establish the distance between the ground and your buttocks.

- Take some flat objects (discs, books, rubber mats, etc.) of approximately one-half to three-quarter inch thickness. In each squat, sit lightly on the lowest one and teach yourself to progressively "melt" to the next lowest until you find the floor rising up to "give you a seat."

- Allow this experiment to work itself out over days, weeks, months. Some squats will sit to the floor almost from the outset; others will remain recalcitrant for years. For the artist or inventor, recalcitrance is the opening to new discovery and is taken as a creative challenge to one's talents, rather than as a limiting barrier or inadequacy. Remember: Body Wisdom is for life, not just until you turn the page.

The
Five
Squats

Series Three:

- As suggested in the illustrations, and starting with the first squat, repeat the up and down squat-glide three times in rhythmic sequence, using a dance-like or interpretive body expressiveness.

- After the three floating squats, do three crescent-like body-yawn stretches, each with a different hand and arm gesture, always using a perfect C-curve.

- Widen the stance about six inches, as many times as is comfortably possible and repeat as graphically illustrated. Please note that as the distance widens, the stretching down becomes more difficult for most of the squats. Stretch only with the help of buoyancy, radiancy, or potency energy or any combination of these feels. Wherever vocal exclamations instinctively "pop out" — like yawning or grunting or calling or expressing a rugged "Oh, it feels so-o-o good" — not only should you use them, but enjoy them. Stretch completely, elastically, flexibly, reachingly, but always with body-yawn "painfreeness" or buoyancy "melting," or both.

- Repeat all the above in this series with each squat position. This series represents a long exercise, but it is excellent progressive "stretch work" and endurance training. Later this series may be used in smaller segments as a change of pace and to fill in breather-breaks.

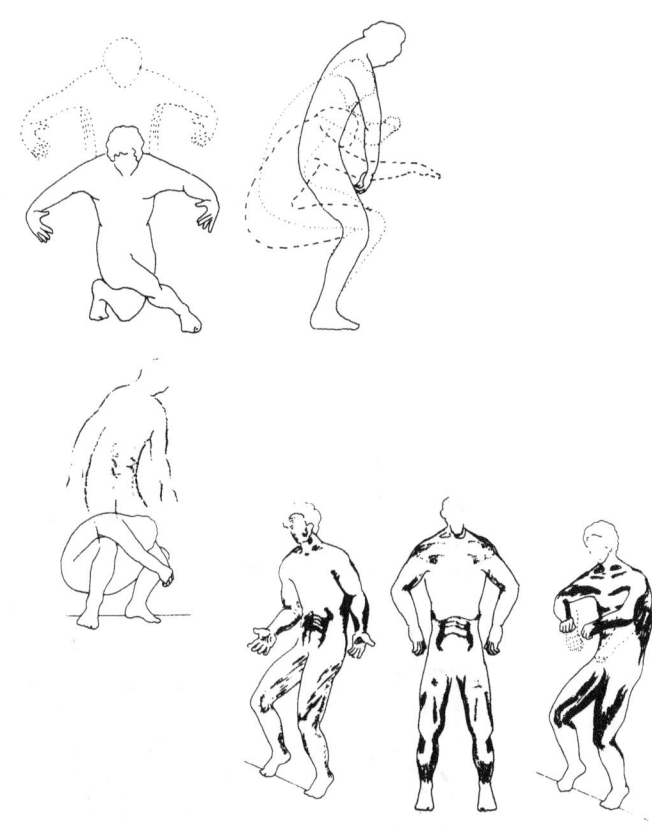

Crescent-like body yawn stretches

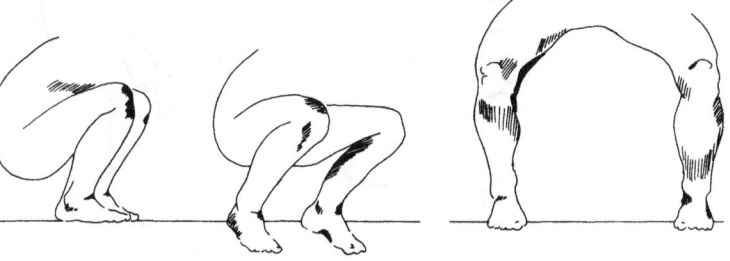

No hands should be used in these workout series, whether squatting down, up, or in the crescent stretch. If you need some help, use a finger-tip control (contact vanishing point assistance) that feels as light as a feather. (See pp. 104-106)

Some Additional Aids:

Tune in often and regularly to the sensation of body respiration and to the perception of its effects on the body.

Become aware of balance control through the feel of anti-gravity urge-extension, especially in the spine, neck, and head when posture and balance seem precarious.

Tune into the rhythm feel, the inner rhythm of the action, and relate and respond musically to that rhythm.

Series Four: **Buddy Squats**

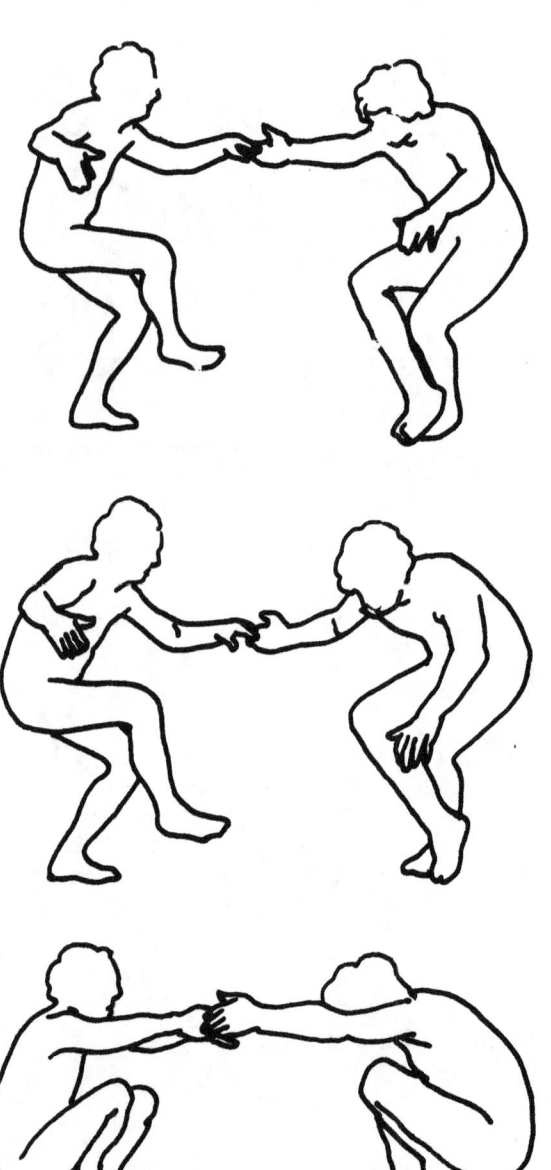

- Do any of the floating squats with a friend or partner. Coordinate the movement of both partners to the characteristic style of whatever energy state is used. While working with a buddy you both become a team of ensemble artists; neither of you functions as spotter, helper or instructor; both of you are follower and leader at the same time and any form of support is imperceptible even to the watchful eye. All that can be sensed and noticed is spontaneity and esthetic functioning.

- Finally, decide which squat takes you to a sitting position in a gentle, undiscerned, graceful manner. If none qualifies as yet, then work on the one you like best or feels most comfortable. Out of the five floating squats, let's achieve weightless, esthetic "sit-down" or "touch-down" on one or two of them; the others will remain a challenging recalcitrance, but subject to progressive exploration. On sit-down, train yourself to rise buoyantly to upright, without use of hands. A little waft and wave loosening, anticipating a weightless, resting-up feel, will help immeasurably. In the sit-down, fetal-like posture, your body becomes a small ball, ready for the next chapter's workout.

Getting the Body into Small Sphere

Certain body dynamics have a catholicity of purpose and can be applied over and over again in nearly every experiment and exploration. Prominent among these is wafting and waving, spanning a spectrum of motion from sustained, flowing movement to a tremulous, vibrating quiver. Within this spectrum, wafting and waving assumes an intra-training function in Body Wisdom. It crosses over and impacts upon body development in such areas as: fear diffusion; "contiguous continuity" or the atom-to-atom discovery of body surfaces; reserve safety-cushions; relaxation strategies; balance and rhythm; and techniques for penetrating the body environment's inner space.

As you explore the five floating squat postures, continue to observe and discover the "inspiring" pleasure of inhaling and exhaling. The gliding buoyancy of wafting and waving in these "body as a small ball" positions adds new dimensions to breathing energy.

Waft and wave in the squat posture on the smallest, resting pedestal provided by your foot position. As you explore the sensation of body balance in this posture, teach yourself the thrill of what we mean by "dynamic balance in movement." This "moving or traveling balance" begins to give you the sense of rhythmic, deliberate, slow motion floating.

In squat postures, you'll explore the contact surface of the body with your feet. As you do so, make every effort to register the feel of subtle "rocking and rolling," in order to pin-point every spot on the foot surface making contact.

Whenever you feel the slightest bit of muscle tension anywhere in the body while doing your squats, exploit the buoyancy experience of the calf muscles, the thigh muscles, and the back.

Summary Observations:

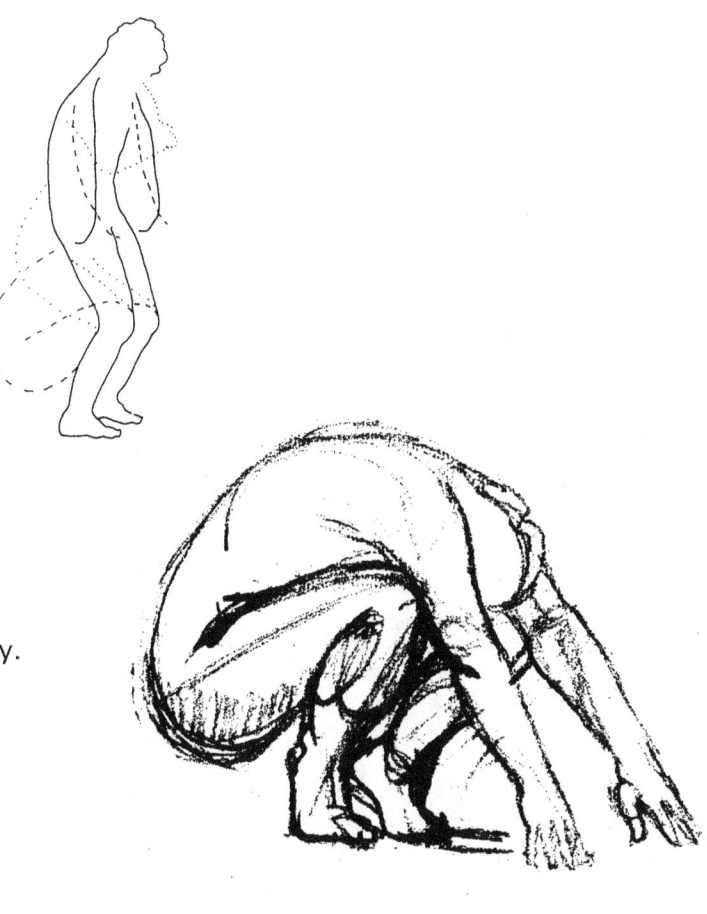

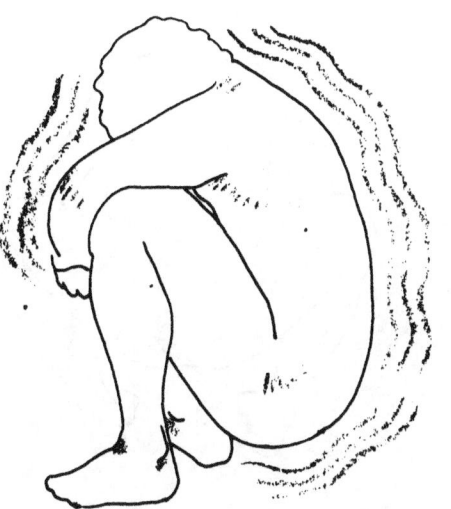

Energy and Relaxation in Movement

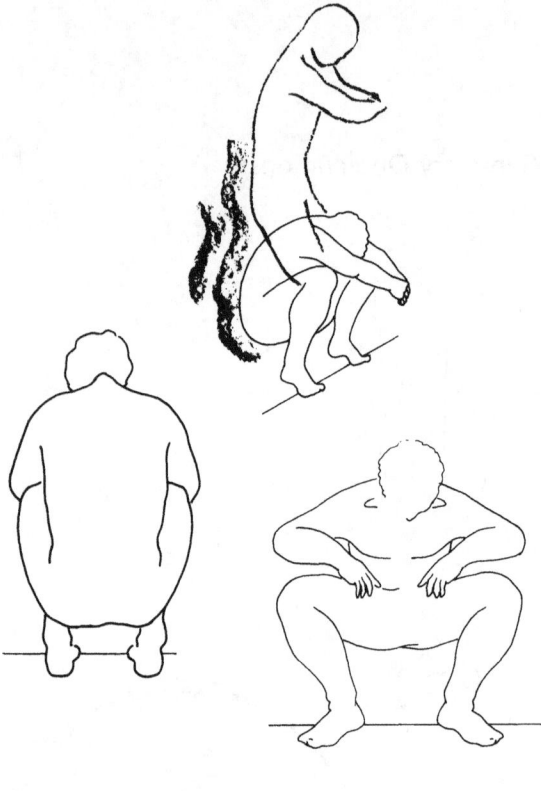

- As you waft and wave, concentrate on softening and melting those muscles, and sigh gently as you rock and roll through graceful, smooth movements. This gliding, mellow feeling of free movement will help to melt those tense muscles. While it may take quite awhile before your squat is comfortably at sitting position, you'll find that the melting, loosened softening of every part of the body through wafting, waving, and increasing body balance assists your efforts in moving gradually lower to the ground. **Reaching the ground from a near sitting position must be so imperceptibly gradual that without the slightest bounce or drop, you suddenly find yourself thinking: "Is that really the ground or is it just my imagination?"**

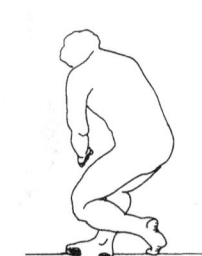

- At the beginning, you'll probably find that squatting and floating down and back to upright position in the criss-cross posture are much more difficult to accomplish than with the other squats. However, the criss-cross position is perhaps the easiest with which to reach the ground in a gradual, relaxed, and quiet, sitting posture.

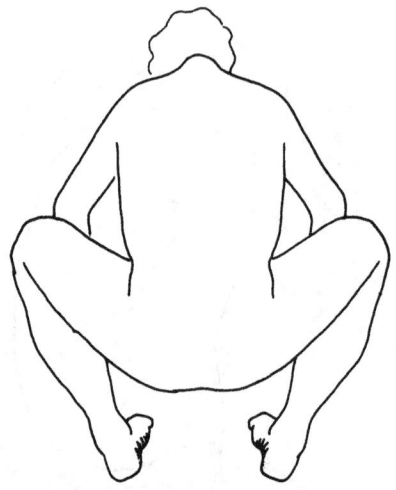

- The two-bladed squat is the one that should be practiced most, because it contributes so much to the others, as well as to other body activities such as walking and running. It also offers a valuable bonus for foot arch improvement and arch support. Another carry-over benefit: When doing some normal walking right after the two-bladed squat work, you'll find a peculiar yet satisfying sense of gliding, a new rhythm. Take special note of this sensation, as it is the beginning of a kind of "leg-wheel rolling" which we'll be treating at length in a subsequent chapter. Also register a new ease in using the proper foot posture (feet straight forward, not turned

Getting
the Body
into
Small Sphere

out) in standing, walking, or running. The two-bladed squat offers us the most subtle, sophisticated body-balance experience of all the squats.

- The flat-sole squat requires a great deal of patience, work, and sensitivity in mastering the ability to touch down to the ground without losing balance. Some of you, with longer body lines from the knees to the pelvis, may have less difficulty than others. But everyone can learn to do it in time. Don't give up. Hire an image and transform your frustration into inquisitive experimentation.

- The most difficult touchdown is from the toe-squat position or from the balls of the feet. Meeting the ground from this squat is well nigh impossible even for most gymnasts and dancers. A key to touching down from the toe squat is to try to expand and extend the toe perimeter to include more of the outer edge of the feet. Like the two-bladed squat, this is almost like figure ice-skating in squat.

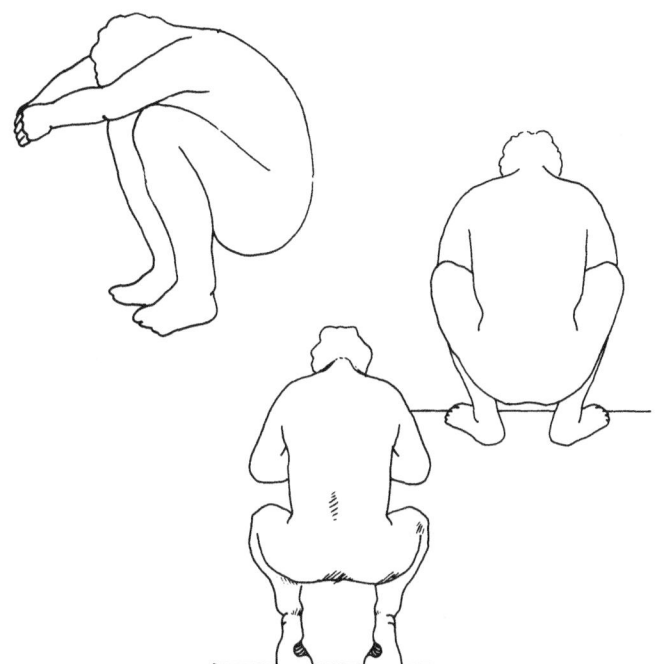

° Work with a buddy and develop squat exercises of your own.

° Invent squat games and squat improvisations.

° Devise "variations on the theme" of squat.

Extra-Curricular Activities

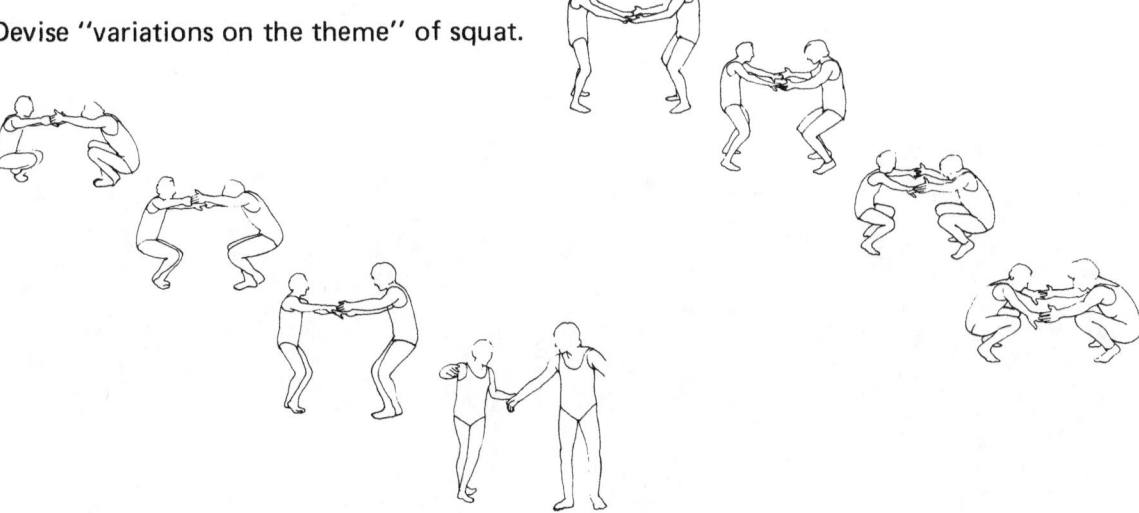

8
THE BODY AS A SMALL SPHERE

As we work our way from "touch-down" to "sit-down" in the five floating squats, our posture gradually enfolds into fetal position, the body coming to feel like a compact ball or egg-shaped orb. This, of course, is what we mean by "the body as a small sphere."

By turning the illustration clockwise and counter-clockwise, you can see how, from sit-down position, the body can move through a fluid series of small-sphere variations, each with its own shadings and nuance. In this chapter, we will work through this series, advancing alternately from sit-down position to kneel-down, low spine back-down, mid-spine back-down, upper spine back-down, shoulder-down, neck-down, left side-down, and right side-down.

Some of these small-ball postures are easy and immediately comfortable. Others will feel strange at first and require getting used to, but take heart. They are all positions a child can do easily and so can we, if we're sufficiently free and "untight." We should always think of our small-body sphere as a spongy, fibrous, porous ball that can breathe, expand, contract, and be saturated; that can curve and roll itself glidingly over firm surfaces; that can swim and float, submerged in water as well as skimming the water's surface. These are the kind of images you'll want to hire, and your task is made easier by the experience you already have with buoyancy, radiancy, foam-rubber elasticity, and body-yawn potency, all of which carry-over into the following experiments.

Consider the work in these experiments as pioneering explorations rather than exercises. In exercise routines the tendency is to drill, imitate, repeat mechanically, and force the body through the activity despite strain or pain. **In exploring** there is always creative challenge of inquisitive searching, of discovery, of self-teaching.

Chapter 8

The Body as a Small Sphere

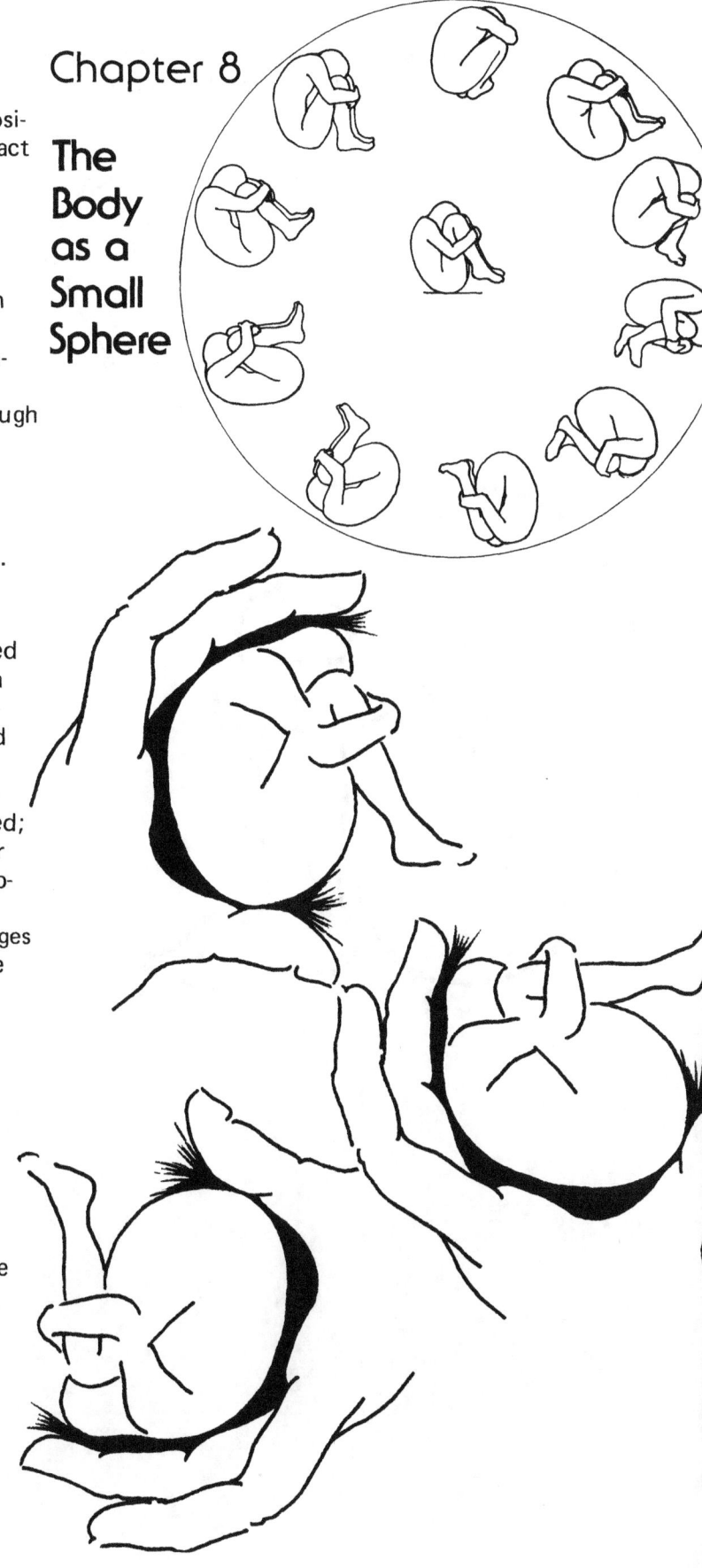

Energy and
Relaxation
in Movement

Experiment One: Breathing Energy in Small-Ball Posture.

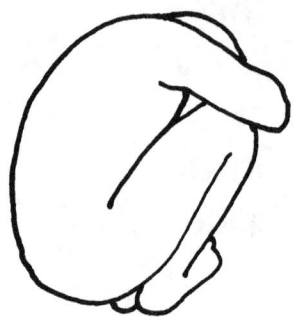

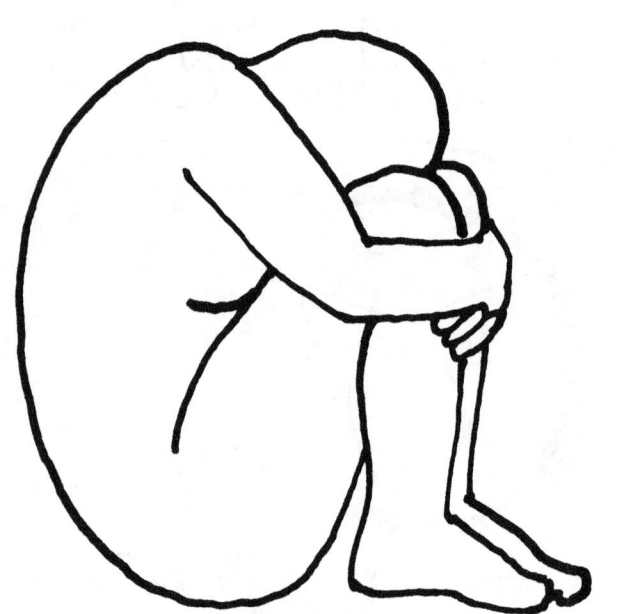

- Using your favorite squat, achieve a touch-down and then, as smoothly as you can without losing the enfolded fetal position, roll and move through all of the small-ball postures, as suggested in the illustrations. Do this with a minimum of flopping, bouncing, and balance-loss.

- As you find the "fit" of your body in each small-ball starting posture, carefully note the degree of facility or difficulty experienced as you "move in stillness" through each of them.

- Maintain each posture long enough to:
  ○ breathe in easily, freely, and fully; then
  ○ hold the inhalation for approximately six counts; then
  ○ exhale slowly, in a relaxed but deliberate way.

- Register your sensations, perceptions, and reactions to the movement of breath energy as it affects your musculature in the different small-ball positions. With smooth and sustained breathing, you should be able to hold the fetal-like posture long enough to observe the accompanying "feels."

- With this kind of natural, instinctive inhaling, the breath flow and muscle activity will move smoothly from the stomach muscles to the side muscles, and then into the lower and upper back "spine-centers," but **not at all into the chest area**. With smooth, gentle exhaling the process is reversed, as the energy flow returns from the back and side muscles to the lower spine-center, and back to the now contracting, grooved stomach, but **never to an expanding, extended abdomen**.

Body as
Small Sphere

Study these muscle contractions and expansions: their direct relationship to breathing energy; their structural dimensions; and the sensations they produce within the body.

- Starting in sit-down position, waft your body gently in slow, small alternating movements and observe its undulating motion. Wafting and waving helps to relieve muscle and body tension.

- Coordinate the wafting with breathing energy and respond to the moving distribution of breath throughout the body.

- While wafting, trace designs, symbols, and perhaps even word spellings with the body, associating the motions with a sense of inner balance and internal rhythm.

- Smoothly waft into kneel-down position and repeat the first three steps in Experiment Two.

- Do the same for each of the other small ball positions.

- Then return to kneel-down position for rest and reflection.

While wafting from posture to posture, you'll begin to "taste" a graduated swinging and swaying that seems to be moving toward a body "rock and roll." Do this smoothly and slowly, without bouncing or flopping; imaging yourself as a sailboat, gently swayed in all directions by soft winds and wafted by floating water currents. Explore these sensations as you waft and sway.

Also note that in spontaneously wafting and swaying, in all directions, your body sphere forms a single curvo-linear motion in continuum. In circular movement, some-

Experiment Two: Wafting and Waving in Small-Ball Positions

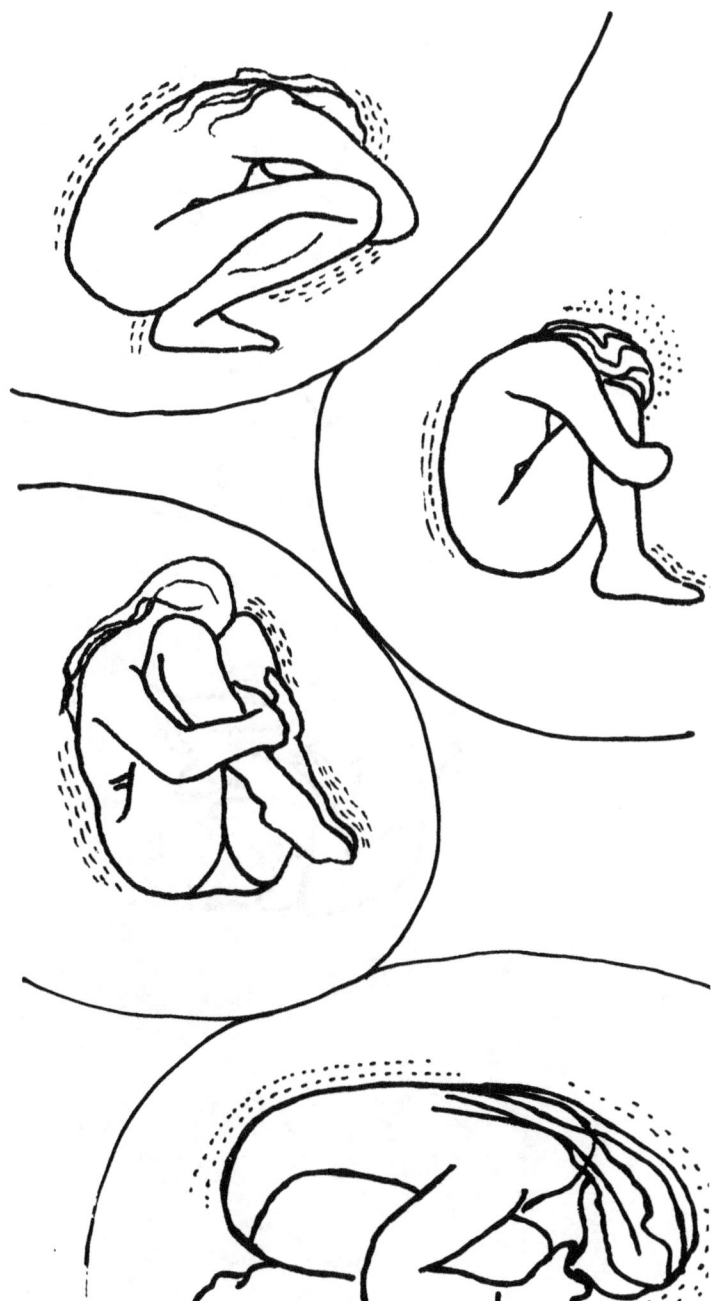

Energy and
Relaxation
in Movement

thing is always moving **forward.** Every move, turn, or roll that your body as a small ball makes is moving in a positive forward direction, constantly "reaching" toward something ahead of you. This is an important perception.

Experiment Three: Atom-to-Atom Discovery and Exploration

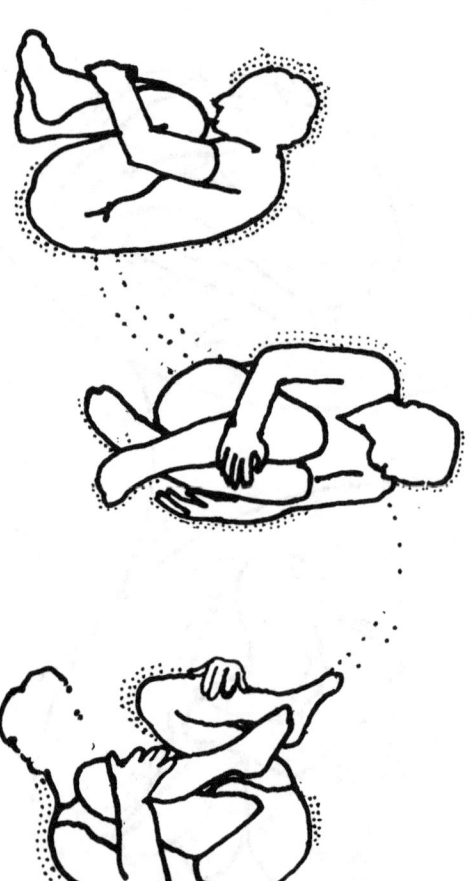

"Atom-to-atom discovery" refers to the "Principle of Contiguous Continuity" and intimately relates to our concepts of forward direction, rocking and rolling, diffusion of the fear of falling, body balance, slow-motion movement, and rhythm. Simply put, "contiguous continuity" means not moving from any one spot (atom) on the body until you successfully experience the feel of its most proximally adjacent (closest touching) spot.

- Start by wafting slowly enough to investigate the particular part of the body in contact with the outside surface. By familiarizing yourself with those body surfaces, perceiving and responding to them, you'll be better able to relate that response to the exploration of the rest of the body.

- Keeping your focus on this one spot, take the opportunity to observe your muscle movement and gentle body expansion in its breathing process.

- Also, respond to your own instructions to soften the muscles; particularly those which are in direct use. Waft and wave in order to sense a muscle-loosening experience. When all the muscles involved cease to feel hard and tight, you are ready to move to the next contiguous spot on the body. Muscle loosening offers a continuity of body surface while you sustain the

Body as
Small Sphere

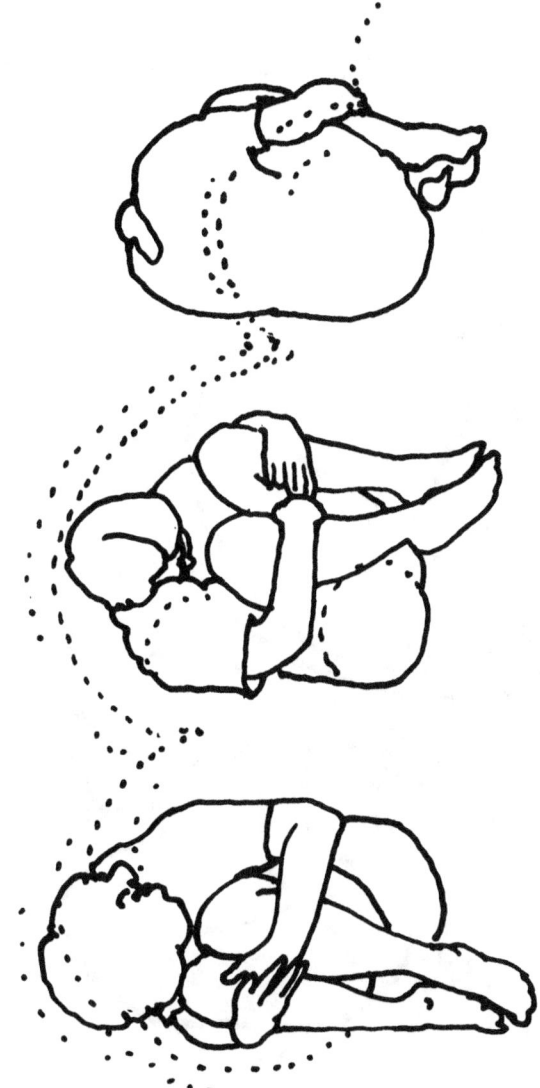

movement and maintain the rolling. You should teach yourself kinesthetically that you can move to the next atom (spot) **only** if the previous atom (spot) is soft and fluid enough to lead the way; this is what I mean by **continuing** the feeling of **contiguous contact** between body-surface and ground-surface.

Contiguous continuity thus involves a deliberate continuum of movement attended by the most conscious, responsive awareness. It is this action that motivates slow-motion skills in rocking and rolling and tumbling, and in the arts of body balance. The principal of contiguous continuity develops both a paramount power of concentration and a sharp awareness of a "moving present," (always in atom-to-atom discovery), into the next piece of "moving future."

The past may be subject to sense memory as a way of recapturing the context of previous experience for purposes of applying it to the present. But once this is accomplished, past and present are disengaged. They no longer stand in **contiguous continuity**. On the other hand, the "moving present" anticipates and is always part of the "moving future." In the grammar of the organic feeling process, with the body constantly in movement, the present is the "progressive forward" tense.

If you appreciate this distinction, you'll understand why we prefer the skills of "slow motion" body control and perceptive motivation to the "thrills of premature body speed" and trial-and-error momentum. Your awareness and appreciation of such engrossed body action will become a great strength for potential body speed, without leaving too much to chance impression. When body-action training is initiated with an agressive, rapid-fire "trial and error" momentum, it too often deters the development of sophisticated control over **de-accelerated** body movement.

Energy and
Relaxation
in Movement

Experiment Four: Slow-Motion Movement

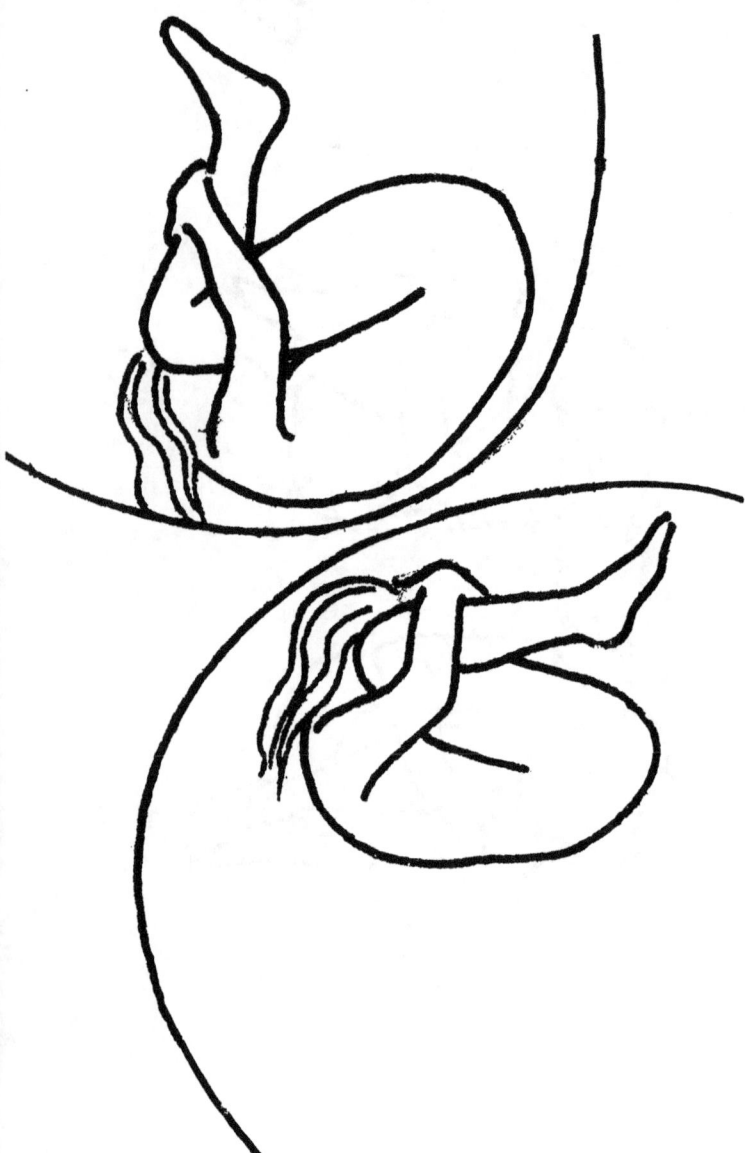

So, as you gently waft and wave, explore the surface area and texture of your body through a continual mapping survey, as with an extremely slow-timed overhead camera. This kinesensic photo survey permits you to experience the double-action feel of stopping and moving at the same time.

Once you discover, atom-to-atom, the body surface area and texture, you'll wonder whether the energy dynamic is that of "balance in movement" or "movement in stillness." All you know is that you feel the body in action and that every particle of the action is positive, forward-directed movement. As you work through the mapping, you'll feel urged to sharpen your sensor system so that it better feeds all those direct images of balance, control, and rhythm that now seem curiously un-related to the "issue of speed." The surprise will come later when you discover that speed, in running for example, is much better produced by your perception of balance and rhythm than it is by blunt muscle-force.

It bears mention that when one little spot on the body surface is "curvingly" bridged to the next little spot immediately contiguous to it, we can fill in those little gaps without getting trapped in bounce-shocks, flopping around, or falling. In other words, when you receive the signal that you are about to lose control and fall, you can call for help on contiguous continuity and convert the fear of falling into a creative opportunity for "muscle-melting." When the body tells you that you are about to fall, say to yourself: "I am a small ball — I never need feel that I am falling — I need only to sense myself **rolling** from one curved body point to another." So that what would have been a "STOP: DANGER" signal becomes an eagerly anticipated, trap-free "GO AHEAD" sign.

Body as
Small Sphere

Introductory references to body shaking appear in Chapter 5 (**Relaxer-Energizers**). Here, and in succeeding work chapters, our concern is to describe and develop these skills as they apply to the evolving body curve, and to increase awareness of energy and relaxation in movement.

In a broad sense, muscle shaking serves as:

◦ a natural relaxer-energizer;

◦ a muscle-loosening and muscle-lengthening activity;

◦ therapy for damaged muscles and physical exhaustion;

◦ both an extrinsic and an intrinsic body vibrator; and

◦ a familiar event for physical vibrato and emotional shaking experience.

In terms of the body energy states you've already investigated, buoyancy wafting and waving might be considered the slowest shake, while radiancy oscillation in the form of nervous vibrato, tremble, shiver, flutter, or quiver would generate the fastest body shakes.

- Select your favorite small-ball position and experiment with such vibrations as the mild mini-shake or quiver. Sense and perceive the rhythm-movement of the quiver.

- Call on the different images of the shiver and the tremble. Tune into the "shake character" and quality of each. Then consciously repeat the action as a shake skill, rather than as a tremble or quiver, and sharpen your sensors to the inner rhythm-feel of each.

Experiment Five: Body Shaking and Vibrating

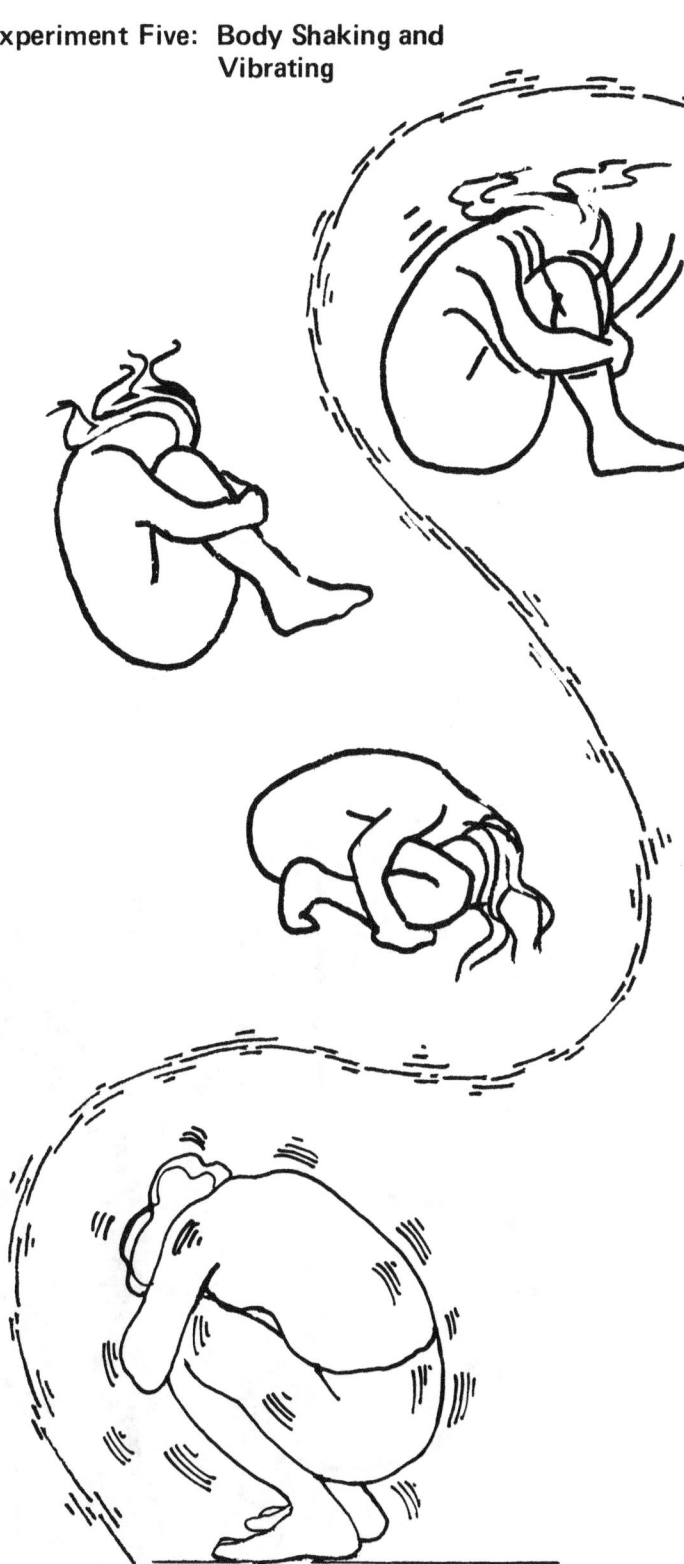

Energy and
Relaxation
in Movement

- Practice vibrating in all other possible manners, using familiar images. Think, for example, of a bowl of shimmering Jello and reflect the rhythm of that kind of shimmering. Or of a closed jar of juice, the liquid being swirled by the gentle shake of an outside force. Or of being vibrated by a moving vehicle or electric pulsating current.

- After sensing your body trembled, shimmered, swirled, jiggled, and vibrated by outside energy currents, winds, or flows, use the awareness of that rhythmic vibration to motivate your body to internally "self-feel" the same experience. In other words, convert the remembered sensation into an organic instruction and apply it to a fresh, familiar event; i.e., the sensation of light, agile dancing — to resonate and vibrate (shake) a tired leg muscle — or the sensation of trembling or shivering after a 'cold water swim' to perceive that 'inner gentle turbulence'. If you do this in a climate of relaxed energy, you will feel a loosening, melting, softening of the musculature that disperses fatigue and helps you move freely and smoothly.

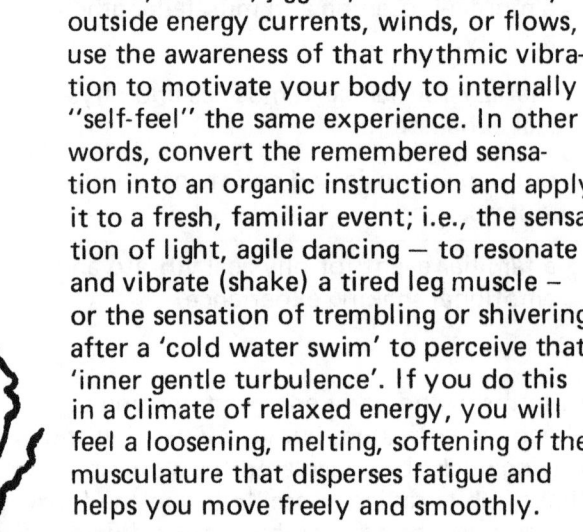

Body as
Small Sphere

Having wafted and waved, swayed, vibrated, and shaken, we are now ready for exploration in preparation of the "roll." Body rolling should not, as yet, be considered a form of tumbling, but rather as controlled slow-motion movement in continuum. Rolling, at this point, should still be considered as uninterrupted atom-to-atom exploration, without the slightest inclination of body-thrusting or body-throwing.

In kinesensic training, we no more "throw" the body in order to reach somewhere than "throw" the voice in order to project it. Hence, body rolling should not be confused with body-momentum. Any accelerated rolling that is not specifically intended as part of a sequenced process of body development would, at this point, only diffuse attention and probably substitute a kind of careless self-indulgence for what should be perceptive awareness. This would simply short-circuit the feeling process.

- Begin by getting into the small-ball side-down position.

- Warm up with a little wafting or vibrating and then proceed to roll slowly in atom-to-atom discovery of first one spot, then the next, then the next, over as much of the body's surface as is convenient and comfortable. The support you require to keep going, to keep the body moving, can come from a neighboring spot on the knee, shoulder, elbow, head, toe, etc. They are all valid and positive as long as they are continuing spots, and as long as you maintain, throughout, the form of the body-sphere.

- Return to sit-down position. Check your breathing and respond to the inhale-exhale sensations as you now direct and sustain your slow-motion movement in a forward-

Experiment Six: Preparing for Body Rolling

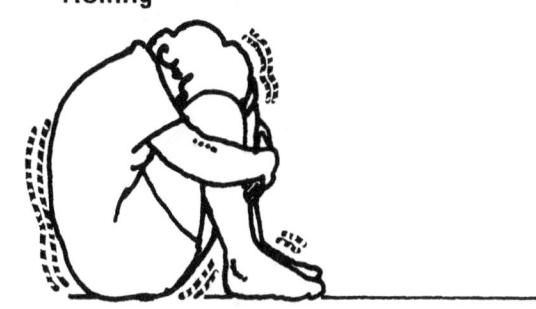

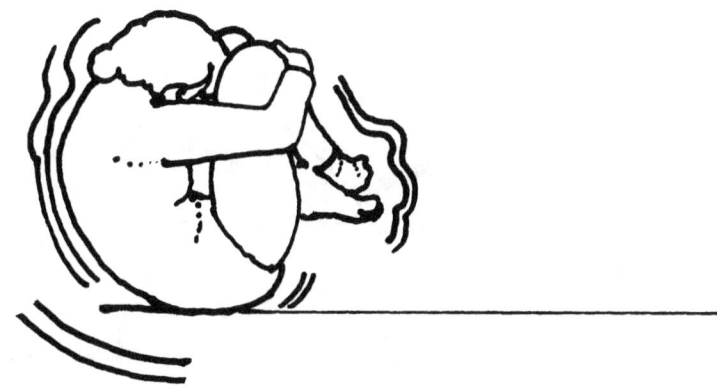

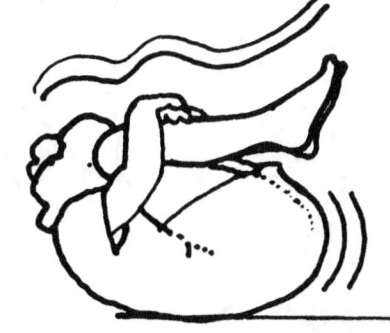

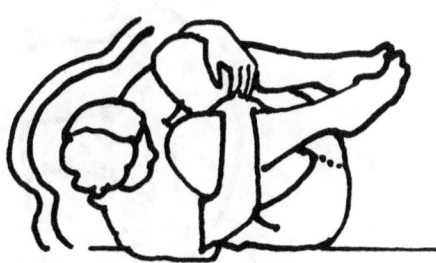

Energy and
Relaxation
in Movement

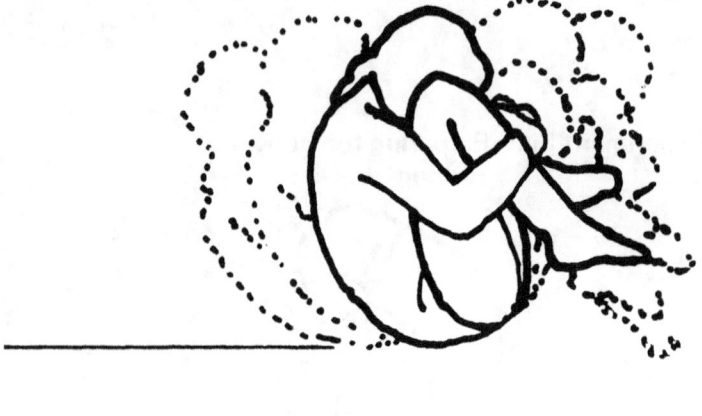

backward action. Register the absence of any sense of pulling at the body, of any force pushing it, of any fear of falling. Imagine yourself as a weightless sphere in gravity-free space. Imagine that gravity-free world as an ocean dense enough for you to rest in (like a fish), enjoying your body rhythm and body balance. Think of your body as a "center of gravity" whose only purpose is to discover and explore new nuances of floating-rolling-gliding experience.

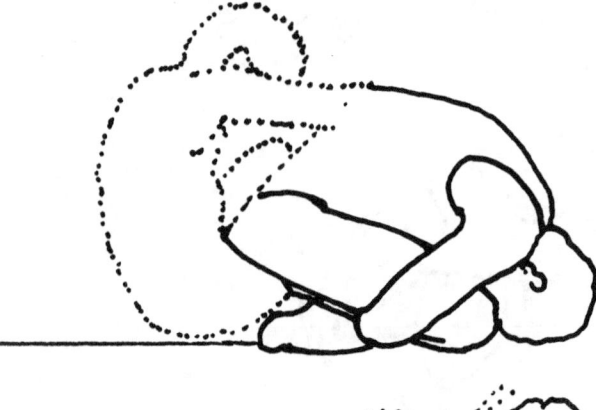

- As you roll forward from the sit-down position, the forward movement will bring your head closer and closer to the ground, until you can gently "kiss" the surface with your head and forehead. As you discover new body surfaces, experience a comfortable rolling and rocking on your knees, elbows, and wrists. And experience, as well, the different rhythm-feels.

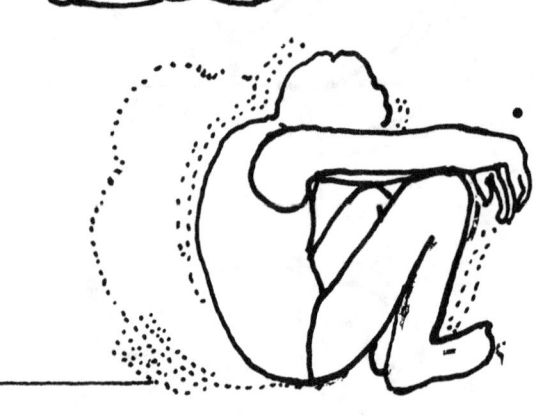

- Then roll back to sit-down position. After a bit of gentle rocking, "waft-roll" backward to a low back-down position. As you sense the new rhythms in this posture, note how the small-of-the-back (which is part of the upper pelvic area and a traditional tension center) feels comfortable, and both relaxing and energizing at the same time.

NOTE: What you are feeling in the low back-down position relates to an earlier reference in Chapter 5 to those traditional body tension centers (lower spine, upper spine, and jaw) that through our training, convert into vital relaxer-energizer centers for the body. These are dominant and dominating body hubs that act also as fulcrums — radiating comfort, vigor, potency, and stamina. The spine centers in particular (more fully discussed in Chapter 9 — The Perception of the Upright) are where most of us experience pressure, strain, and pain leading directly to headaches, neck stress, jaw tension, and a multitude of back problems.

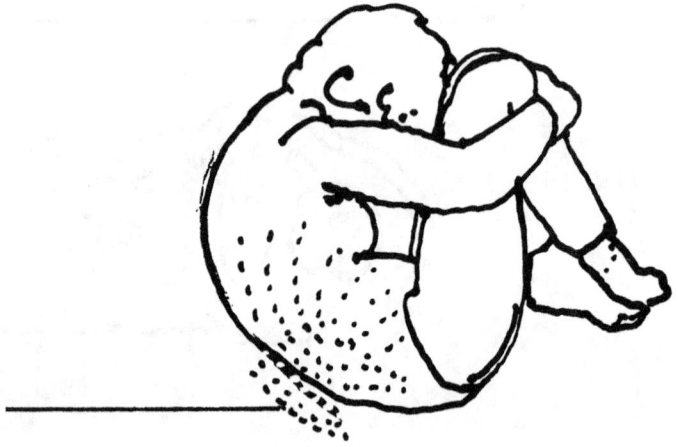

Body as
Small Sphere

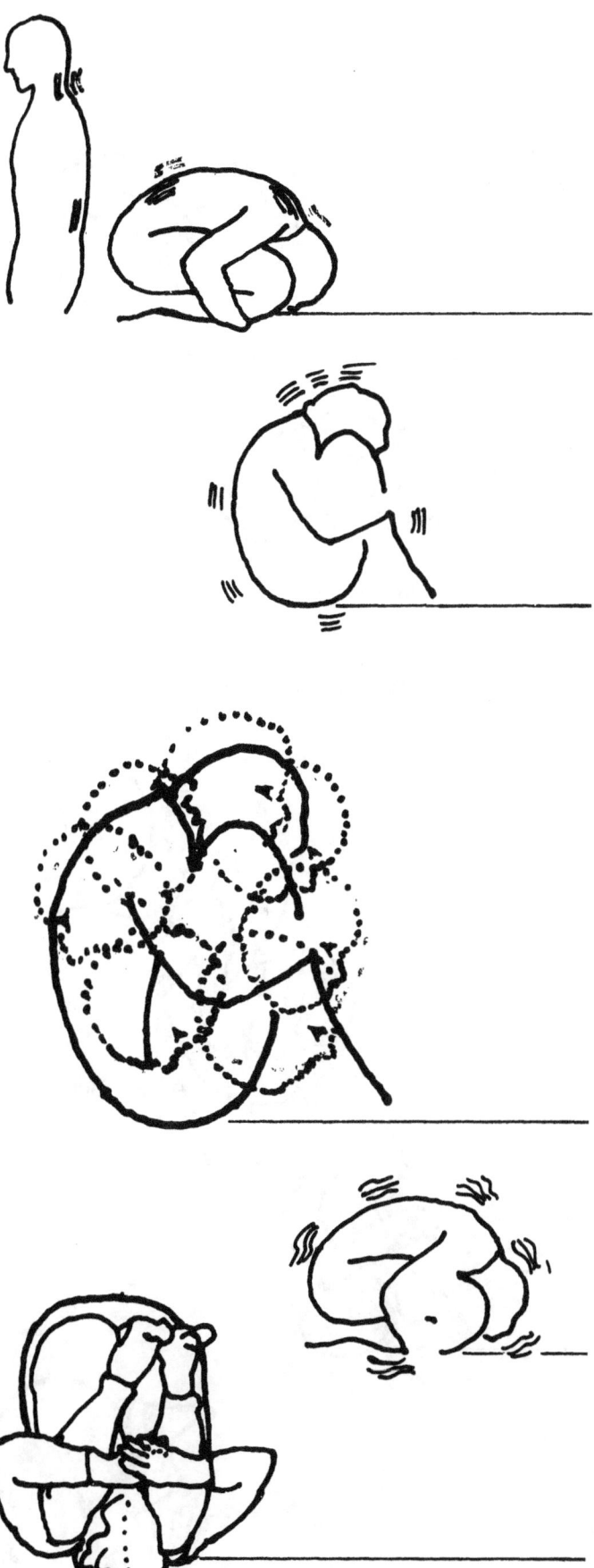

So as you waft, breathe, rock and roll on your spinal surface, in this experiment as a small ball and later as an "expanded sphere" or elongated crescent curve, recognize that the lower and upper centers are part of a natural (convex) body curve — what we refer to, throughout, as the C-curve.

- To become more familiar with the **vital lower-back center,** gently rock and roll from sitting position to lower and mid-back, right on through toward the upper back position. As you move through the entire shaking, breathing, atom-to-atom discovery process, tune in to the full range of rhythm sensations. Your shaking movement could be forward and backward, sideways, circular and diagonal, all of these. Note how backward and forward rolling present different experiences from side-rolling, even though the procedure is the same.

- Now explore the resilience and elasticity of the **vital upper spine center,** where the upper back, shoulders, and neck form a single unit. There is more nerve tissue in this energy-giving center than in any other part of the body, except the brain. Let the rock and roll take you from the crown of the head to each shoulder, down to the area around the shoulder blades. With wafting, waving and gentle rolling, the upper spine region, generally so tight and tense, begins to expand and free up. It is important to keep this energy-producing center strain-free, yet strong, agile, and dynamic.

NOTE: If, while in the neck-shoulder-head position, with its new experiences in breathing and shake activity, you can speak quite freely, clearly and with resonance — then your body is doing a fine job of staying loose, light, buoyant, balanced, and comfortable. Ordinarily, this position would induce a cramped, tightening throat, producing considerable vocal abrasiveness; but exploring your breathing, wafting, and atom-to-atom movement with the neck-shoulder-head position will

Energy and
Relaxation
in Movement

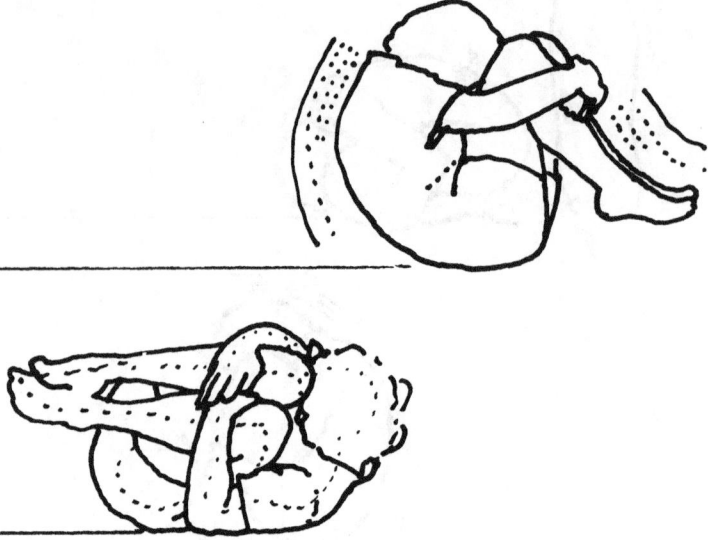

offer an objective example of the "just noticeable difference" between body and voice training.

• The final exploration in this section prepares the way for our experiments in balance. Repeat the entire cycle from breathing, vibrating, and shaking to atom-to-atom discovery; from wafting and waving into rocking and rolling; and then, at any point of atom-to-atom experience, **hold the body-movement in absolute, though vibrating stillness.** Practice this several times, each time holding the movement in stillness at different points of the spectrum.

Experiment Seven: Rolling and Tumbling

By now you have probably managed several full body rolls without even knowing it. You have certainly made a great deal of progress toward the achievement of complete rolls. Now, let's make the conscious effort to rock and roll the body through a full cycle. In our next chapter we will deal with "rolling" and "tumbling" more specifically.

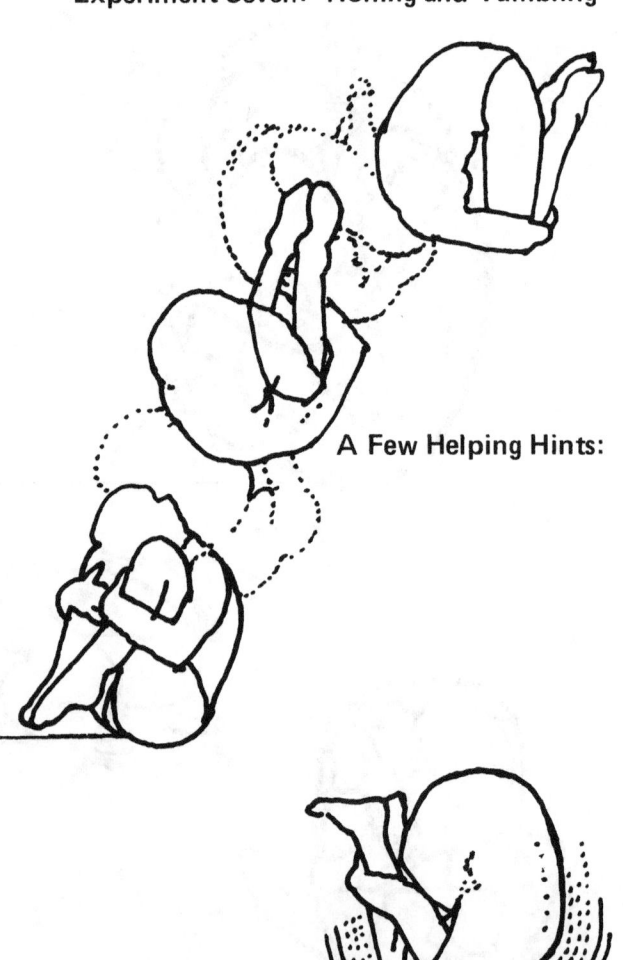

A Few Helping Hints:

○ If you find yourself stopping just short of a complete body roll, then gently rock or roll back to where it last felt comfortable and reactivate the cycle from that point. A specific steering or direction of the "roll" is much less significant than the completion of "full cycles" **in any direction**; as long as atom-to-atom exploration prevents the body from falling, you are working and exploring creatively and esthetically.

○ Wherever it is difficult, waft and wave a bit and then continue on to the slow rocking and rolling.

Body as
Small Sphere

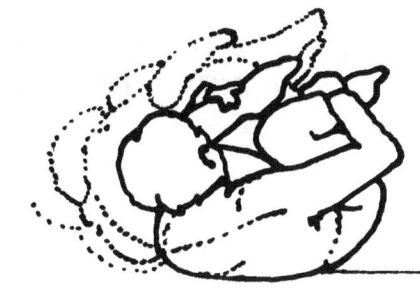

° You should have little difficulty with side rolls and diagonal shoulder rolls. The full forward roll will come easily with exploration. But the back rolls may prove more complicated to maneuver into a complete cycle. At the point where you feel the cycle breaking down, always go back to discovering and concentrating on atom-to-atom surface discovery, assisted by perceptive wafting and waving. This may be all that's required for that extra glide and extra rhythm to help your follow-through with the roll.

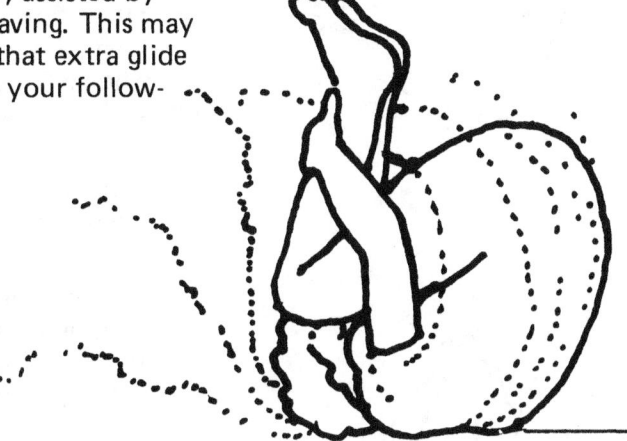

° Negotiating specific rolls, i.e. forward roll, shoulder roll, back roll, etc., is not important — so do not let yourself become anxious about it. The only significant body event, at this time, is continuing slow movement **toward** the full cycle regardless of an unintentional change in direction. As long as the movement is **contiguous and continuous** you are moving properly in a **forward direction.**

° In order to simplify initial attempts with a full forward tumble-roll, cross your feet and let your hands support the upper spine energy center.

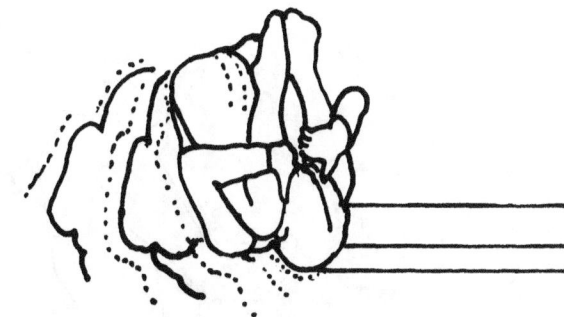

Once you have completed any of the body rolls, in full cycle, have fun with it: respond to it, relax with it, feel its esthetic qualities, rhythms, and energy-giving behavior. Fully enjoy it and remember, you are using it to develop expertise in converting the body's dead weight into simultaneously relaxing and energizing live weight.

Energy and
Relaxation
in Movement

BALANCE IN MOVEMENT — MOVEMENT IN BALANCE

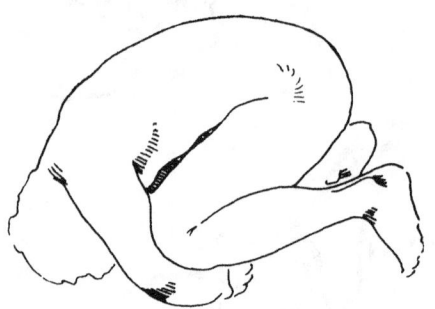

From whatever vantage point you view a piece of dynamic sculpture, you will undoubtedly come up with a different point of view. "Balance" is just such a dynamically sculpted art form of Body Life. No single definition or explanation will suffice or do it justice. We need to move all the way around it, perceiving it from every viewpoint to realize how each is vitally connected with the other, how all together form a network of organic inter-relationships that constitute the whole. To illustrate and prepare for the work of the next three experiments:

- When you become aware of any form of dynamic stillness, you experience balance;

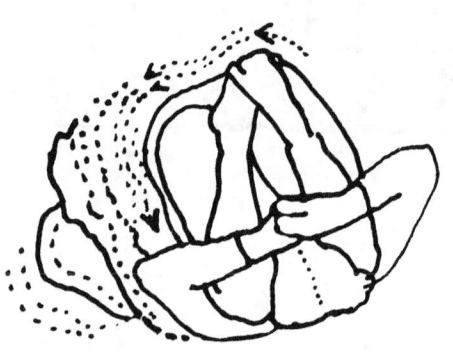

- When you convert dead weight into live weight, and sustain its "vibrating stillness" in a given position for a reasonable duration, you experience balance;

- When you explore atom-to-atom discovery in such slow motion that movement is no longer visible, you experience balance;

- When you feel the combined climates of Radiancy, Buoyancy, and Potency in any psycho-physical behavior of the body in movement, balance or equilibrium can be taken for granted;

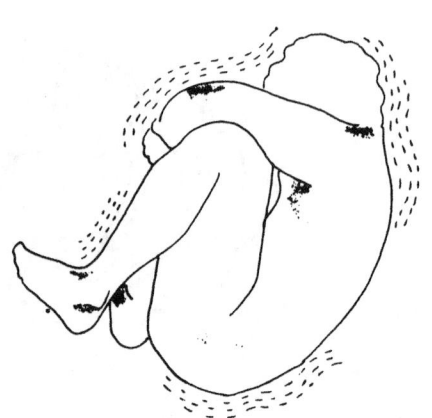

- When the body feels as if it were a center of gravity — floating, swinging, resting, extending in what seems a gravity-free space field — the body is in balance;

- When the body experiences "balance and rhythm" as a single entity, the body allows for falling; turns falling (with its attendant fears) into creative movement and puts the element of play back into the work of physical tasks, the "labor of love" of which we spoke at the outset.

Body as
Small Sphere

In kinesensics, there are three major classifications of body balance:

1. **Pedestal Balance** — where the "resting base" offers little or no security problem;

2. **Pin-Point Balance** — where the resting base is precariously small; and

3. **Moving** or **Traveling Balance** — where the balance is part of slow-motion movement and accelerated body skills.

The following experiments explore these classifications as they relate to our body work in the various small-ball positions.

Pedestal Balance takes its cue from the Potency energy-state with its body-yawn-lift extension and its anti-gravity urge feel. The sit-down position, with feet slightly off the ground, offers one example of pedestal balance. The other small-ball postures also depend upon pedestal balance; that is, they feel as though the body, filled with air (breath), is resting comfortably on a pedestal base.

Experiment Eight: Pedestal Balance

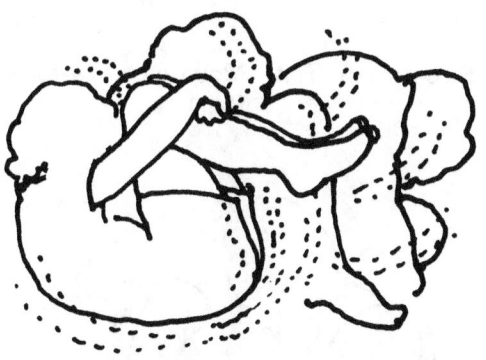

- Starting from any small-ball position, waft-wave-roll. Whenever the inclination strikes, hold the movement for several seconds interrupting the slow, gradual glide. Use these intervals of relative stillness to register the accompanying vibrations and sensations. Repeat the process, each time varying the small-ball starting position.

- As you move through each cycle, holding the movement just long enough to interrupt the gliding action, feel the rhythm response to pedestal balance. Check with the Illustrations.

Energy and
Relaxation
in Movement

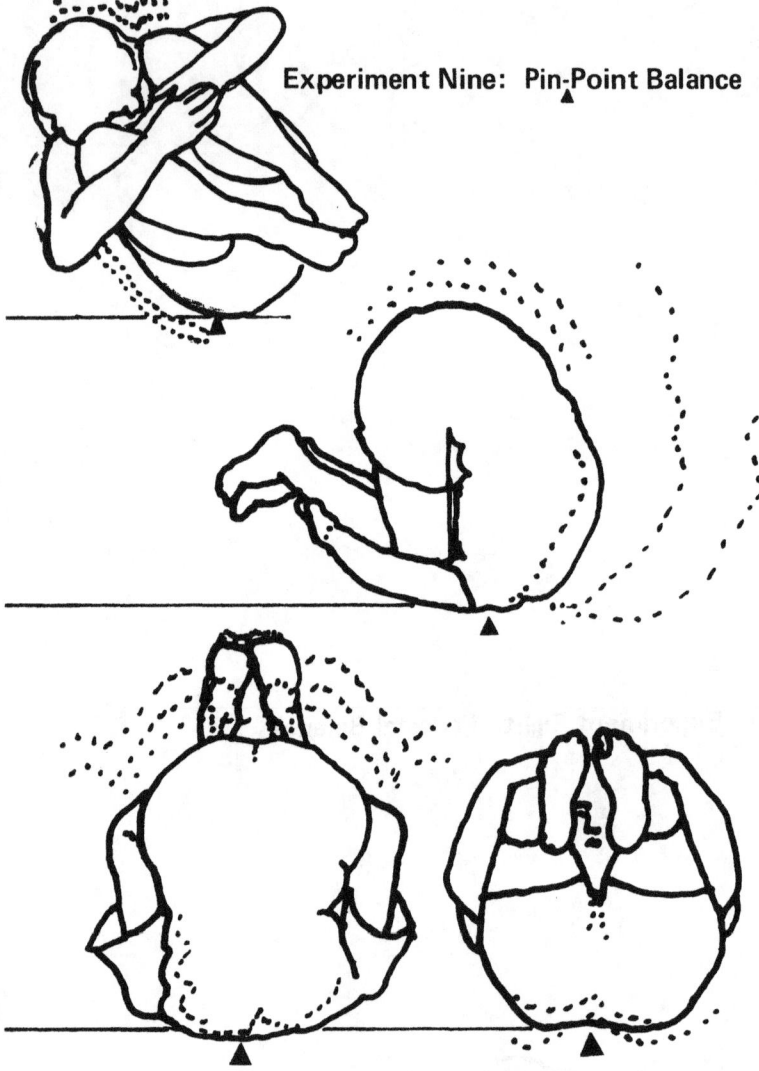

Experiment Nine: Pin-Point Balance

Pin-point balance takes its cue from the Radiancy energy-state in combination with the anti-gravity urge of Potency.

- Glide or roll from small-ball position, so slowly and deliberately that you can take mental pictures, along the way, of any number of pin-point balances. Your mental screen will be particularly active, in this regard, as you move through one side of the pelvic bone or through the shoulder, the small-of-the-back (lower spine center), or the neck area (upper spine center). The emphasis must be on **the adventure of exploring, not on the routine of drilling.**

- Add the body-vibrato of Radiancy energy and expansion-extension breathing activity. You'll know that pin-point balance is present when you feel your body about to be borne spaceward, as though by thousands of little helium bags attached to your skin, hair, muscles, bones, and nails.

- Feel the rhythm energy of pin-point balance and respond with self-teaching perceptions.

Experiment Ten: Moving or Traveling Balance

Moving Balance, while the body is traveling, takes its cue from the Buoyancy energy-state, with coordinated assistance from both Radiancy and Potency. This is especially true when the body is involved in accelerated activity such as running, dancing, leaping, vaulting, etc. At this stage of training, all of your experience with moving balance still takes the form of atom-to-atom discovery.

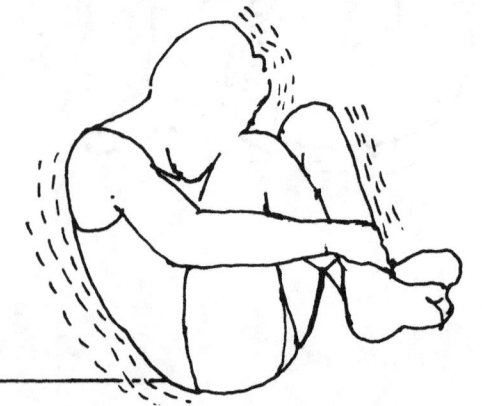

- Repeat the very first wrist-pressing experiment, but now understand it as an example of moving balance in just the arm.

Body as
Small Sphere

- Apply the principle of contiguous continuity (the image of atom-to-atom discovery) beyond the small ball activity to your everyday walking, writing, running, eating, or other familiar movement. Tune in to the new rhythm-feel of each activity. If you perceive a change toward developing sensations of buoyancy or radiancy in these actions, then rest assured that you are activating the concept of moving balance.

We will be working more on balance as a major esthetic as we evolve the body into an "expanded sphere" and "upright posture" in subsequent chapters. For now, it is sufficient to perceive balance, with its three classifications, in terms of the rhythm and energy dynamics of the different small-ball positions.

As you've already discovered, the "buddy system" is an initial step in ensemble or team training. It is also an advanced step in fear diffusion and so relates directly to our work with the body as a small ball.

The present experiment involves two fundamental principles: "Finger-Tip Control" and "Just Noticeable Difference."

Finger-Tip Control refers to the **adding of bodies in circuit** without disturbing or breaking the fluidity of kinesthetic/nerve energy currents. The actual connecting points, where additional bodies "join" the circuit or make contact, whether with the finger-tips or with any other body surface, are sensed and perceived as firm and gentle coupling without the slightest feel of push-pull pressure or weight stress.

Just Noticeable Difference refers to any degree change in sensation that feels, or is psycho-physically perceived, as almost similar but not quite identical to a preceding sensation or feel.

Experiment Eleven: Buddy Work in Small-Ball Activity

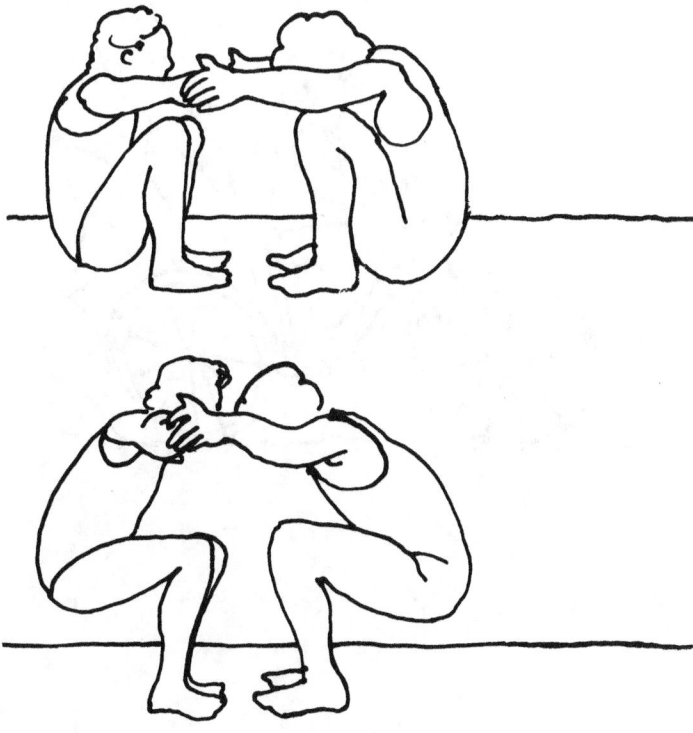

Energy and
Relaxation
in Movement

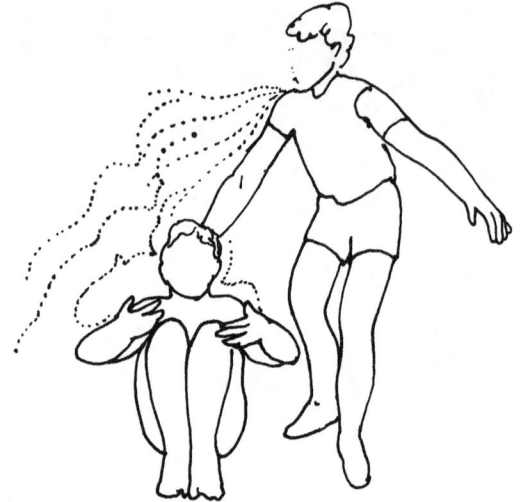

In drawing up a partner by holding onto a hair on the head, or lifting your buddy from squat position by the tender placing of a hand beneath the base of the skull, or teaching a child to ride a bicycle by running behind it but not really holding onto the bike or child, (rather just barely touching the back of the seat with the tip of the finger) — in all these activities, we use "finger-tip control" as an esthetic approach, and "just noticeable difference" as part of the esthetic process. The buddy suddenly removes the sense of fear by becoming another and larger part of the whole, sharing the body esthetics and reinforcing the creative effort through ensemble support.

- As your partner wafts, waves, and rolls in small-ball position, assist him or her with finger-tip control. Remember, only finger-tip contact is needed.

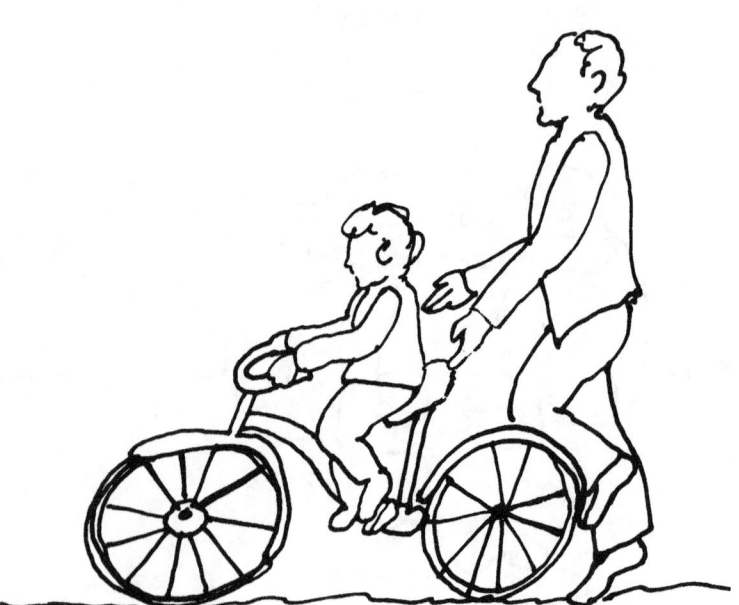

- You can spontaneously influence your buddy's movements in any and all directions, constantly changing the direction the way air currents cause a glider to gently float or cruise through space. Don't think of yourself as a spotter, but as an intrinsic part of the experience — a creative part of the whole picture that adds style, image, rhythm, balance, and creative body expression to the developing event or "happening." Remember, both of you are leader and follower at the same time, giving and receiving cues and signals, perpetually passing between you the rhythm and balance dynamics of different energy-states.

- Continue with the wafting-waving-rocking, and with contiguous, continuous rolling. Change the rolling directions as you wish. Remind yourselves that if the ensuing movement is not as smooth, fluid,

Body as Small Sphere

or buoyant as it should be, you may easily return to the waft-wave-rock action and work your way back, as a team, to the roll. Pretend you are playing a "hoop-and-stick" game, with the tip of the finger as the stick, and your buddy's small-ball body sphere as the moving, rolling hoop. You can roll the buddy-ball all over the floor in any direction, but never press, push, force, or actually lead it. Should you both feel a danger of falling or bouncing, the system of organic cues you've established will allow you to sense this and esthetically signal to each other the desirability of an alternate direction. Picking up "cue feels" provides both of you with clear information, but remains imperceptible to others watching. Completing full "roll"-cycles feels easier, simpler, and downright fascinating.

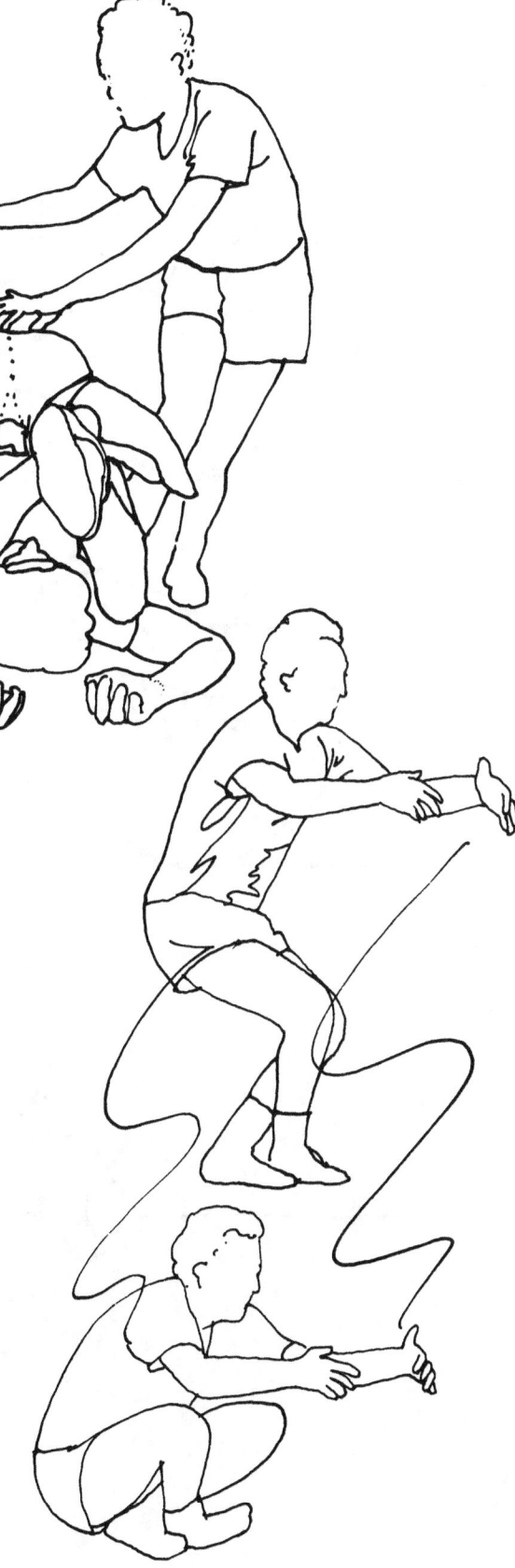

- Now change partners and repeat the same steps. Both buddies should "play" the rolling ball, assisted by finger-tip control of the other. Explore this several times, alternating partners and playing with the free-form coordination that is built into your mutual system of organic cues. As you develop and refine the skills for anticipating each other's esthetic cues and signals, the exploration becomes ever more interesting and inventive.

- With yourself as the rolling ball, and your buddy assisting with finger-tip control, cross your feet comfortably and easily so that while rolling, you may gently and gradually glide, roll, and waft yourself into a criss-cross squat. Then, inspire yourself with breath energy that buoyantly floats you to upright posture.

Energy and
Relaxation
in Movement

- Repeat the same "finish," but now float to upright from one or two of the other more comfortable squat positions and then float back to sit-down posture.

- Now, from sit-down position, comfortably balanced with feet slightly off the ground, open up the small ball — allowing the body sphere to gently expand as though blossoming out (See Illustration).

You are now ready to work with the body as an "expanded sphere."

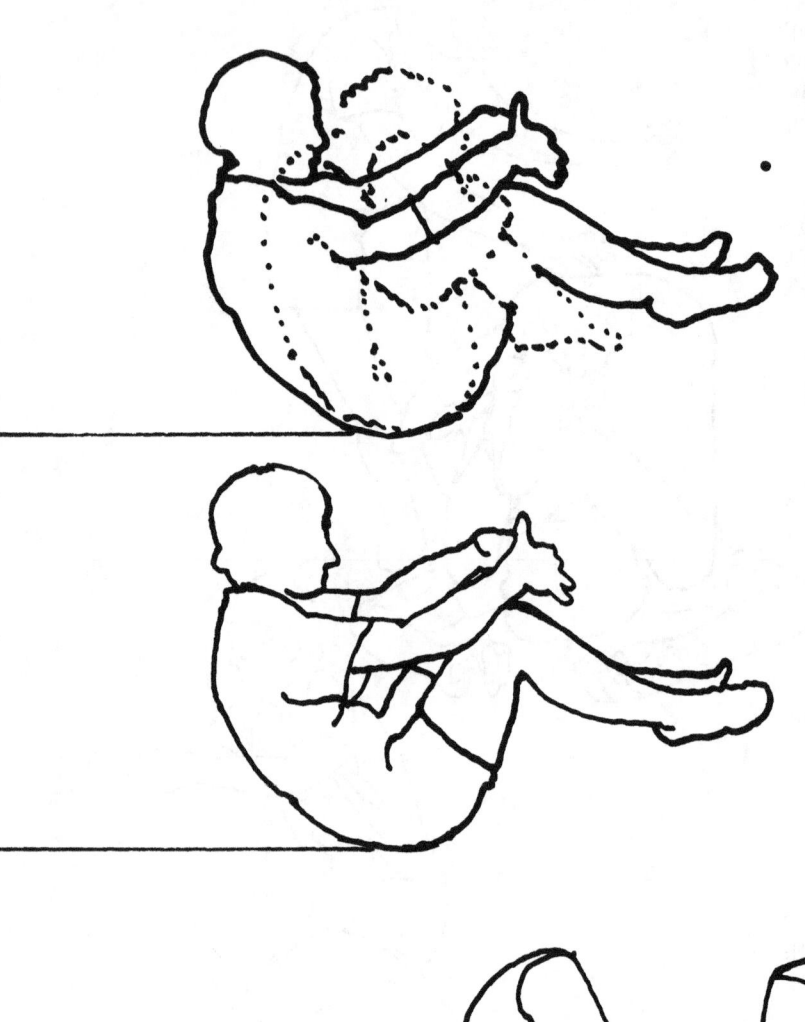

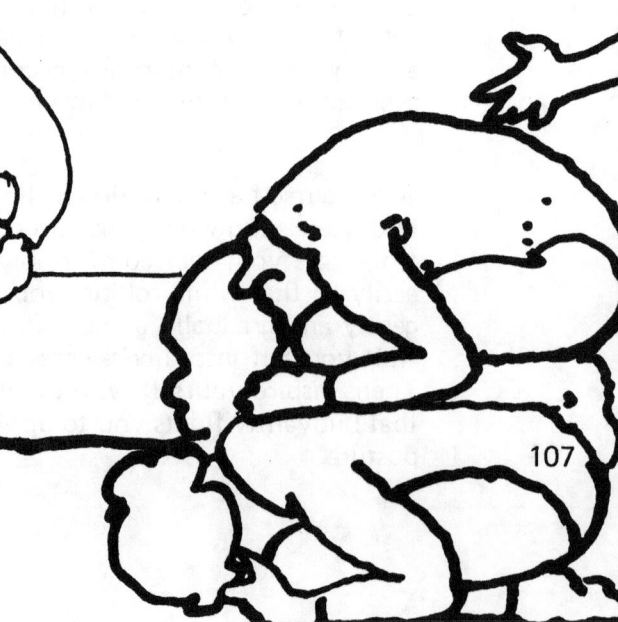

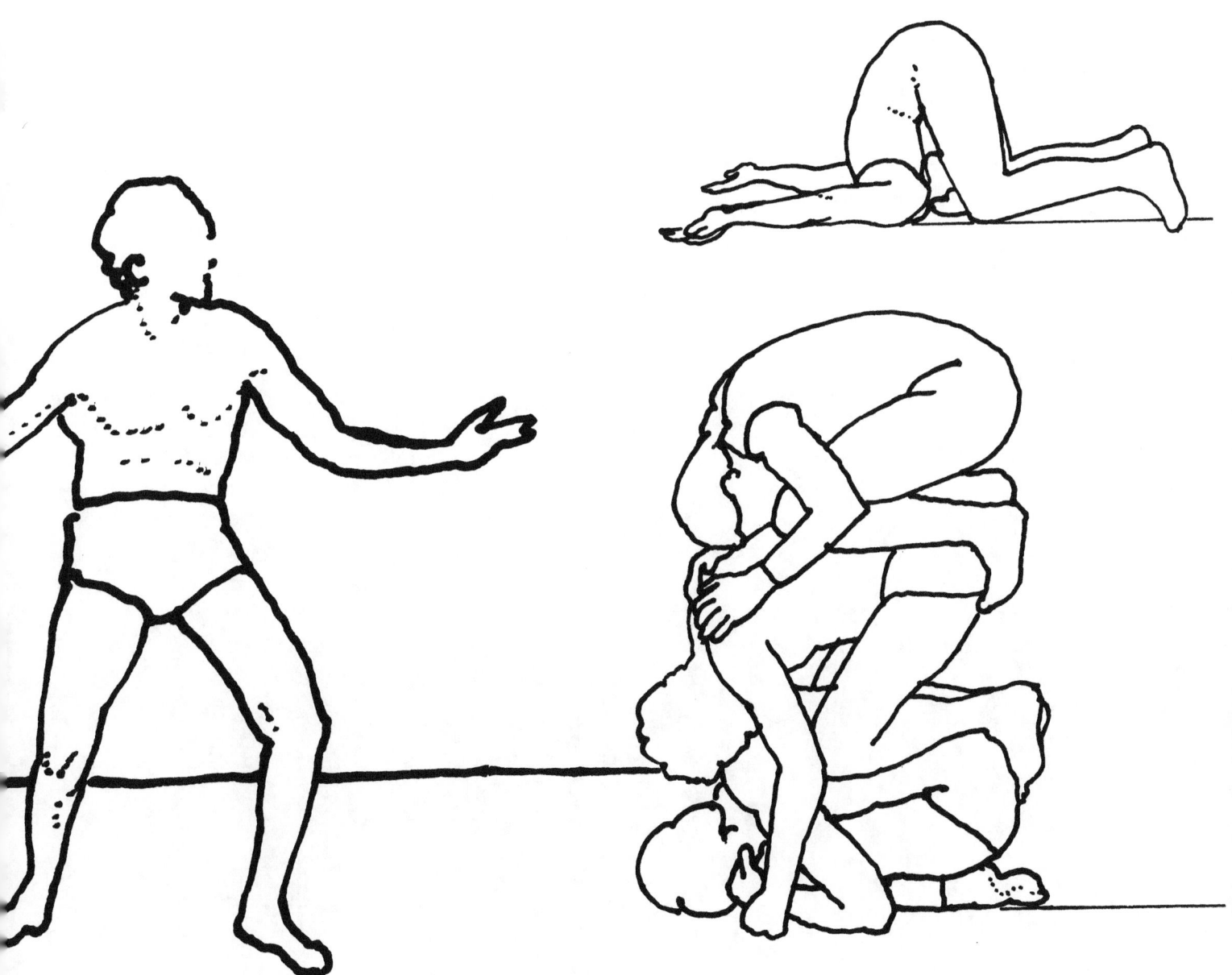

9 THE BODY AS AN EXPANDED SPHERE

Chapter 9

The Body as an Expanded Sphere

With the unfolding of the small ball into an expanded sphere or hemisphere, there develops not only the feeling of larger curves, but also an awareness of the **inside** of those curves. The image of the small compact ball changes to that of a sphere with hollows and spaces; with expanded fields, currents and tides. The fluid concavity of the body as an expanded sphere is fashioned by the unfolding areas of the legs and thighs, as well as by the expanding "crescent" shapes of the shoulders, spine, and back.

Four significant concepts are also unfolding, which may be summarized as follows:

1. An awareness of the body evolving;

2. An evolving growth potential within the feeling process, itself — i.e. after reviewing and retasting the different energy states, we actually feel the process "moving" and unfolding;

3. A recognition that each body curve has a set of different needs — that joints and hinges that help to create structural curves have their own set of needs; that curves that depart from the body's natural "sphere contour" induce unnatural body activities and hence, unless understood kinesensically, are inevitably done incorrectly; and

4. **A self-generating notion that we are, each of us, both the subject and the object of our work — that as both subject and object, we learn how to perceive and how "to do" at one and the same time.**

To clarify, particularly point three, let's take the example of the body evolving into upright posture. As we continually expand the body curve into a crescent-shaped, upright standing position, we abandon the spherical condition where good, full natural breathing is instinctively determined as a natural event. We have clearly two choices. We can accept this unnatural state, as we

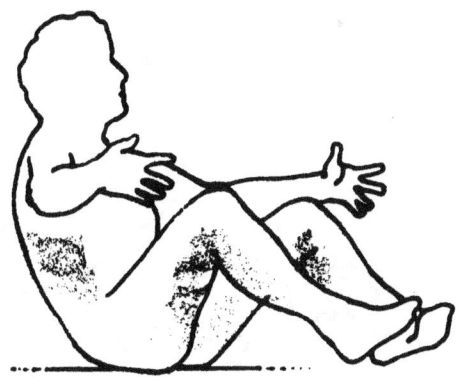

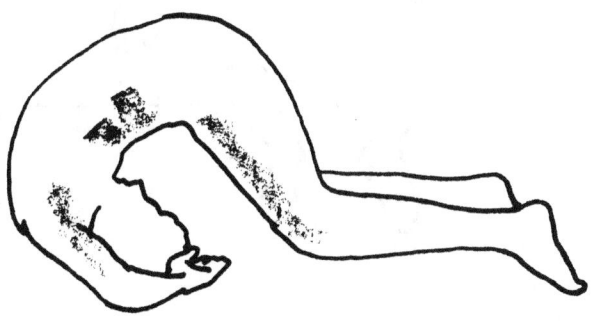

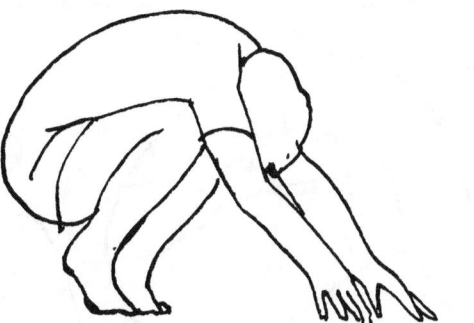

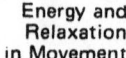

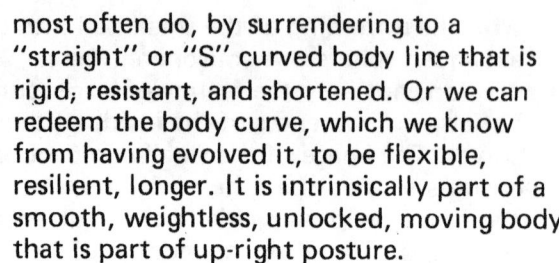

most often do, by surrendering to a "straight" or "S" curved body line that is rigid, resistant, and shortened. Or we can redeem the body curve, which we know from having evolved it, to be flexible, resilient, longer. It is intrinsically part of a smooth, weightless, unlocked, moving body that is part of up-right posture.

To accomplish the latter, we need only recall the earlier curves, postures, sensations, and comfortable breathing of the body as a small compact ball. Only now in its expanded — its fully expanded state — the curves of the body, particularly in upright posture, will have their own set of needs. The wider curves of the back need a correspondingly larger circumference in the front, as though the larger curves **require** more filling in. The longer spinal curve, with its joints and hinges, needs to be more organically engaged with its structural sphere in such a way that any body movement — be it leaping, standing, walking, running, tumbling, or rolling — induces a double-action feel: as the arms, shoulders and side-muscles expand the back and body sphere horizontally, the pelvis, thighs and legs (along with the neck and head) expand them vertically.

In our expanded sphere activities, accept the image of the body curve "asking to be recognized," that it may offer more salutary experience to your body systems and to your conscious awareness of sensory learning. As you proceed, your own body intelligence will steadfastly remind you that a curve never wants to feel friction, heaviness, tightness, or abrasiveness; that all it really wants is the sense of "formation-extension-expansion" within the perception of one or more of our energy dynamics.

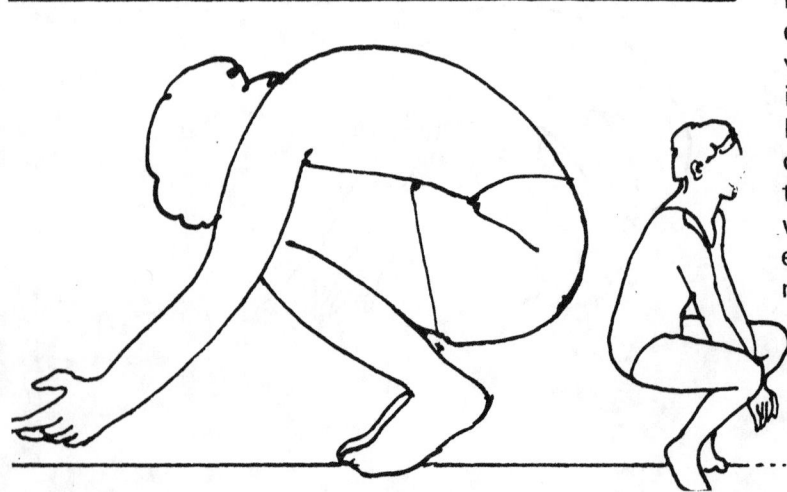

Body as Hemisphere

The following experiments continue our approach to the body as a small compact ball, but are now applied to evolving the body as an expanded sphere.

Throughout, we progressively develop the exploitation and refinement of:

- breathing activities and explorations;
- rhythm and balance perceptiveness;
- wafting and waving — swinging and swaying — rocking and rolling;
- loosening exercises — quivering, shaking, vibrating;
- "quieting" those pulled-tight or rock-hard muscles;
- atom-to-atom contiguous continuity and discovery — softening, spreading, and melting muscles involved with "surface contact;"
- identifying sensations, qualities, and characteristics of Buoyancy, Radiancy, and Potency energy states; and
- expanding our repertoire of body dynamics and our perception, response, and awareness of such kinesensic principles as Contact Vanishing Point, Finger-Tip Control, Just Noticeable Difference, Resting Up and Resting Down, Balanced Muscle Tonicity.

While working with the body as an expanded sphere, enjoy the esthetic image of a crescent moon floating on clouds or moving like a graceful sailboat over the flowing water; or a "glider" breezing through air; or a skater skimming the icy surface. All such images, as well as any original variations, will work. Remember: hinges and joints naturally curve the body parts by bending in the direction(s) of their **natural**

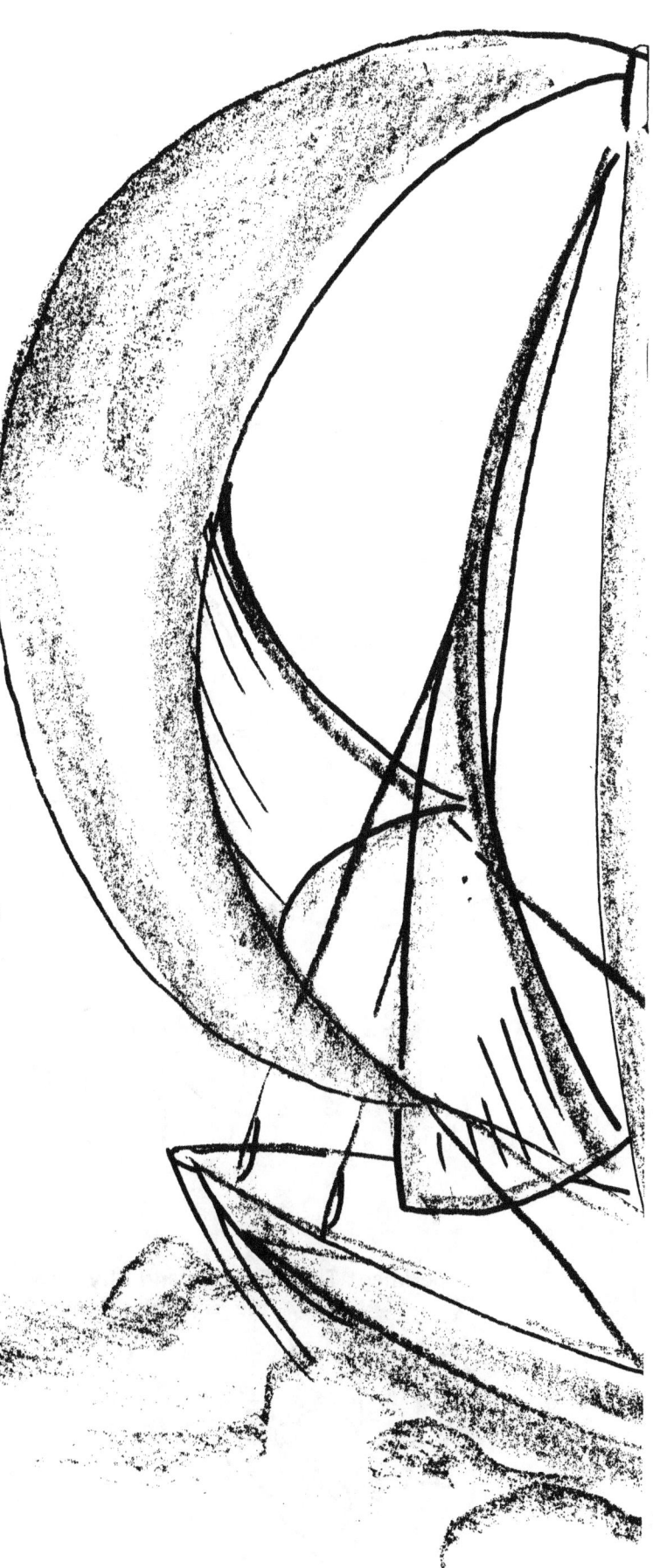

Energy and
Relaxation
in Movement

structural inclination. To bend or turn them any other way requires that we teach ourselves, through kinesensics, the consummate skill of 'doing the incorrect thing correctly.'

Experiment One: Moving Into the Expanded Sphere

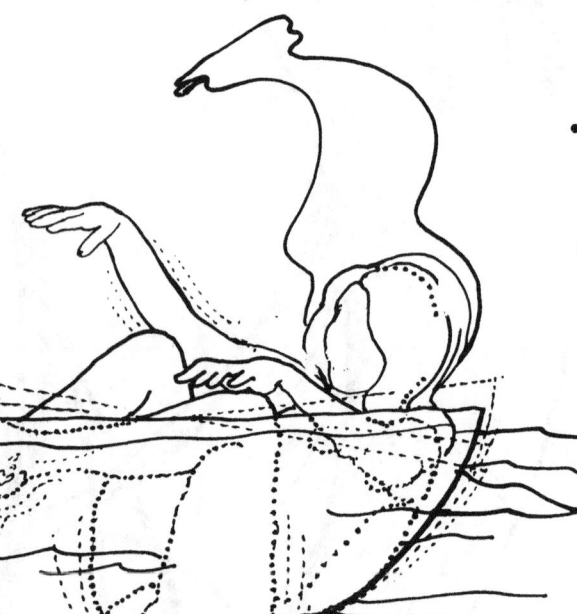

- Starting from the sit-down squat position, gradually "unfold" yourself so that arms, shoulders, and legs assume the appearance of a round-bottom sailboat, as suggested in the illustration.

- Gently waft and wave to get the feel of the size and shape of your expanding body hemisphere. Take special note of the body lines that form the new spherical contour and **register their feel**: the arms, legs, hands, head, and feet completing the convex rim of the sphere along with the back and side surfaces of the body; the stomach, groin, and chest composing the inside, concave space of the sphere. All together, the "feel-image" is like the earth-sphere itself, with changing oceans of water, tidal-flows, wind and weather filling the outside hollows, gaps and spaces; while thermo-dynamics, chemistry, electricity, breath-spirit and nerve-spirit fill the body's inside spaces, structures and thru-ways.

- Once in the expanded sphere position, repeat the breathing activities of the compact ball experiments. Recall the water image to re-experience water buoyancy and breath buoyancy weightlessness, with its almost inevitable floating of arms, hands, legs, and feet. Using breath energy, tune into the sensations, perceptions, rhythms, and equilibrium of the expanded body sphere.

Experiment Two: Balance and Rhythm in the Expanded Sphere

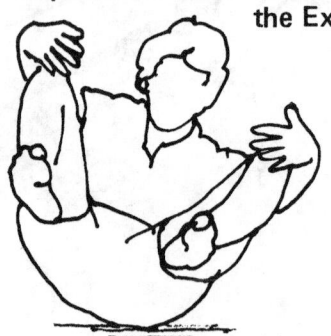

- In the expanded sphere, which now is really a hemisphere, rock gently but fully as far as the body **wants** to go, without bouncing, all the while exploring contiguous continuity or atom-to-atom discovery. If

111

Body as Hemisphere

your rocking takes the body into a roll-over, go with it as long as it feels light, loose, resilient, and comfortable — and only if you continue the movement in deliberate, slow motion. Feel the pleasure of the roll-over in whatever direction, without push, force, or pre-planned movement. Your body must move easily enough to sense the experience of slow-motion, "moving balance."

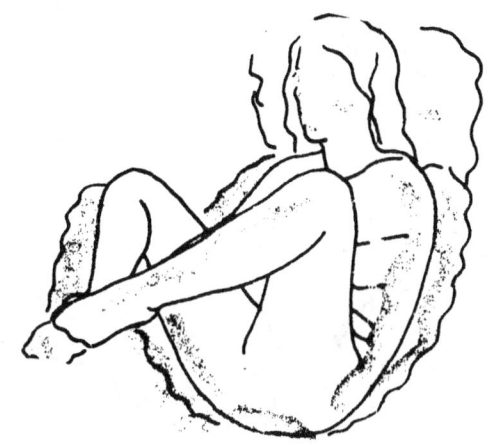

- Whenever tension or heaviness develops in your rolling, practice shake-radiation — from sophisticated quivers to larger vibrating shakes. Feel the different internal rhythms of the various shakes. Check the illustrations.

- Return to atom-to-atom discovery as you roll and rock in any direction. If shaking doesn't completely eliminate the stall to continuous movement, then use contiguous continuity to advance you through the roll-over; i.e. continue the rolling but concentrate only on finding the next atom of body surface, even if support comes from the fingers, elbows, head, toe, knee, or shoulder. And as you discover each new atom, add buoyancy, radiancy, and elastic-stretch potency to the rolling movement.

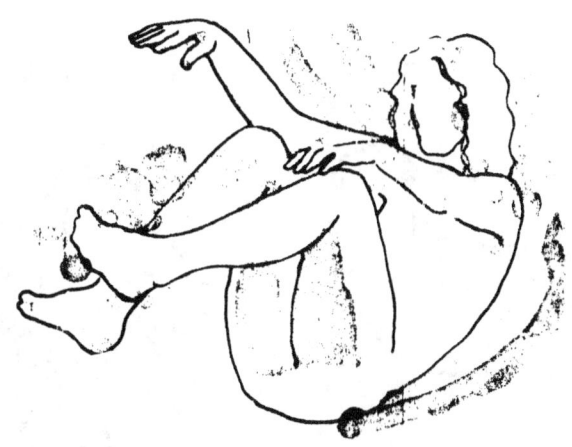

- Finally, explore the rolling movement sideways, forward, backward, and diagonally, following where the body wants to go without flopping, bouncing, or pushing. When you have rolled yourself into the neck and shoulder position — one of the traditional tension centers that for us functions as a major relaxer-energizer area — soften, loosen, quiet, and lengthen every strand of muscle fiber. Muscle-crowding in this vital area makes it almost impossible to breathe, speak, or use the voice freely. But once you loosen and uncrowd the muscles in the neck and shoulder, you'll be able to breathe easily. You'll discover that even in this strange position, good vocal resonance goes hand in hand with balanced muscle tonicity.

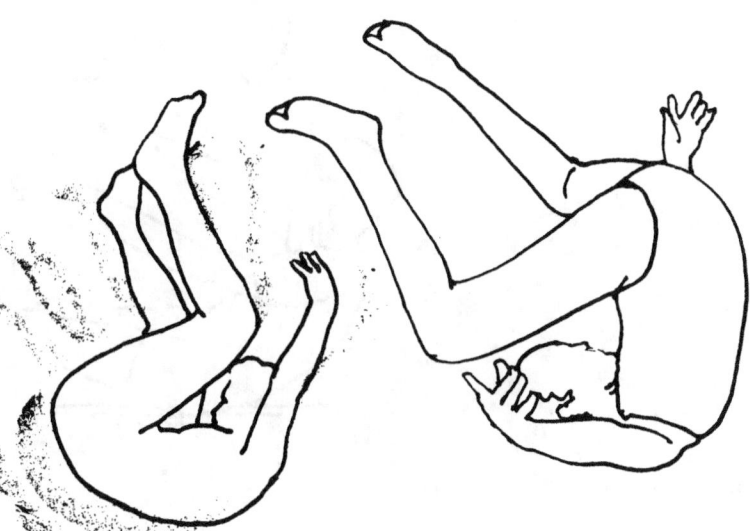

Energy and
Relaxation
in Movement

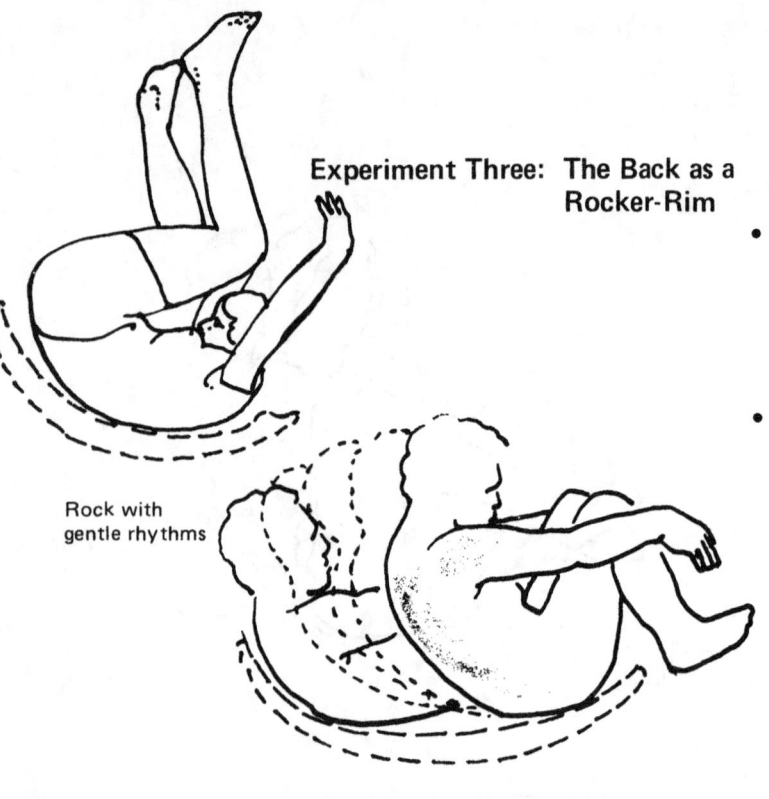

Experiment Three: The Back as a Rocker-Rim

Rock with gentle rhythms

Follow the illustrations and:

- Using your back as a rocker rim, and with open, extended arms and legs, roll-rock from sit-down to shoulder position and back again. Repeat the rolling-rocker, back and forth, several times.

- Repeat this rolling-rocker, back and forth, until it feels natural and smooth enough to gently roll into the softened neck area and on to the head. Don't fall back defensively on momentum. Rely instead upon energy-motivated — mostly body-yawn — consistency and constancy. Unless the complete "roll-over" takes place inadvertently, easily, and naturally, do not anticipate it or attempt it; the controlled "complete roll-over" is still a bit premature.

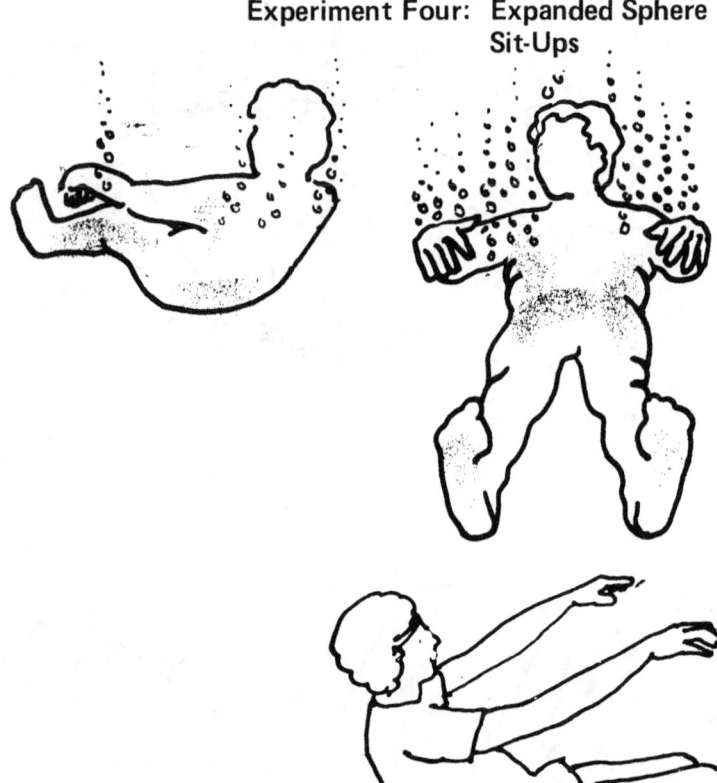

Experiment Four: Expanded Sphere Sit-Ups

The difference in sensation, perception, and function of the following sit-ups will depend upon your response and awareness to the various body energy states.

- **The Buoyancy Sit-Up**

In this breathing-buoyancy action, start with a comfortably loose and lightly flexed, lying-down position. Using your breath energy, float yourself up to sitting position with arms reaching forward.

Feel free, at any time, to "stay" the body and feel the bouyancy-balance in this position. The image is that of breath-energy coursing through the veins and arteries, inspiring and vitalizing the organism.

The rhythm feel of water buoyancy, and super-lightness out of water, appear to take charge of the body in place of the muscles. It is almost as if the muscles and bones were hollow and infused with helium, directing the dynamics of this floating, buoyant energy state and making the body lighter than air. It is the rhythm of floating — of gliding up and gliding down — of reaching and extending in weightless, dreamy legato. The rhythm feel of buoyancy in the expanded sphere position reinforces your sensory skill to distinguish between a depressing body heaviness and an inspiring body lightness.

- **The Radiancy Sit-Up**

    The feel of this energy state, as you know, is that of electricity and sparkle; it is one of **lambency**.* As you imagined breath-energy coursing through your veins and arteries during the buoyancy sit-up, now imagine radiancy energy conducted and pulsated through your nerve networks. Repeat the sit-up, and concentrate on "lighting up" your inner environment with vibrato-like radiancy "spirit" that energizes the entire organism.

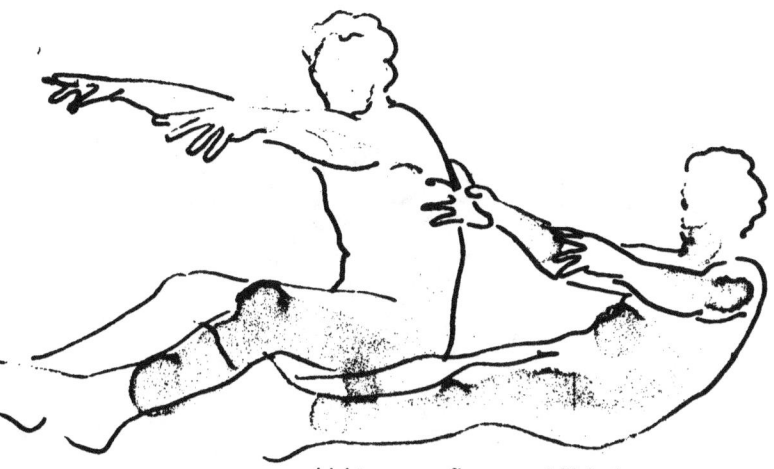

Light up your fingers and flick them lambently as you do the Radiancy Sit-up

Without any sense of tightening, do the radiancy sit-up with darting, pulsing muscular agility and eagerness. Sense yourself anticipating a new quality of reaching forward with flick-like flexibility and elasticity. Like a delicate coil-spring, trigger your body from lying-down to sit-up position with arms **lambently** reaching forward with electric current.

- **The Potency Sit-Up**

    In this action, the body feels as if its muscles were fed by a magnetic force. The muscles dominate in the form of a body-yawn stretch and feel supercharged. The body literally yawns itself, through its every fiber and muscle cell, from the lying-down to the sit-up position; at the same time, the back, shoulders, and arms extend forward as if reaching with a fierce, deep intensity, a feeling of unlimited potency. Try it and feel for yourself the different sensation produced by potency energy, when applied to the sit-up.

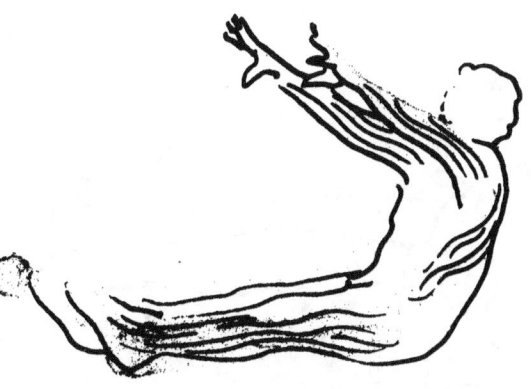

***Lambent:** (1) Characterized by lightness of touch and brilliance, as lambent wit and humor; the lambent style of a mime or clown; (2) playing or moving lightly over a surface; touching sprightly, gliding smartly, wavering, flickering, as the lapping, licking tongues of flame; (3) Brilliantly playful; dealing gracefully with a subject; (4) Soft, bright or radiant — as the lambent eyes of a child.

Energy and
Relaxation
in Movement

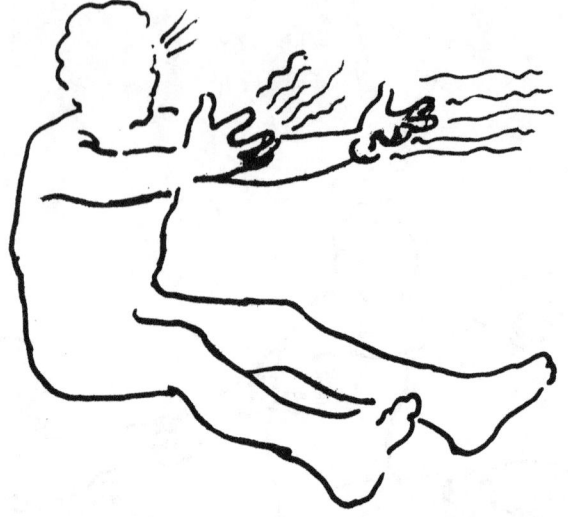

- **The Inter-Involvement Sit-Up**

    This is the action of motivational vitality agitated by the emotional experiencing system in 'self to other' communication. In the inter-involvement sit-up, the role of the muscles is pre-empted by a deeply involved, intense communicating and inter-relating system, like an infant in its crib reaching out to its mother. The vigorous, vital muscular system, no longer the primary agent or body intelligence, appears instead to have taken on a semi-voluntary function, while the emotional experiencing system, communicating an intense message of emergency, need, or assistance, takes total command of all voluntary physical actions. Do a series of "emo-tivated" sit-ups, fed by any emotion or drive or excitement that works for you.

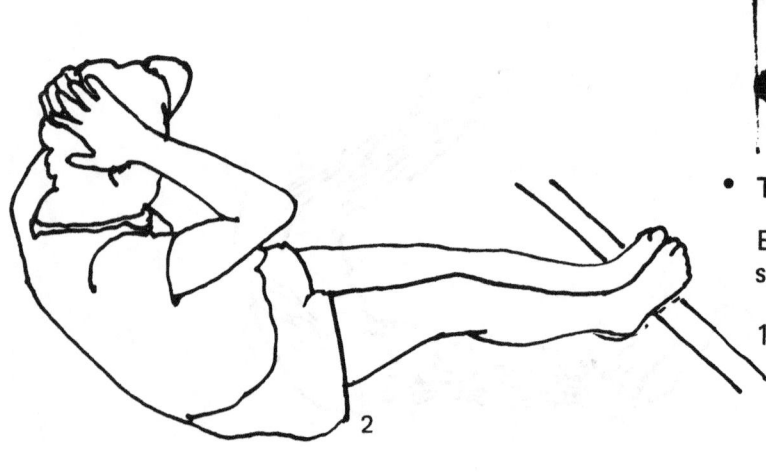

- **The Toe-Tip to the Wall Sit-Up**

    Experiment with three variations of this sit-up as graphically indicated.

    1. Lying down so that your toe-tips gently but barely touch the wall, repeat the buoyancy, radiancy, potency, and inter-involvement sit-ups already set forth above.

    2. In the same toe-to-wall position, but now with hands behind your head, (though not touching the head) do a "curl-up" sit-up, unfurling every vertebra from the neck down to the coccyx. Since this sit-up is deliberately gradual, stop at any point, waft and continue.

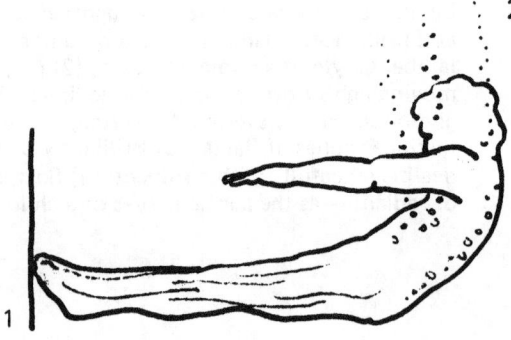

115

3. From the same position, do a buoyancy sit-up with your back and rib cage, while at the same time introducing a potency energy current through the thighs into the toes, and through the toes into the wall.

Vary this with the conventional "hands-behind-the-head" sit-up while maintaining the 'toe-to-wall' position. Don't press your hands into the back of your head, but rather feel a gently contiguous contact of hands to head (or hair) while doing this sit-up.

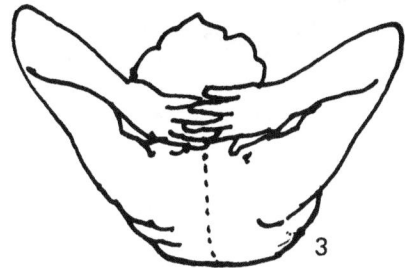

Follow the instructions for each leg lift in the series and check the illustrations whenever necessary.

Experiment Five: Expanded Sphere Leg-Lifts

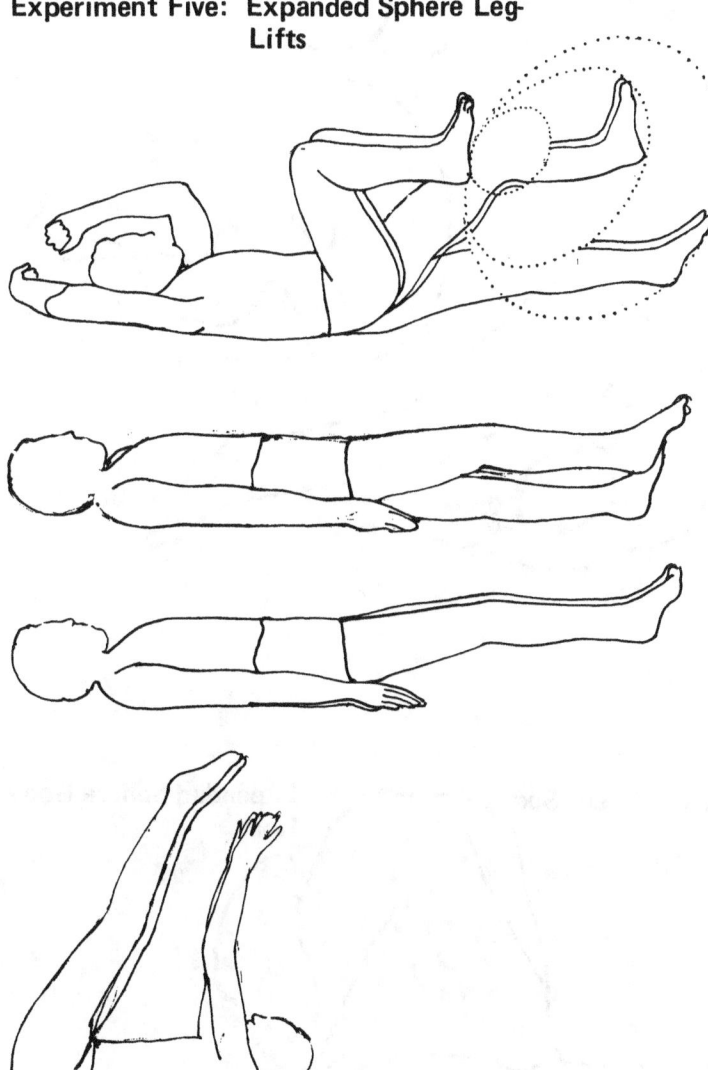

- **The "Paddle Wheel" Leg-Lift**

  Feet together, bring your knees to your chest and proceed to make small paddle wheel circles with your legs; gradually increasing the size of the paddle wheel until the forward return is negotiated with the legs almost fully extended.

- **The "Buoy-Float" Leg-Lift**

  As if floating and resting in water, first lift one leg, then the other. Then lift both feet together, a few inches from the ground. "Float" both legs progessively upward, always maintaining the water image.

- **The Buoyancy Leg-Lift**

  Repeat the buoy-float action, but this time adding breath-buoyancy energy.

- **The Radiancy Leg-Lift**

  Now add the lambent sparkle of radiancy-alert to your leg lifts.

- **The Potency Leg-Lift**

  Now infuse the leg-lifts with muscle-yawn body stretch power. Muscle-yawn from

Energy and
Relaxation
in Movement

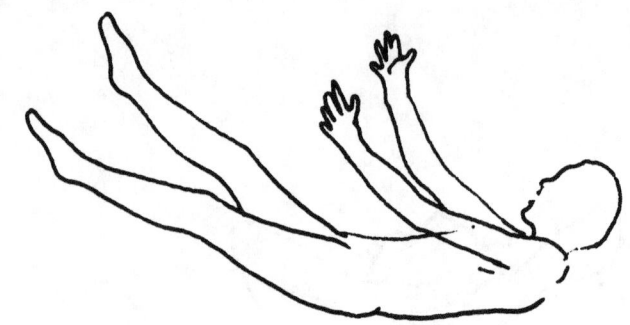

your waist into your thighs, calves, feet and toes; simultaneously muscle-yawn from your back into your shoulders, arms and fingers.

- **The Inter-Involvement Leg-Lift**

  Do a series of "emo-tivated" leg-lifts. Help yourself by taking a full breath **before** the leg lift. Hold the breath during the leg lift. Then, exhale gradually with the return of the leg, timed so that the complete exhalation and touch-down of the heels to the floor occur simultaneously. For each leg-lift, reach above the head with the opposite arm extended while communicating meaningful and expressive information with both, 'leg→toes' and 'arms→fingers.'

- **Leg-Lift Flip-Over**

  Do a body-yawn leg-lift and let the ongoing dynamic potency-feel take you easily and gradually all the way up and over, as far and as close to the ground as is comfortable. As you continue experimenting and exploring the "flip-over" you will come to rest with toes touching the floor or hands touching your toes as illustrated.

- **Combined Energy State Leg-Lift**

  Start with any of the energy state leg-lifts: potency, breath-energy, radiancy, buoyancy, or inter-involvement. Then follow in sequence with the others, using any combination you wish. Then introduce the paddle wheel and follow with the floating leg-lift. Do them all in a complete series before returning the feet to the ground.

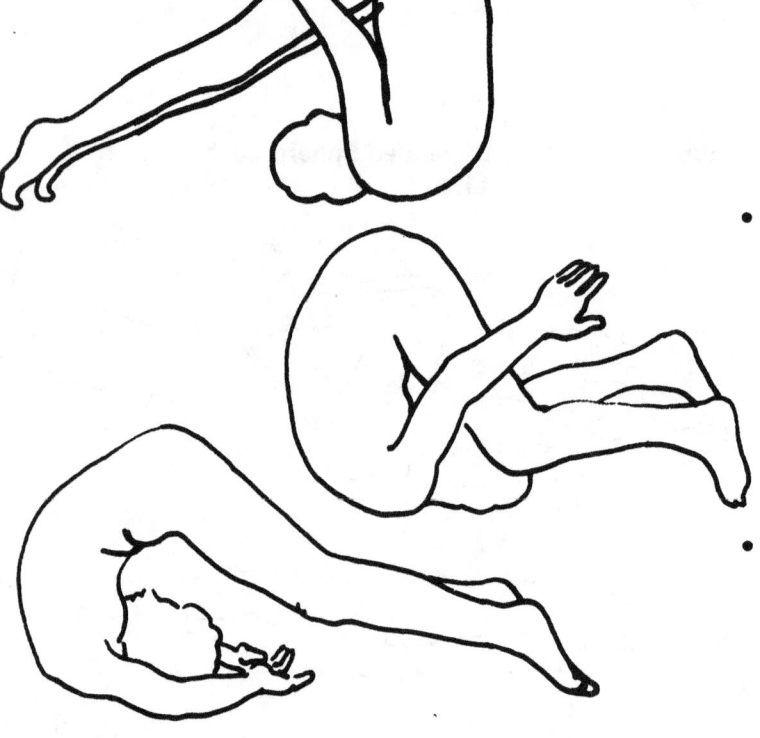

Experiment Six: **Expanded Sphere Body Rolls**

- **The Backward Single Shoulder Roll**

  Checking the illustration, roll to neck and shoulder position, and then place your arms conveniently on the ground. Loosen, soften, and quiet the neck and shoulder muscles. Then, roll easily onto one shoulder joint

Body as Hemisphere

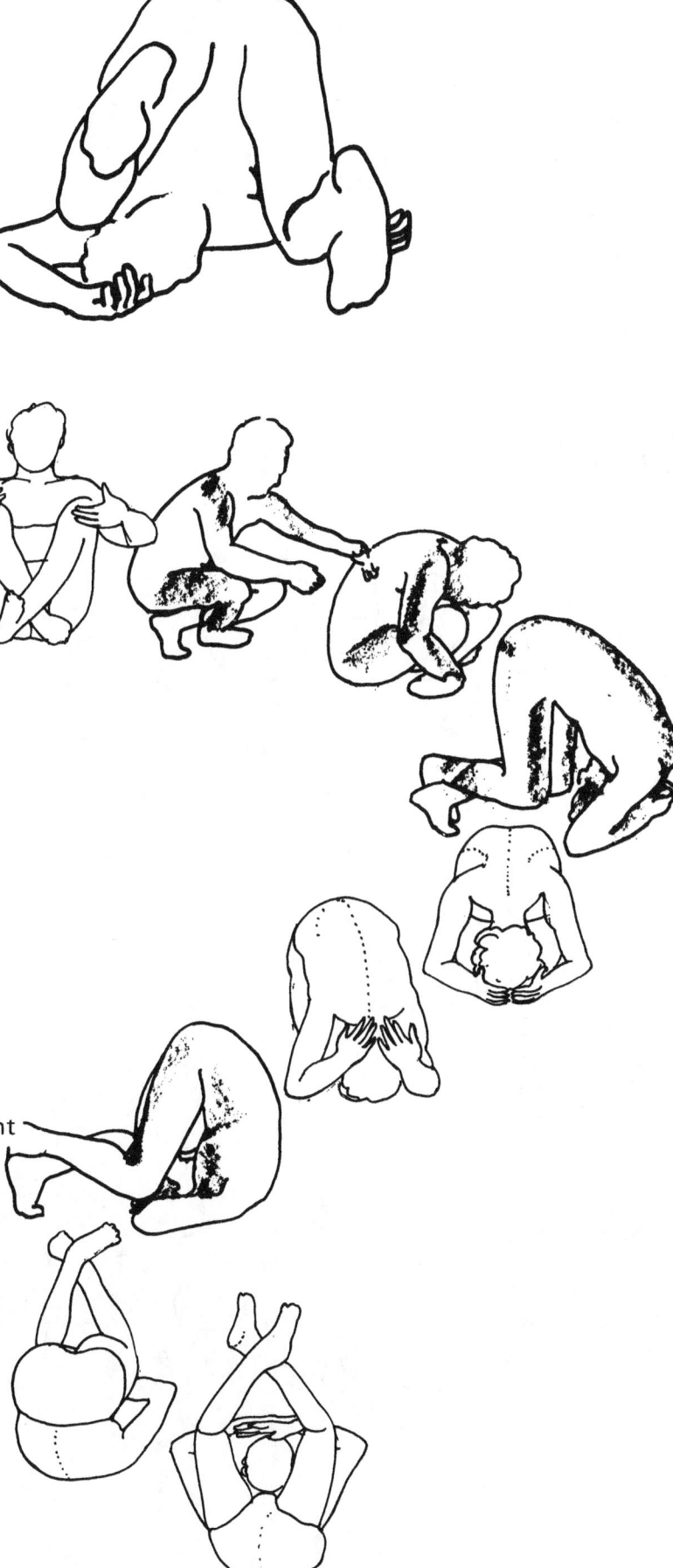

and continue contiguous movement, relying for support on atom-to-atom discovery. Feel your knee gently kiss the ground inside your arm. As soon as your knee touches and your toe comes lightly to the surface, you are ready to complete the shoulder roll. That's really all there is to it. You've probably already achieved this shoulder roll a half-dozen times during the course of your expanded-ball rocking and rolling. Experiment with the single shoulder roll, alternately rolling to the opposite shoulder and knee.

- **The Forward Roll**

  This is the simple, old-fashioned "somersault" that children do so easily and naturally well. Begin in sitting position. Bring your feet into "criss-cross squat" position. Balance yourself by wafting and waving forward until you rest on the squatted, criss-crossed legs. Then continue forward movement until your head floats gradually and gently toward the ground.

  Use your arms, hands, and fists to give you additional surface support. Place your arms in diamond-shaped position on the ground, so that your cupped hands can securely cover and support the back of your neck and upper back as you roll forward. Notice how this offers you additional support for a gradual, easy, slow motion.

  Your arms, from elbows to hands (with hands cupped) should be moving out in front of your head. Continue the roll until your head and elbows seem to provide the leverage needed. Atom by atom, proceed to inch, walk, or roll your way forward to the point where your hands make contact just below the collarbone. You'll know you're there when you feel no weight on the head. Roll continuously into your arms and hands. Once you return to sitting position, you will have completed a forward roll.

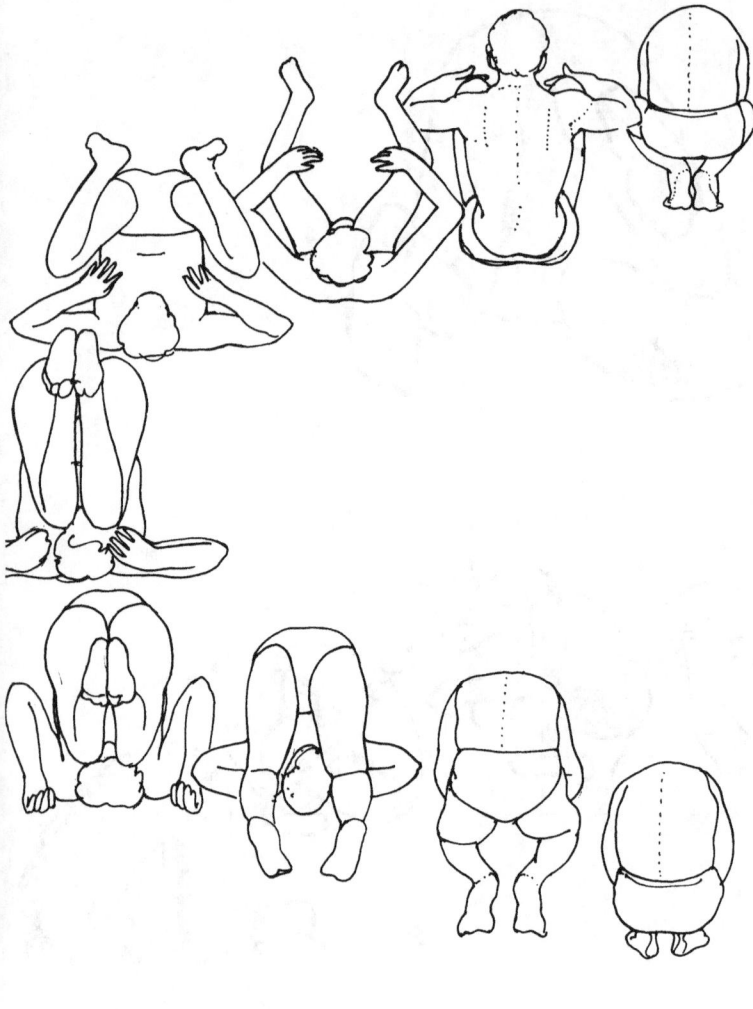

Practice the criss-cross forward roll until it feels comfortable. Then try it with the legs uncrossed.

- **The Backward Roll**

  This is similar to the backward single shoulder roll, except the roll here is over the neck and head.

  As illustrated, start with the combined, flip-over leg-left. Using your open fist knuckles as balance supports, quiet and soften the neck and shoulder muscles. Your toes and knees will come to rest, touching or getting quite close to the ground. During this action, the head weight feels more lightly balanced, permitting a graceful roll over as you nudge and peel yourself slowly and rhythmically, with total equilibrium, off the ground. This is a surprisingly comfortable backward roll. If you get stuck, don't fight it. Just waft and wave, then continue. Remember: no pressure or heaviness; no flopping or bouncing around.

- **The Shoulder-Girdle Roll**

  This is a variation of the backward single shoulder roll except that here we add the forward single shoulder roll in continuing movement.

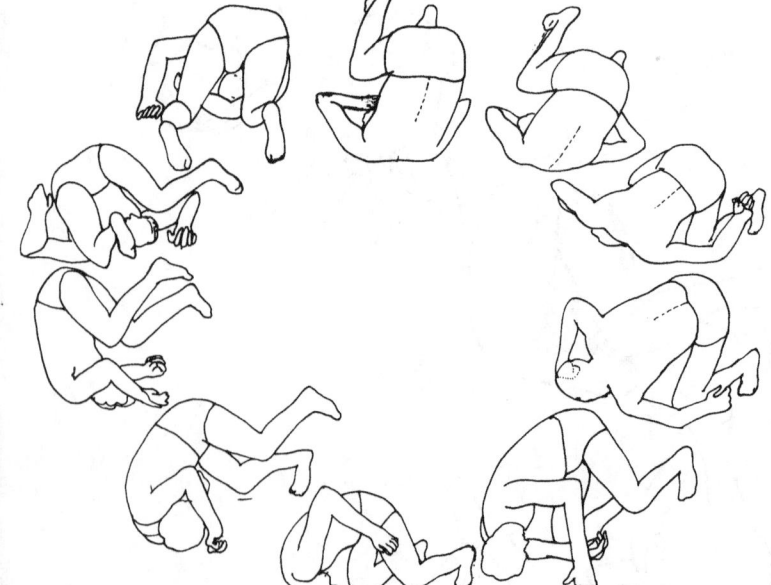

Start with the backward shoulder roll and move onto your left shoulder. As your left knee and foot make contact with the ground, roll diagonally on your left shoulder until your right knee and foot make contact with the ground. Then keep rolling, as illustrated, until you have maneuvered yourself into a right-shouldered forward roll. Follow this immediately with a "girdling around" to the left shoulder and continue rolling. Practice, alternating the direction by starting each roll on opposite shoulders. (specific instructions p.120, para. 3)

Body as Hemi- sphere

- **The Diamond-Shaped Shoulder-Girdle Roll**

    Start with the expanded-sphere neck and shoulder position, with legs high forming a diamond shape as indicated.

    Then, with atom-to-atom balance, do the shoulder-girdle roll retaining the leg diamond throughout. Keep circling in a neat, easy "round." When you stop, alternate the starting direction and repeat the procedure.

    Note in the illustration the deliberate "balance points" from left shoulder to left arm, elbow, forearm — to left knee and toe — to shoulder girdle — to right toe — to right knee — to right wrist and forearm — to right elbow — to right shoulder — and so on.

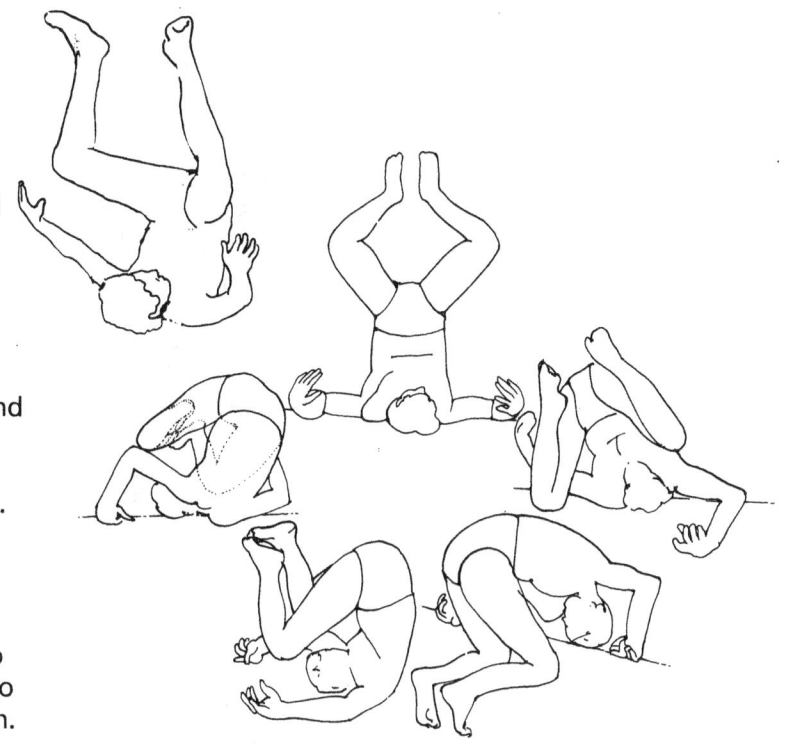

Check the instructions with accompanying illustrations and start with the expanded sphere head-down position.

- Do a head-roll neck expansion, making **absolutely certain** there is no heavy weight on the head during the light, gentle neck-muscle-stretch. This is achieved by sharing the body mass — i.e. by distributing the weight to every contact-point such as knees, toes, and fists. By so doing, the actual weight-volume is nowhere consciously experienced, but only registered as a general sense of balance.

- Continuing the gentle neck-extension head-rolling, tiptoe lightly toward your face, with knees relatively close to the ground, until your toes feel a light, balanced "lift-off." Your cupped hands, (or flat palms if loose fist knuckles pose problems), along with your head, now form a "tripod" resting base. This cupped hands knuckle-position can strengthen your wrists. Since it offers a different kind of balance experience, practice using both the knuckle and flat palm hand positions, padding your knuckles, if need be, with a pair of old socks or gloves.

Experiment Seven: The Tripod-Headstand Balance

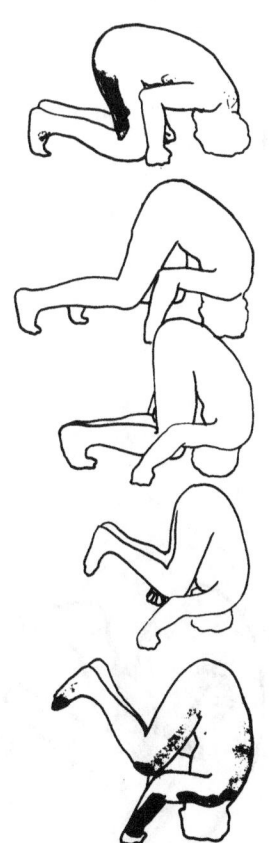

Energy and
Relaxation
in Movement

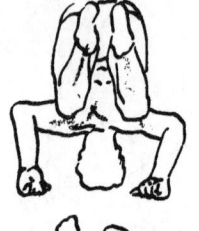
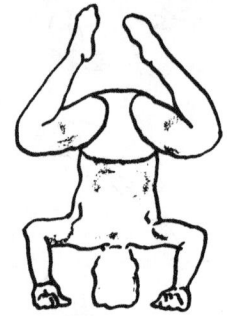

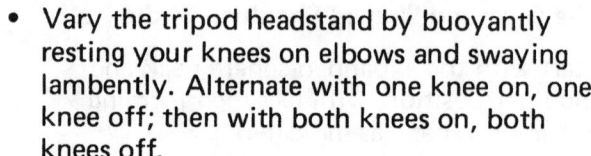
- Vary the tripod headstand by buoyantly resting your knees on elbows and swaying lambently. Alternate with one knee on, one knee off; then with both knees on, both knees off.

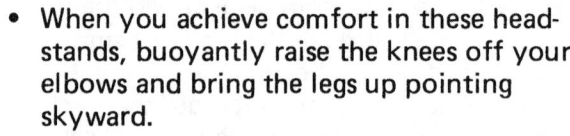
- When you achieve comfort in these headstands, buoyantly raise the knees off your elbows and bring the legs up pointing skyward.

- Finally, when really secure in the balance of these headstands, explore different forms and shapes with the legs.

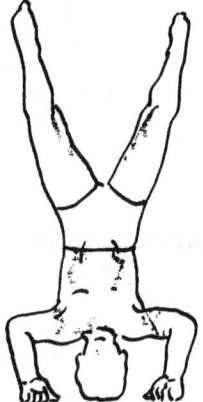
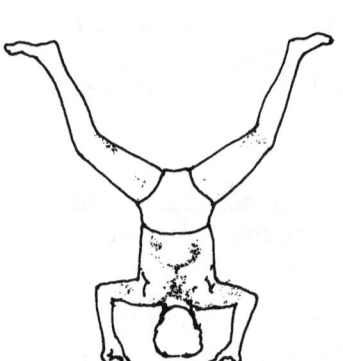

Experiment Eight: The Yoga Headstand Balance

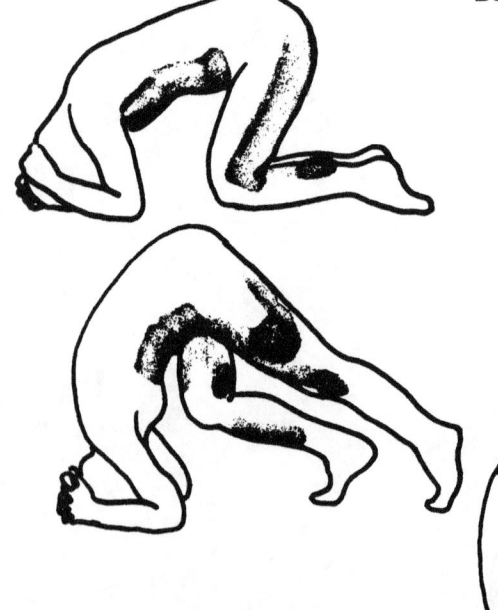

In reality, this is a variation of the tripod headstand, only with the elbow-forearm-head forming the smaller, base triangle. Check with the illustrations.

- Start with the elbow-forearm-head-down position, as indicated. Using radiancy energy, tiptoe (with knees low to the ground) toward your face until you sense a lift-off at the toes. If you find yourself going backward "out of balance," recall this feel as the perfect backward roll, and either use this familiar event to experiment with body balance in the new position or very gently complete the backward roll.

- When you have explored body balance with the lift-off at the toes and possibly through the backward roll, you are ready for the Yoga headstand. If your move-

Body as Hemisphere

ment on the way up is gradual and balanced, simply continue until your legs stand straight upward. If your balance is not so secure, then "scissor" the legs (one back, the other forward) until balance is achieved.

- Discover and tune into the accompanying rhythm component, its particular feels and rhythm-perceptions. Try to identify the different body energy states at work in the Yoga headstand and respond to their different characteristics. Experiment in Yoga headstand with mini-shakes, vibratos, and other radiancy explorations. Remind yourself of the Just Noticeable Difference, the Contact Vanishing Point, the Finger-Tip Control, the simultaneous Resting Up and Resting Down, and all the Relaxer-Energizers that are now activated. And isolate the three basic balance experiences in the Yoga headstand: Pedestal Balance, Pin-Point Balance, and Moving (Traveling) Balance.

Some of these activities apply the buddy work of the preceding chapter ("The Body as a Small Sphere") to the evolving curves of the expanded body sphere. Others extend our experience with the sit-ups, leg-lifts, tripod, and Yoga headstands of this chapter to ensemble teamwork. The accompanying graphics provide most of the guidance both of you will require.

- Using various expanded-sphere positions, adapt and improvise upon the Hoop and Stick Game — alternating hoop and stick roles, establishing an organic system of cues and signals, and changing direction(s) as required to negotiate the rolling hoop in constantly moving balance.

- As an ensemble, do a series of coordinated, double body rolls in expanded-sphere postures: backward single shoulder rolls, backward rolls, shoulder-girdle rolls.

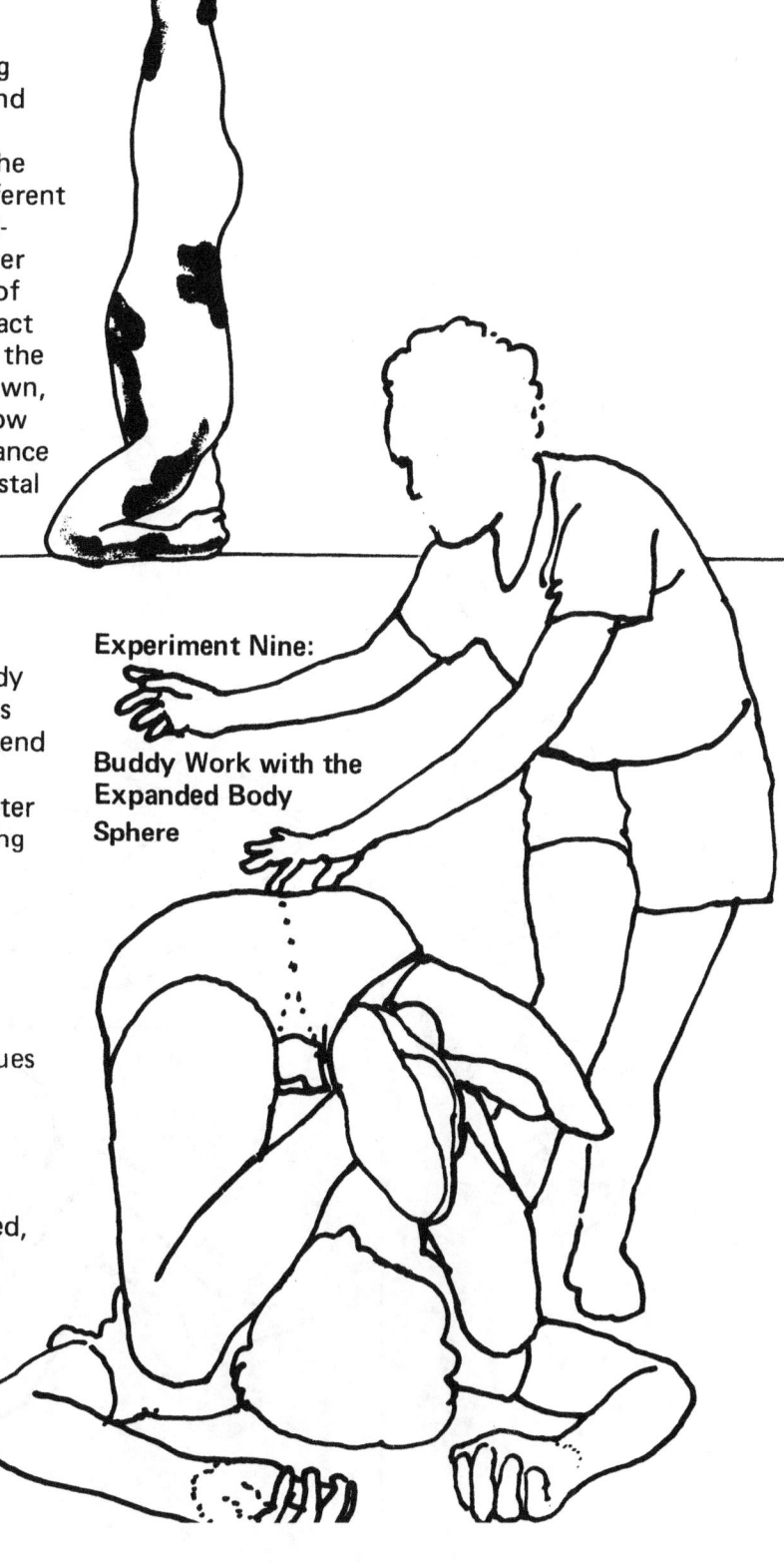

Experiment Nine:

Buddy Work with the Expanded Body Sphere

Variations and improvisations.......

122 a

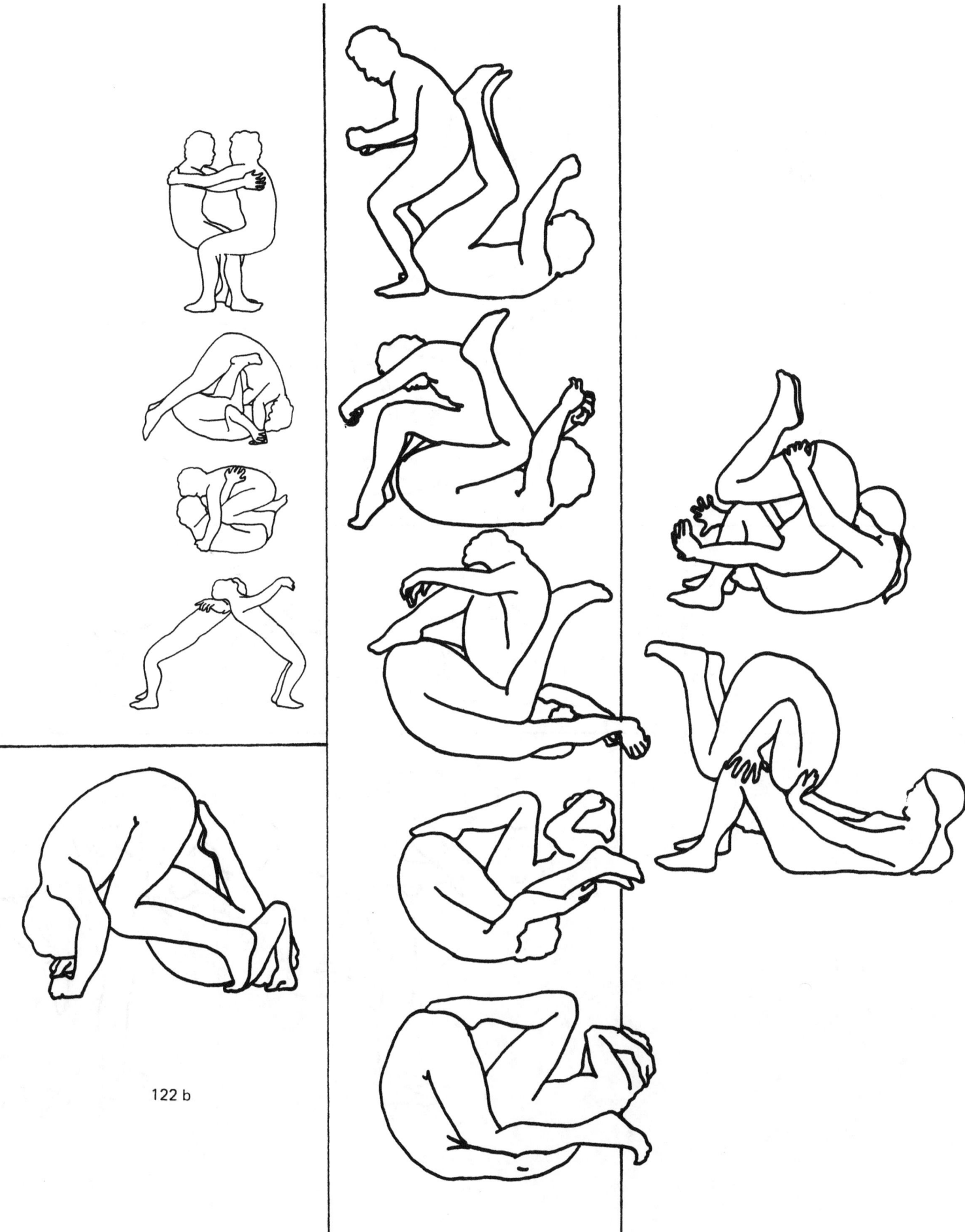

122 b

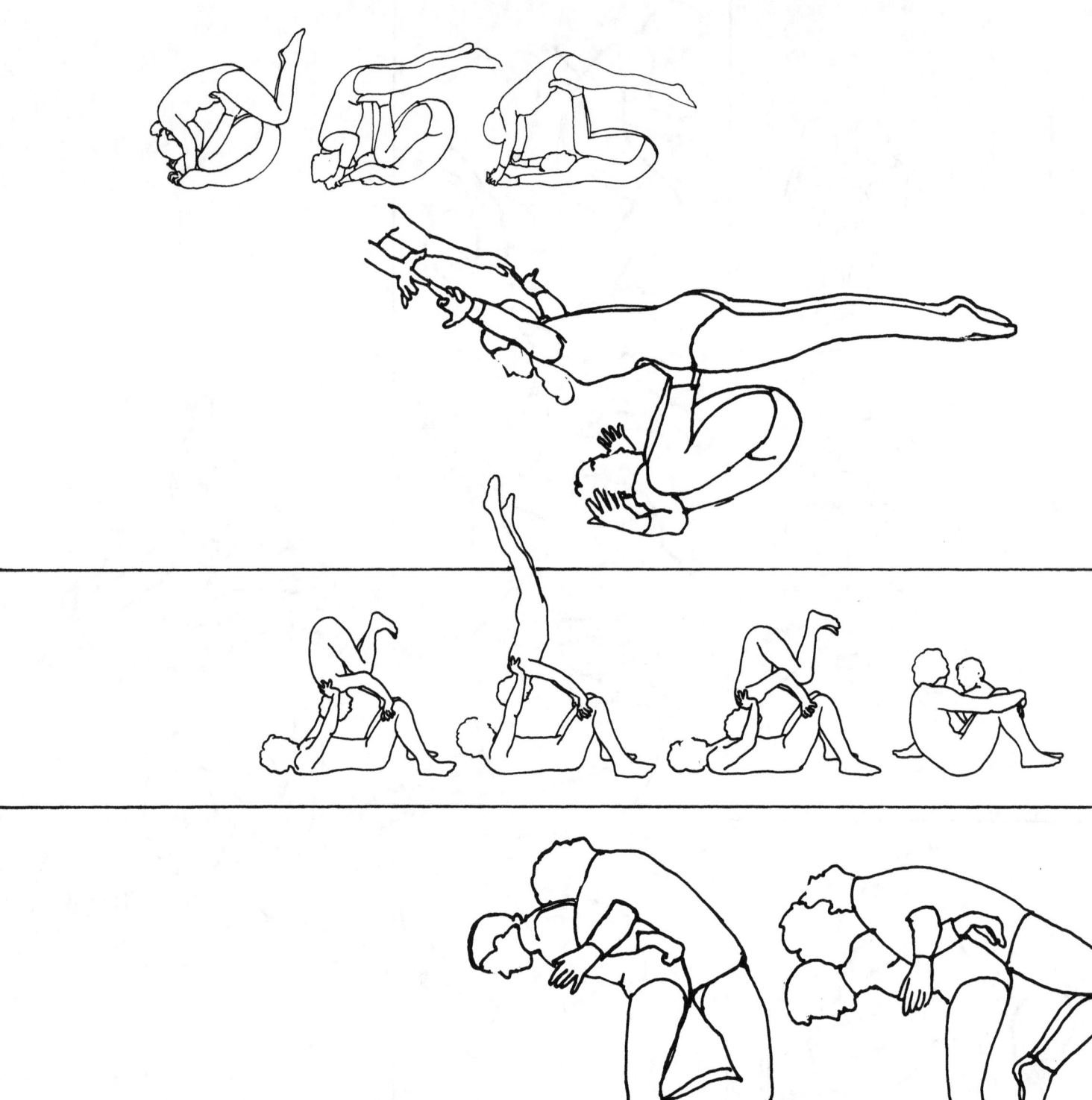

122 c

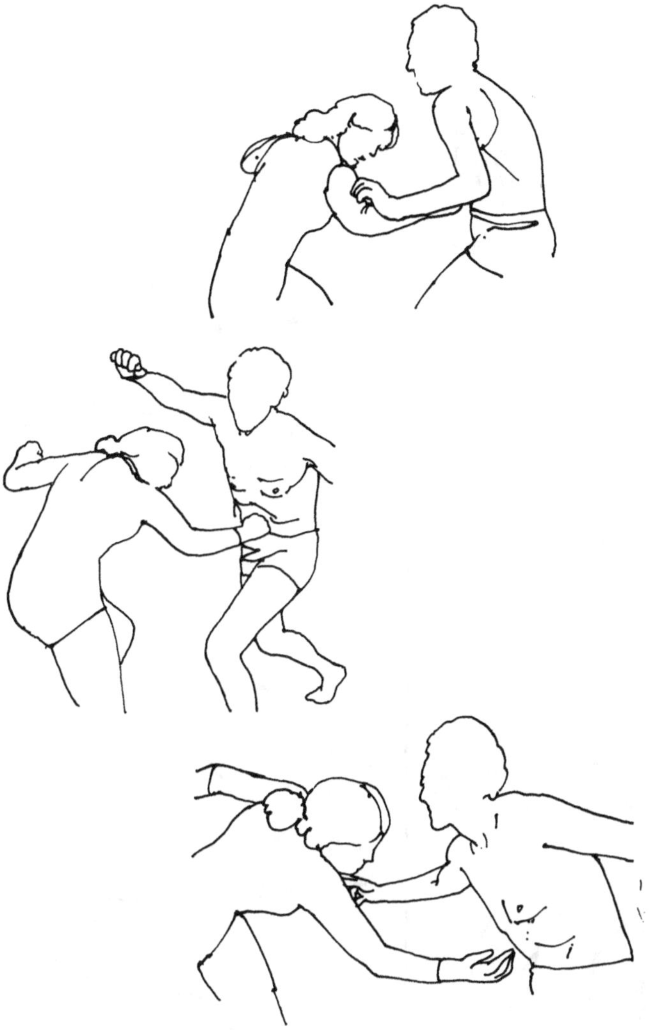

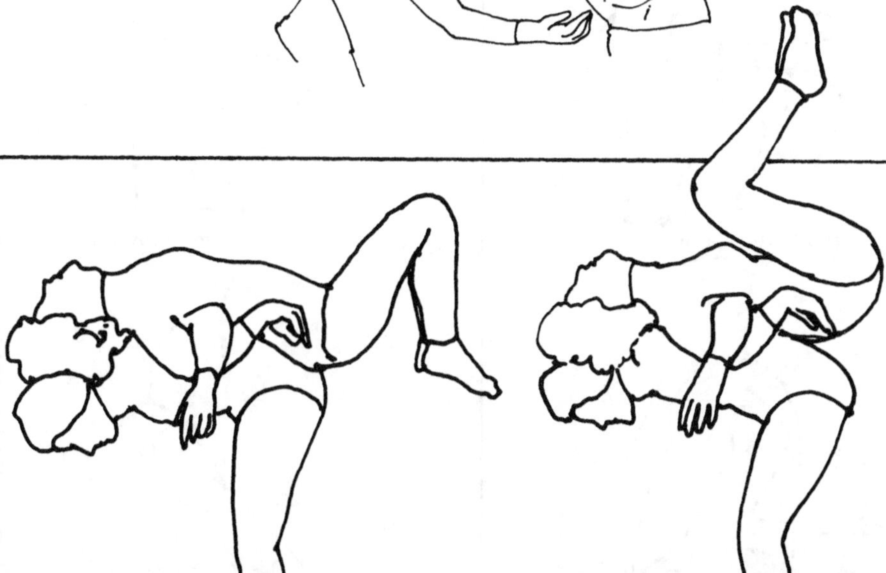

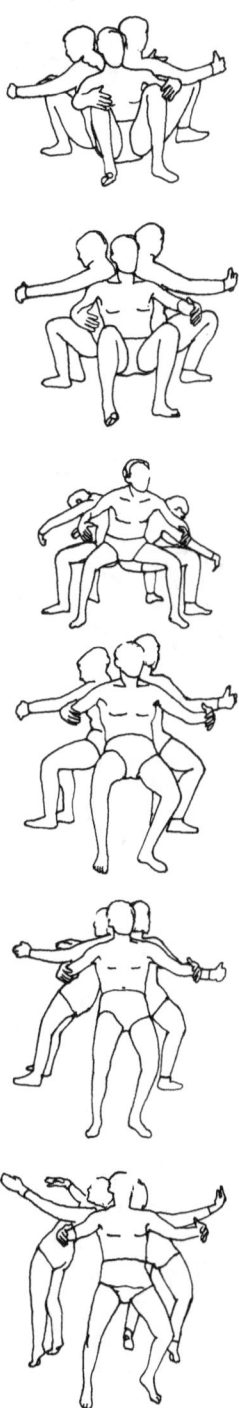

122 d

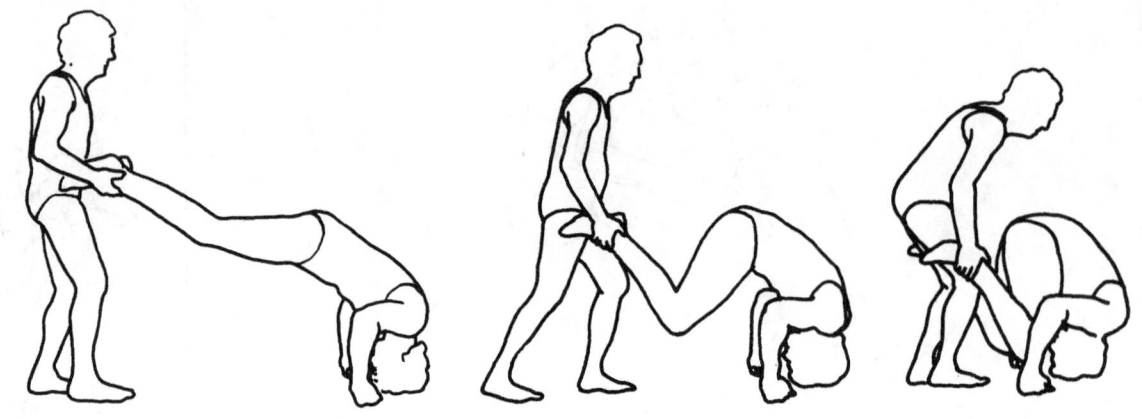

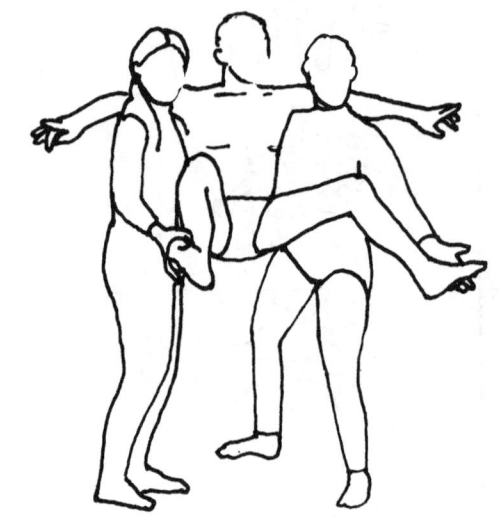

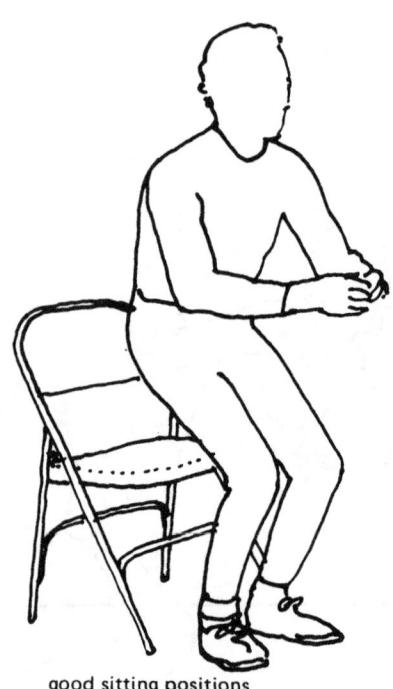
good sitting positions

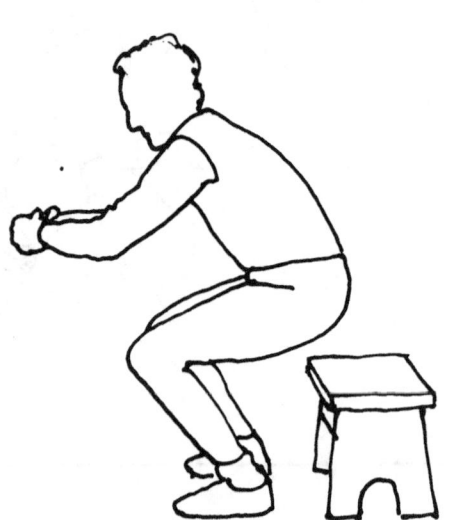
good sitting positions

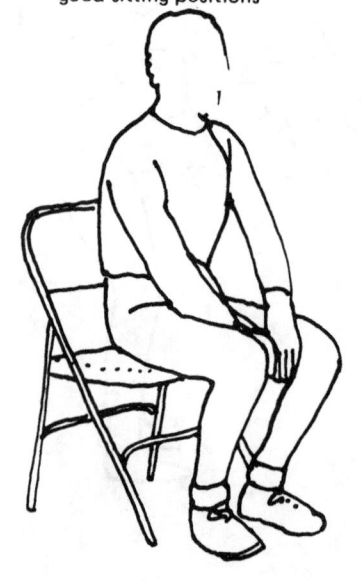

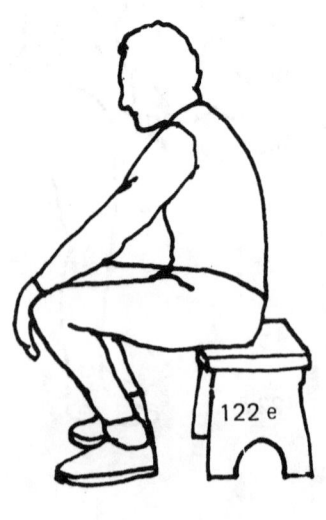

122 e

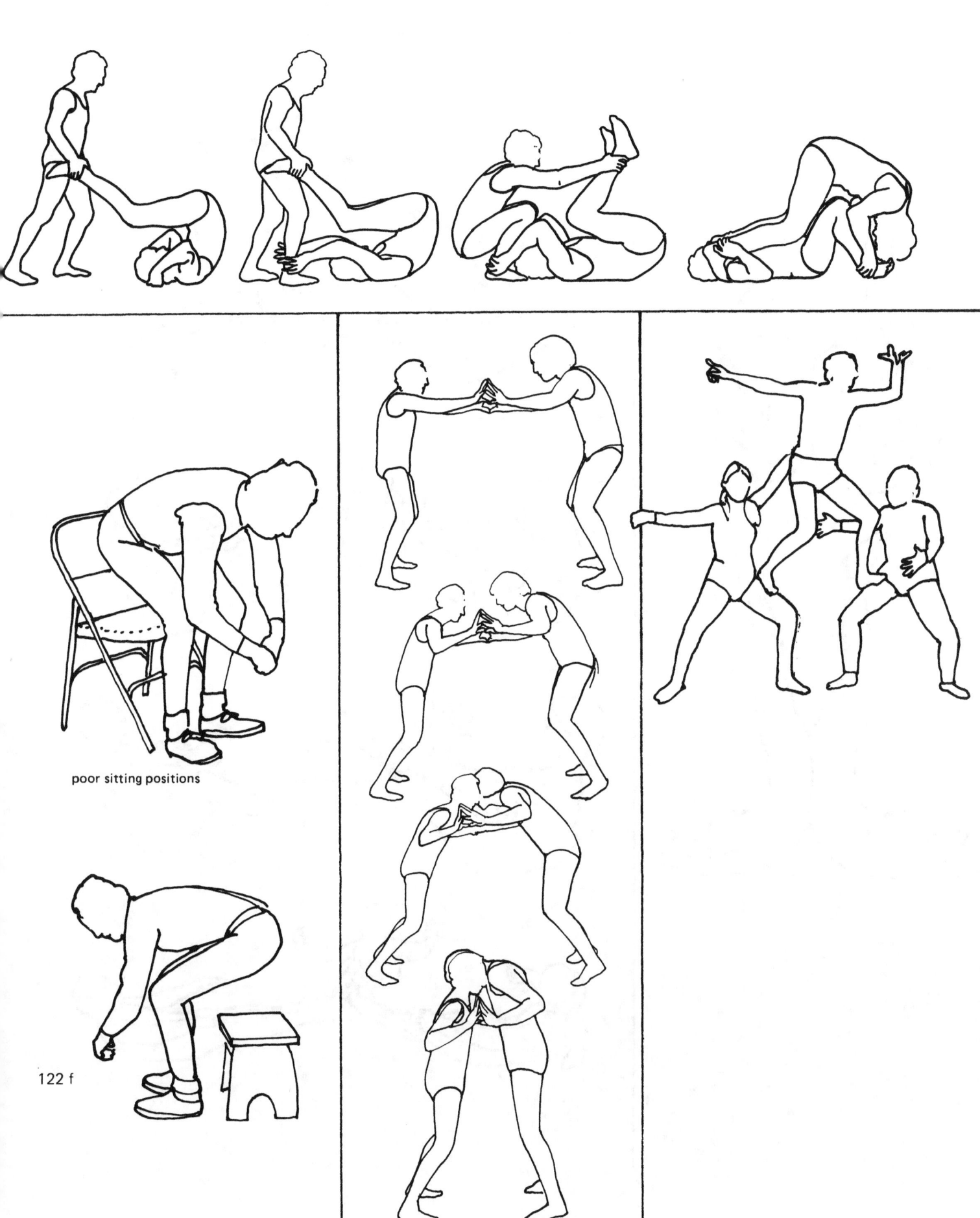

poor sitting positions

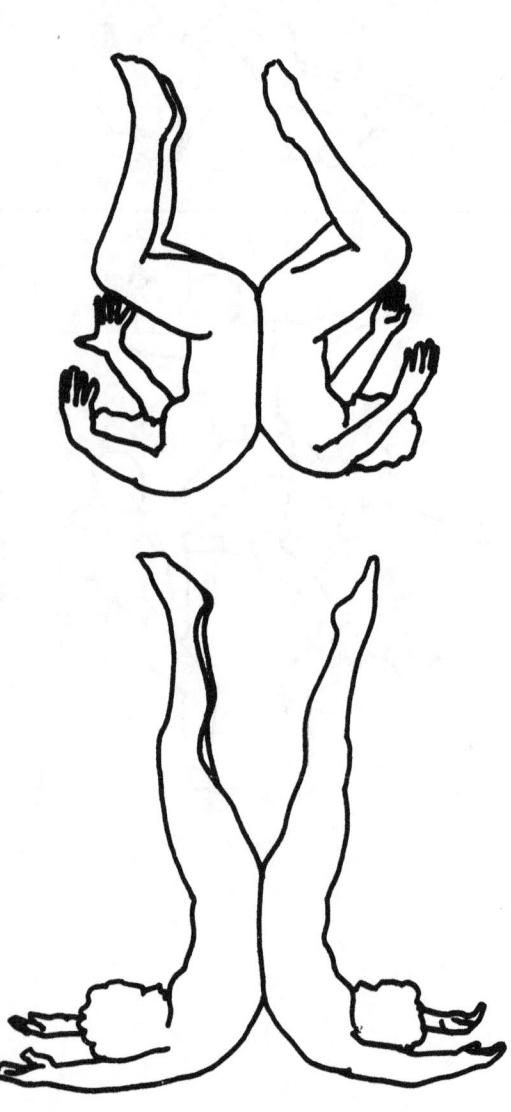
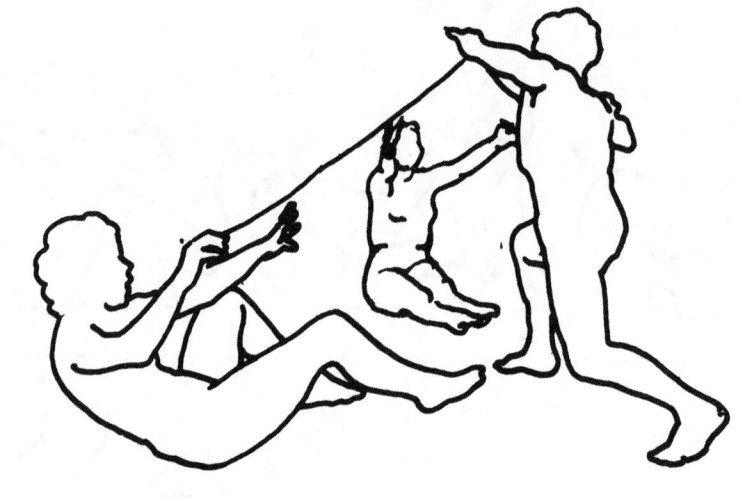
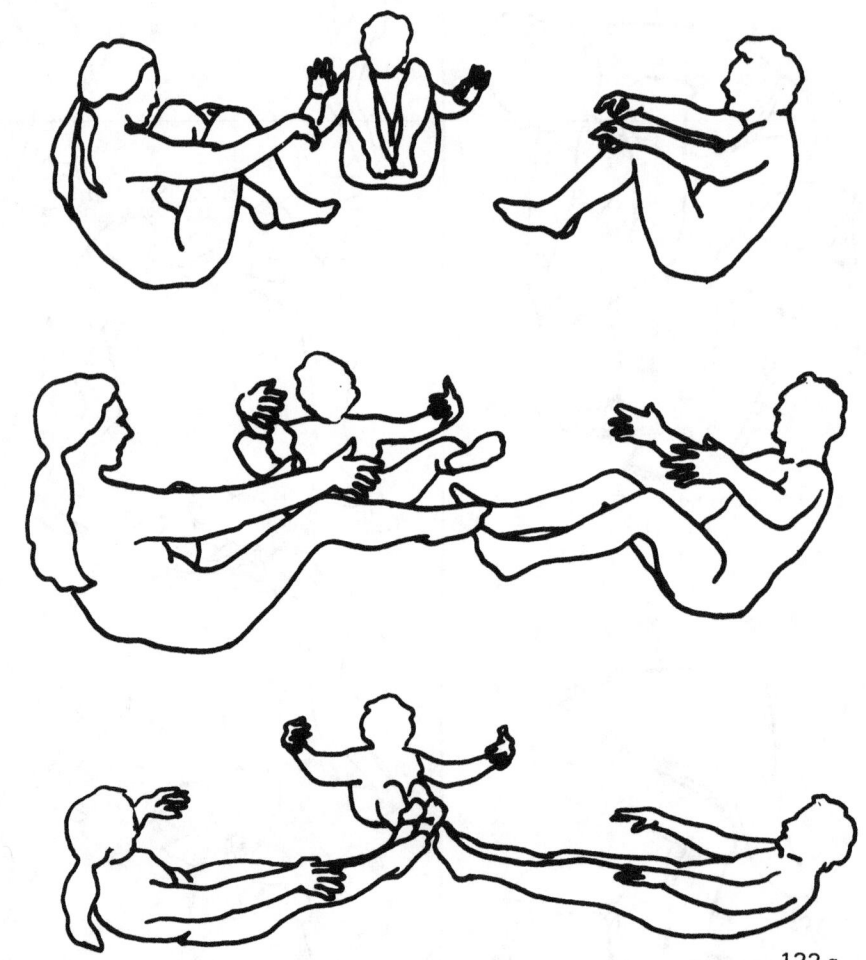

122 g

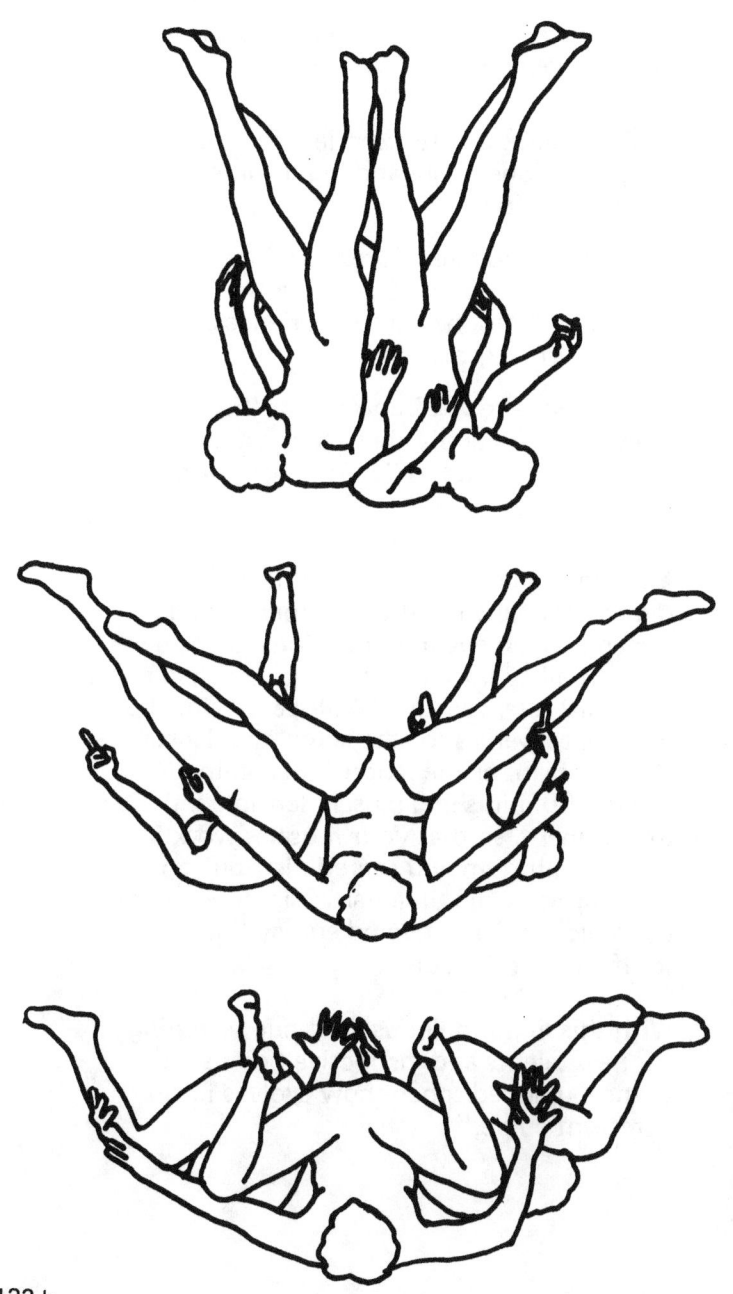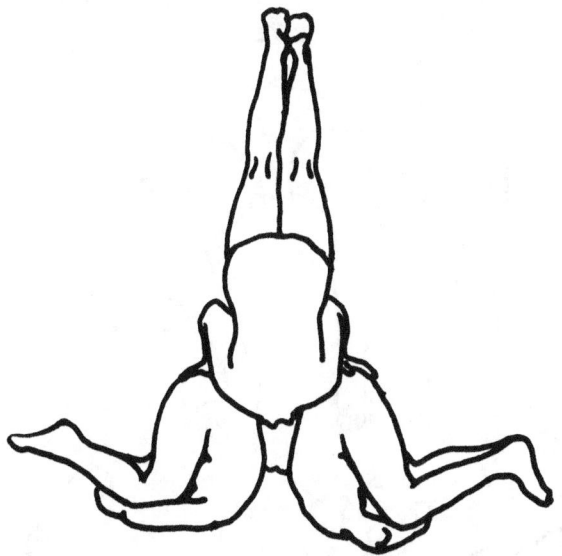

122 h

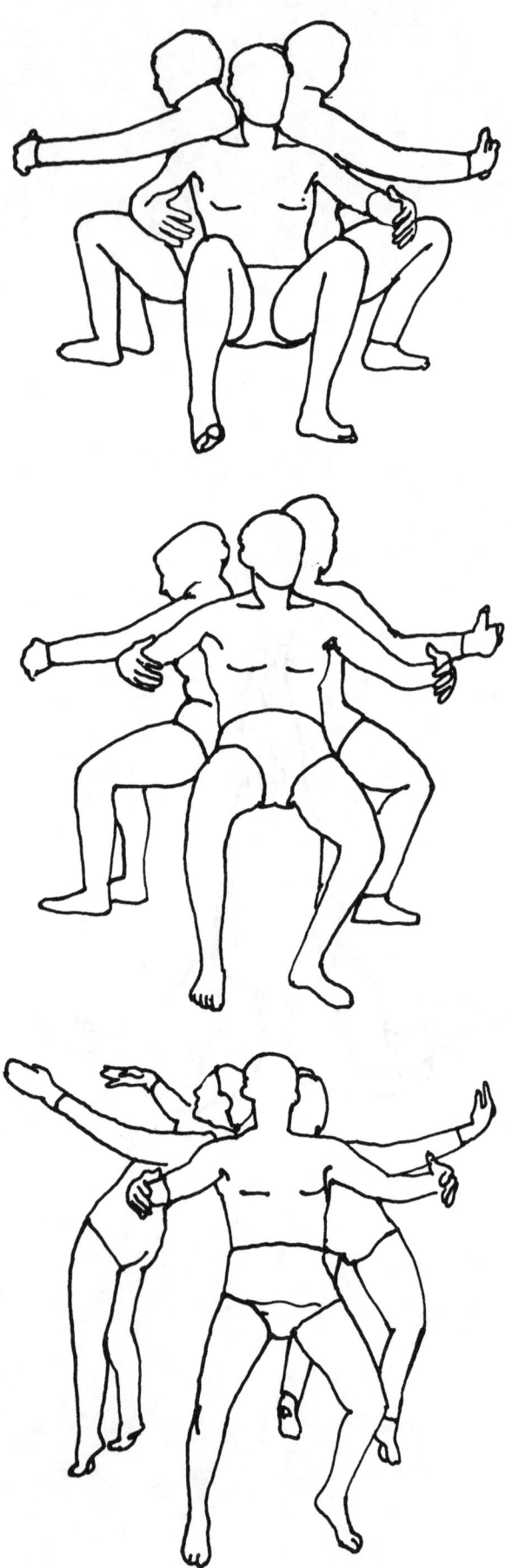

- Repeat each of the experiments with expanded-sphere sit-ups, leg-lifts, tripod headstands, and Yoga balance stands as a a duo — leading and following at the same time, giving and receiving organic signals without dictating or imposing direction upon one another's continuous, atom-to-atom movement.

  ◦ Experience and re-experience all the applications singly and in multiple combinations.

  ◦ Explore and re-explore the variations that arise from introducing different body energy states, balance experiences, and free-form expressions.

  ◦ Discover and re-discover your "familiar events" and apply them to expanded sphere activities as "unique behavioral events."

Your involvement with the motivational dynamics of the emotional experiencing system, which channel traditional muscle responsibility into a follower rather than a vanguard role, is a key "skill-secret" for the athlete, as well as for the actor, the dancer, the musician, or the laborer. Becoming aware of diminishing muscle tension and involvement, so that your muscles work in total equilibrium and shared distribution, while at the same time harnessing the potent dynamics of "emo-tivated energy," is in itself a major TALENT.

With this in mind, let us continue searching for new talents and instinctive body skills as the expanded sphere now evolves into a "crescent curve."

10
THE BODY AS A CRESCENT
LYING DOWN

We first perceived the body as a **small compact ball,** and our activities set out to discover and explore the outer surfaces of the body sphere. Next, we perceived the body as an **expanded sphere,** blossoming out like a budding flower into an open hemisphere with hollows, bends, curves, and loops. We are now ready, in the third stage of this evolving strategy, to perceive the body as a **crescent,** as a crescent-like section of the open sphere that can extend to a fully elongated body curve, much like an unstrung Indian bow.

The convex, bow-like body curve should be understood as an organic and structural consequence of the small ball and expanded sphere. It becomes the organic alignment of body structure for such fundamental activities as sitting, reclining, standing, crawling, walking, running, climbing, hopping, and dancing. The crescent may bend into a full C-curve, as in rolling, running, crawling, and sitting, or extend into a mild "parenthesis curve," as in standing and walking. Compare illustrations.

The important thing to remember is that whether bent into a C-curve or extended into a "parenthesis curve," the convex line of the spine remains constant. It is, for us, the natural carry-over of body-sphere esthetics with its distinguishing characteristics of curvo-linear and spatial movement.

Our experiments with the body as a crescent begin where the exercise activities of the last chapter left off, with the body hemisphere on the floor ready to elongate into reclining posture. These experiments consist mainly of cylinder rolls, peel-ups, push-ups, and conical rolls, and serve to further develop four concepts already familiar, but essential to evolving the body curve from the expanded sphere through the crescent to the eventual upright structure. These include:

Chapter 10

The Body as a Crescent - Lying Down

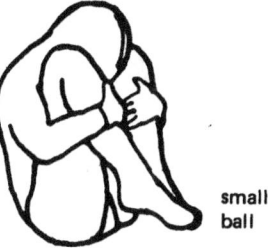
small ball

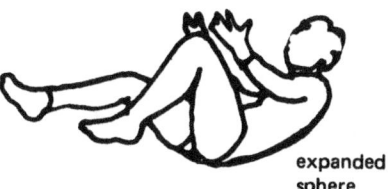
expanded sphere

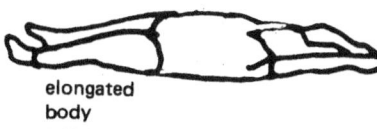
elongated body curve

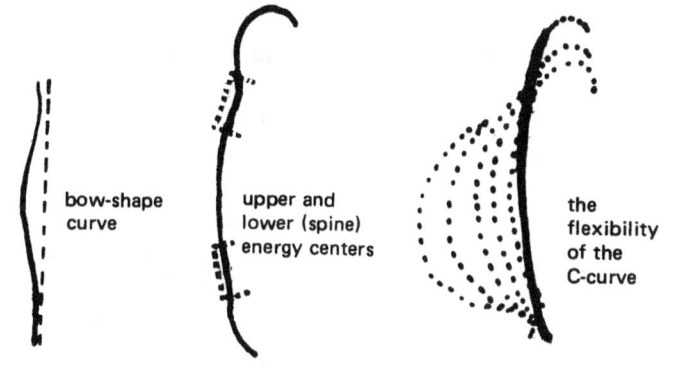
bow-shape curve

upper and lower (spine) energy centers

the flexibility of the C-curve

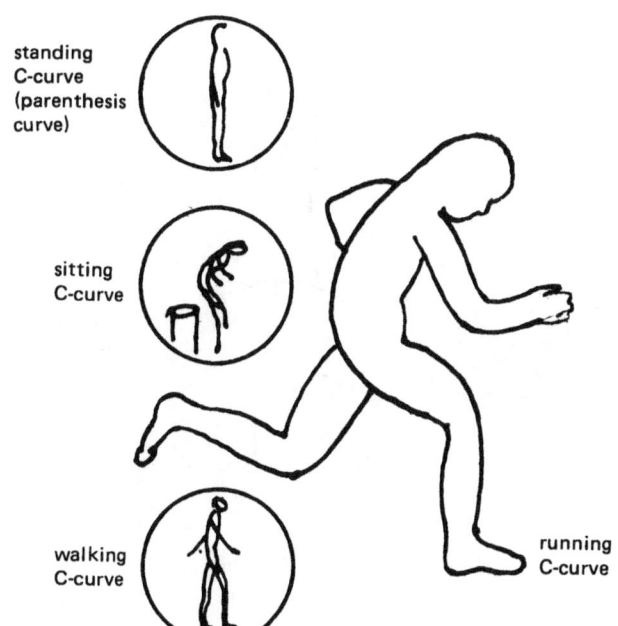

standing C-curve (parenthesis curve)

sitting C-curve

walking C-curve

running C-curve

Energy and Relaxation in Movement

1. The notion of the back as the functioning "locus of awareness" for all body movement;
2. The outer spine-line as a convex, parenthesis-like curve which while not always apparent, is nonetheless consistently felt;
3. The body's curves, following the natural direction of its joints and hinges, as potentially stronger, more flexible and in terms of body ecology, more esthetic than the rigid, straight lines we are conditioned to impose upon the body; and
4. The challenge of converting the lower and upper tension centers, characterized by low-back pains and a host of headaches, into vitalizing relaxer-energizer centers.

Experiment One: Coordinated Breathing with the Body as a Crescent Lying Down

- In reclining posture on the floor, elongate the expanded sphere into a curvo-linear, parenthesis-like side position. Hire the image of the parenthesis-curve,")", (which we use in writing, or associate with the shape of a cigar or frankfurter), and image it in horizontal position. The dorsal (back) surface must always feel convex, while the frontal area consistently fulfills and justifies that dorsal curve by responding to its inside concave shape. (See illustrations) Your posture includes resting the extended neck and inclined head on one outstretched arm, while the other arm rests conveniently top-side. Check for looseness of every body joint and hinge including vertebrae, pelvic, shoulder, knee and finger joints, but especially those in and around the lower- and upper-spine centers.

Remember: if vertebral joints or hinges of the spine should incline toward the unnatural articulating of "concave bending", the resulting "S-curve" spinal movement will disturb the body's crucial nerve-center network and block its pathways to the rest of the body.

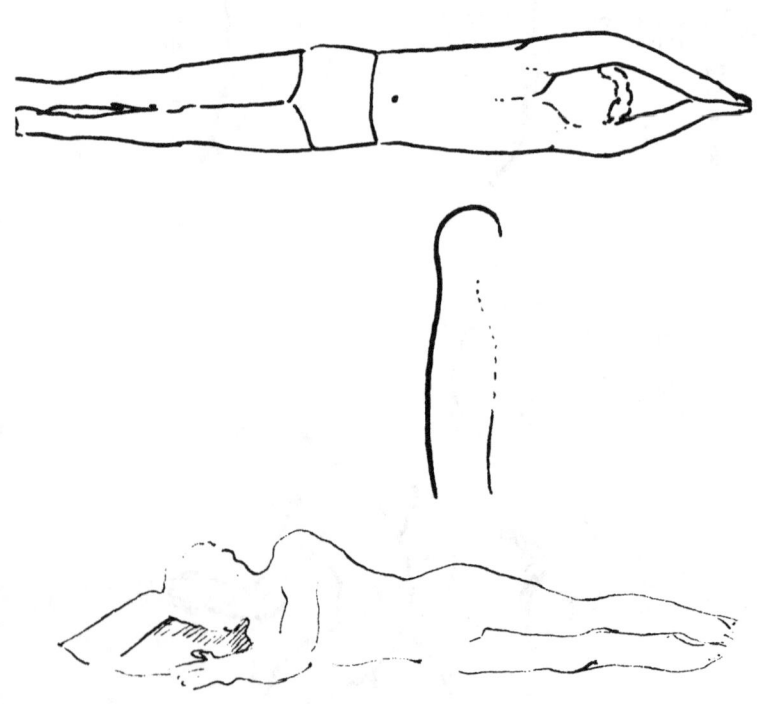

The
Evolving
Body
Crescent

- As you enjoy this comfortable reclining and sleeping position, breathe easily but fully. Observe the additional body comfort that this inspiring brings to the back, especially to the lower "back-center."

- Waft yourself, with atom-to-atom discovery, to prone position. Adjust your arms and head as illustrated, and continue the breathing that inspires the convex shape of the lower back center and now also begins to vitalize the mid-back area.

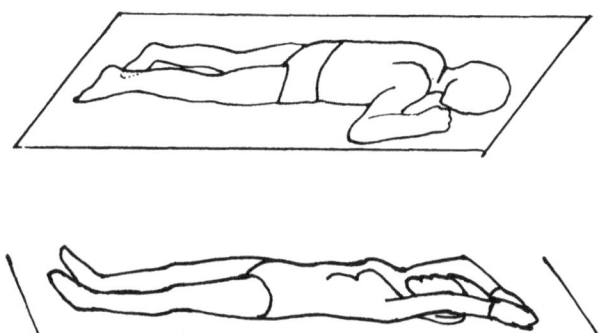

- Waft to your alternate side and, after tasting the sensations of the parenthesis curve in this new side position, move onto your back with arms and head extended as illustrated and repeat the breathing-vitalizing process. The low-back is under serious test here, so loosen your knee and pelvic joints, and "melt-spread" your muscles so that they help to sustain the dorsal curve. As you enjoy this reclining posture, mentally classify body sections into "empty" blocks: head-neck-shoulders-back-chest-stomach-pelvis-thighs-knees-calves-ankles-feet-arms, as illustrated.

- Starting with either the top or bottom block, and moving on to each contiguous block, suggest to yourself the image of all weight "oozing out" of the block. The block, becoming empty and light, thus feels more comfortable on the inside and more expansive on the outside, while it quietly rests **on** and **off** the floor at the same time. As you concentrate on each block, explore and exploit the optimal outside space latitude of each as well as the inside extension potential **between** each block. You will begin to feel all contact points of the body vanishing; the body becoming so relaxed that all you feel is contiguity of body to floor, with no conscious awareness of where body surface begins and

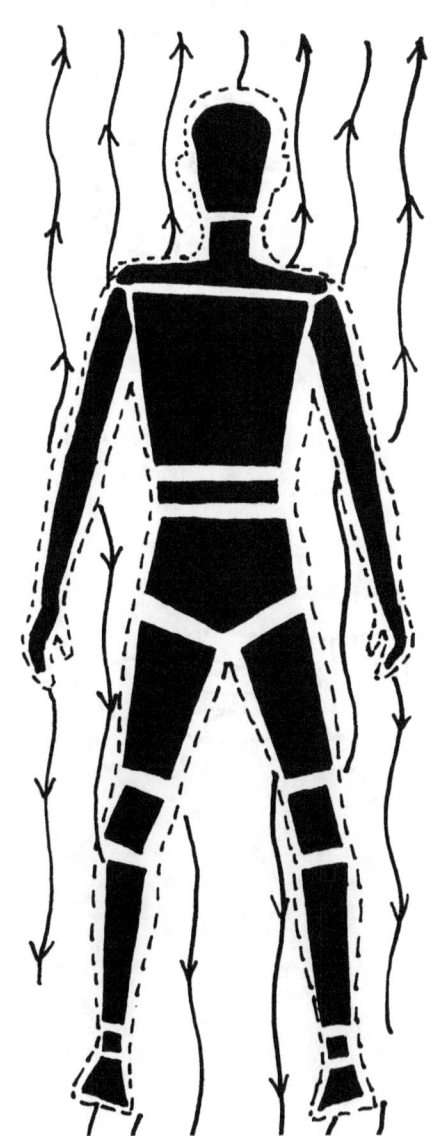

Energy and
Relaxation
in Movement

floor surface leaves off. Note especially the position of the feet: straight up, with no path-of-least-resistance flopping that would only induce a harmful, twist pressure on the knee-joints. By using the inner, rather than the outer, cushion of the calf muscle, you have oriented the feet to a new sense of balance. Without knowing it, you have also achieved the most natural body alignment which, if stood on a vertical axis, would produce an upright posture with perfect structural integration of back and front curvo-linear relationship. And that's precisely what we're working toward.

Experiment Two: Cylinder Rolls

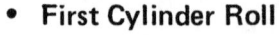

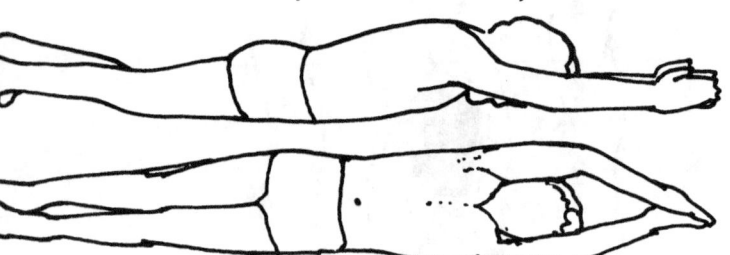

• **First Cylinder Roll**

Starting in prone crescent position, with both arms outstretched, palms together, and breathing to inspire the convex shape in the lower back center, gently vibrate, waft-wave from side to side and then roll two or three times in both directions using atom-to-atom discovery. See Illustrations.

• **Second Cylinder Roll**

Elbows flat to the chest, fists under chin, adjust your arms and hands as indicated and start by gently vibrating and shaking the body, using the heels and crown of the head as pivot points as though you were in a hammock of your own skin. Experiment with this radiancy sensation in crescent — prone, side, and supine positions, but especially on the back as this is the central experience.

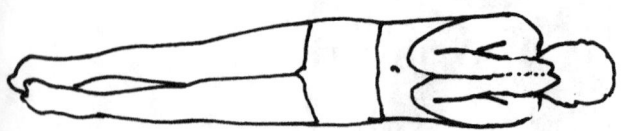

Now repeat the cylinder roll, elbows flat to chest, fists under chin, etc. If you sense a stall in the continuity of rolling, return to the waft-wave-shake and breathing activities, and then pick up where you left off. Do not bounce, flop, propel, or drag the body as you roll. As a cylinder, you roll as a whole not in parts. Be careful not to lead with your chest, shoulder, head, or feet. If you sense this occurring, go back to waft and wave until your whole body resumes its continuous side-rolling. Assisted by the instruments of buoyancy, radiancy, and inter-involvement energy, you are in artistic control of your wafting and waving. You can mold, blend, and glide with it until your body feels the equilibrium that permits you to complete the full roll in either direction with deliberate, exploratory, slow-motion movement.

Experiment Three: Body Peel-Ups and Roll-Ups

These are pre-push-up activities that involve potency stretching, radiancy extending, and buoyancy rocking and rolling on joints — particularly the knee, elbow, fist, and toe joints. The illustrations and captions provide all the self-teaching guides you will need.

- **Elbow-Knee Series:**

    a. elbow peel-up;

    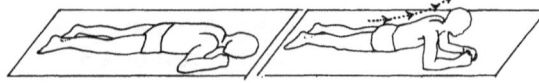

    b. elbow and knee roll-up; "kissing" the ground with forehead, nose, chin;

    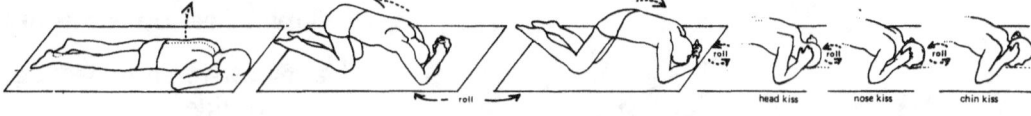

    c. advancing elbow roll-up and return;

    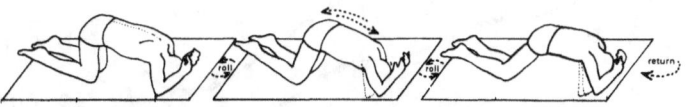

    d. advancing elbow roll-up plus "head-kissing;"

    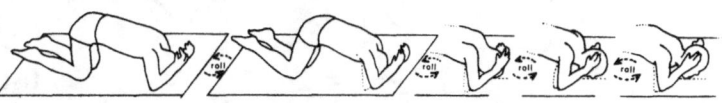

    e. advancing elbow-fist tripod.

    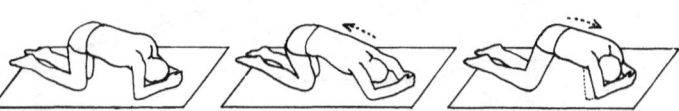

Energy and
Relaxation
in Movement

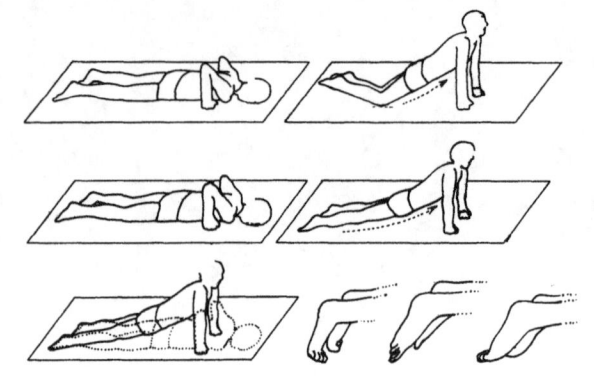

- **Fist Peel-Up Series:**

    a. peel-up on fists to the knees;

    b. peel-up on fists to the toes;

    c. peel-up on fists to the toes and roll on toes.

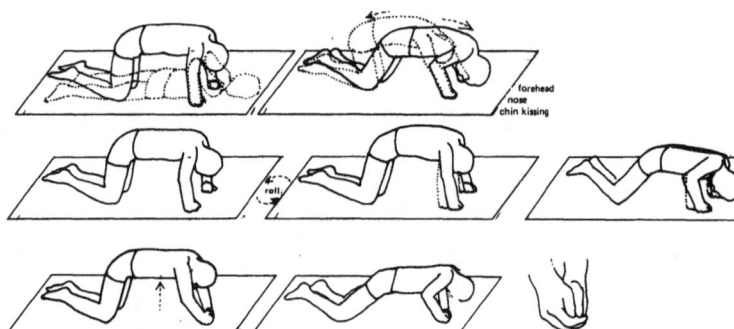

- **Fist-Knee Roll-Up Series:**

    a. fist-knee roll-ups; with forehead, nose, chin "kissing" the ground;

    b. fist-knee roll-ups with advancing fists plus "head-kissing;"

    c. when able, fist-knee roll-up with clasped fists as fulcrum, with or without advancing fists.

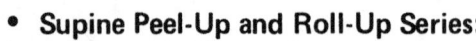

- **Fist-Toe Roll-Up Series:**

    a. fist-toe roll-up; gently "kissing" the ground with forehead, nose, chin.

    b. fist-toe roll-up with advancing fists;

    c. fist-toe roll-up with advancing fists plus "head-kissing" in each of the fist positions;

    d. when the body is ready and able, do the fist-toe roll-up with clasped fists in "fulcrum" position.

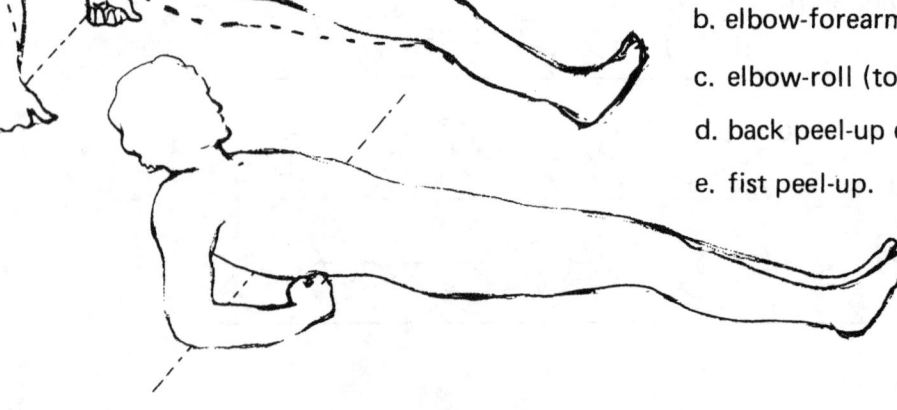

- **Supine Peel-Up and Roll-Up Series:**

    a. elbow-forearm peel-up to pelvis — shake and slide;

    b. elbow-forearm peel-up but off the pelvis;

    c. elbow-roll (to fist on floor), peeling;

    d. back peel-up on elbows;

    e. fist peel-up.

The
Evolving
Body
Crescent

- **Non-Surface Contact Push-Ups:**

   a. Mime-like version of "push-up" using the direct image of body-yawn energy exerted against "open space;"

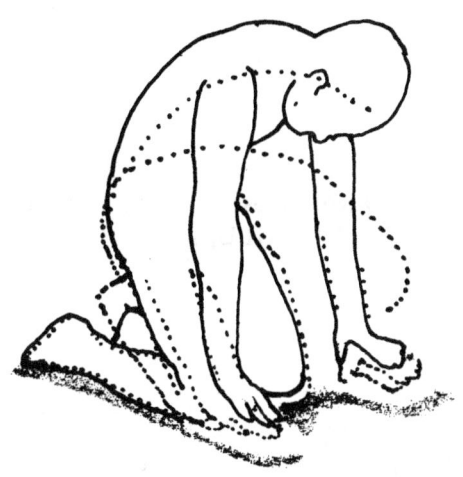

We call the next five rolling exercises "conical rolls" because the changing position of the arms creates a progressively increased rim circumference at one end, forming the shape of a cone. While dorsal contact with the ground is about equal for all conical rolls, prone (on stomach) contact is considerably less and much more challenging. That is, the more the front of the body is turned toward the floor, the more the body is lifted **off** the ground. Follow the illustrations for step-by-step instructions.

Experiment Four: Conical Rolls

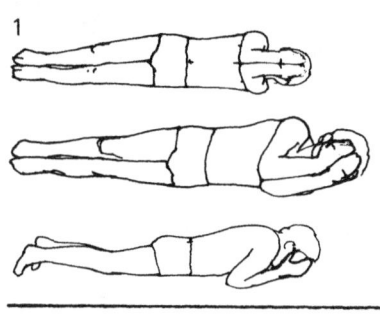

- First Conical Roll: hands cupped, elbows together; knees off the floor;

- Second Conical Roll: hands crossed to shoulders, elbows together, knees off the floor;

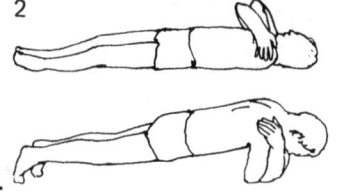

- Third Conical Roll: elbows apart, hands just above elbows; on your toes with knees off the floor;

- Fourth Conical Roll: arms in circle, hands at wrists; on toes, knees off the floor;

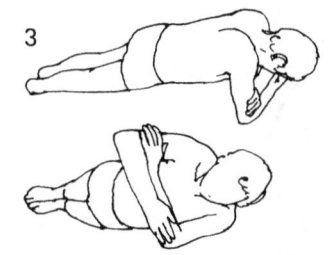

- Fifth Conical Roll: arms in full circle finger-tips touching; on toes, knees off the floor.

This last conical roll is rather difficult and may be left for much later. The back of the hands, the wrists, and the lower forearm should feel like a single rocker-rim curve. No sudden wrist-jerking or forced pressure on the wrists should accompany the roll.

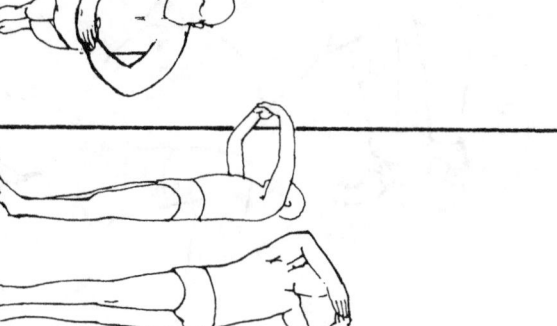

Experiment Five: Crescent Push-Ups and Lift-Ups

Work with the illustrations as you move through each of these exercise activities. Some of the push-up activities below may be too difficult — if so, just pass them by. Doing every one is not important — doing them well, is!

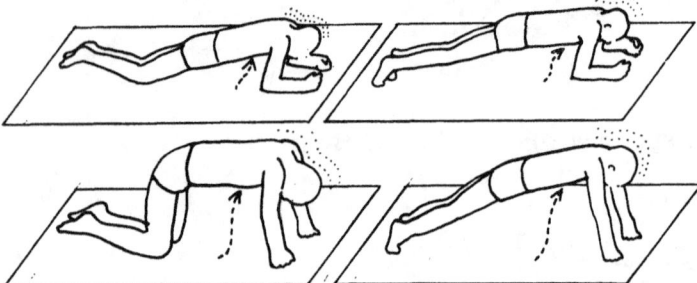

Basic Push-Up Series:

- elbow to knee push-up and roll;
- elbow to toes push-up and roll;
- fist to knee push-up and roll;
- fist to toe push-up and roll.

• **Push-Ups in Supine Position:** (See illustration bottom of page 129)

- elbow-heel push-up and roll;
- fist-heel push-up and roll.

• **Single Hand Side Push-Ups:**

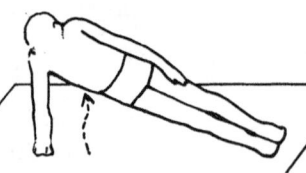

- single hand right-side push-up;
- single hand left-side push-up.

• **Partner Push-Ups:**

- buddies: head to head;
- head to head with alternate changing;
- buddies head to toe:
- one buddy pushes up by holding onto ankles; second buddy lifts up at his partner's ankles;
- double cylinder roll, alternating positions.

• **Buddy Wheelbarrow Push-Ups:**

- in place;
- walking;
- dumping the wheelbarrow.

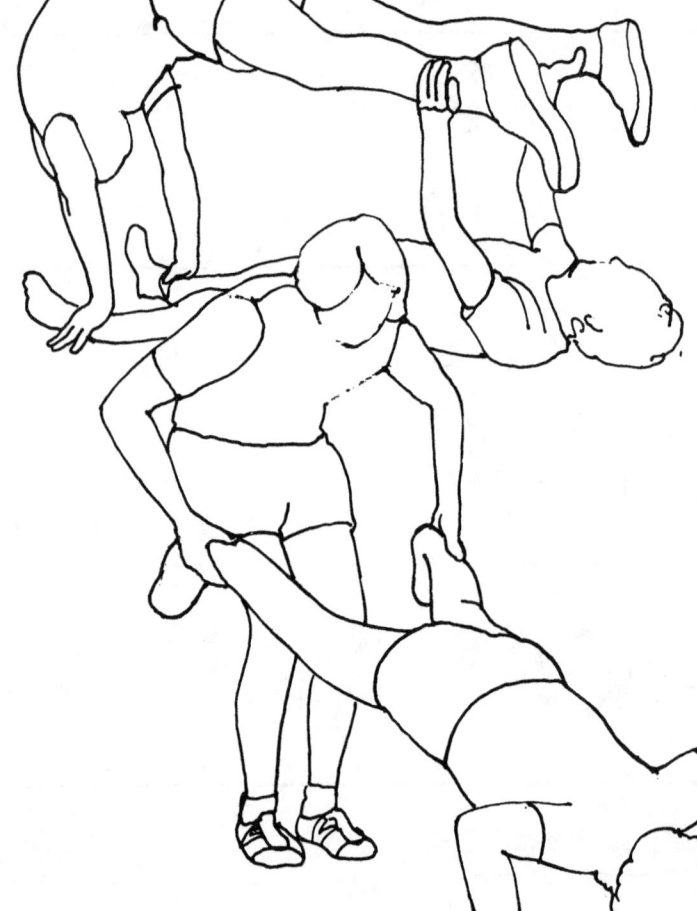

The
Evolving
Body
Crescent

- **Buddy Hand-Stand Push-Up and Lift-Up:**
  - alternate positions, with choice of hand-holds if buddy's weight and height are at extreme variance.

Self-Teaching Aids and Notes:

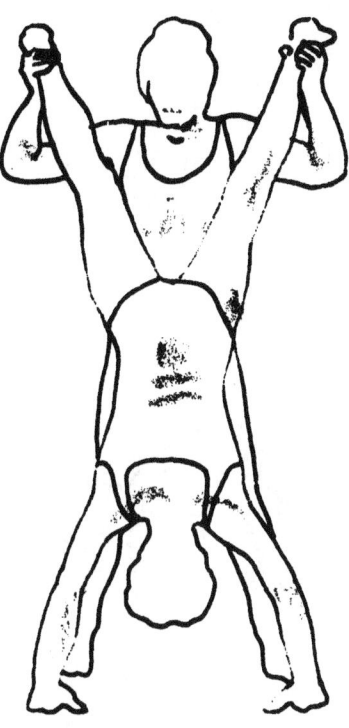

1. In all of these experiments, remain open and incessantly receptive to signals that guide you toward conscious development of a convex, bow-shaped spine-line, especially around the relaxer-energizer center of the lower spine.

2. Although exercises involving walking in handstand position can more easily be performed with flat-open palms, note a preference in all of our floor work for cupped fist-knuckles. Why?

    - Because it provides an excellent technique for strengthening the wrist joint, while offering a new experience to explore;
    - Because, unlike the flat-open palm, it respects the natural direction and articulation of the wrist joint;
    - Because it adds extra distance and height between body and floor surface, and reaches into many more, different muscle groups;
    - Because it lends itself to more instinctive walking, loping, running, and other animal-like body behavior;
    - Because it helps in taking falls and tumbles, and thereby assists in fear diffusion;
    - Because all of our concentrated work should precede the walking hand-stand event.

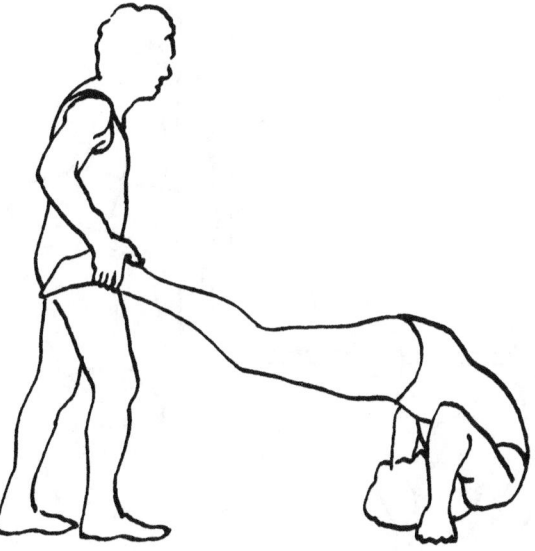

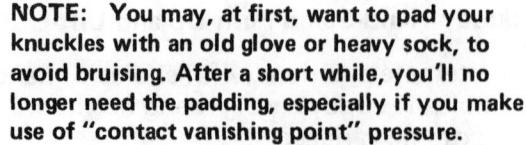

NOTE: You may, at first, want to pad your knuckles with an old glove or heavy sock, to avoid bruising. After a short while, you'll no longer need the padding, especially if you make use of "contact vanishing point" pressure.

Also, avoid recklessly propelling your body weight onto your wrists. They are probably still too weak to withstand such onslaught. Before long, you'll find yourself developing firm, flexible, strong wrists — particularly if you earnestly explore the exercises in this chapter. You'll become accustomed to the lovely balance skill that strong wrists afford the body, and you'll appreciate the perfectly graceful line they give to hand expressiveness and general body communication.

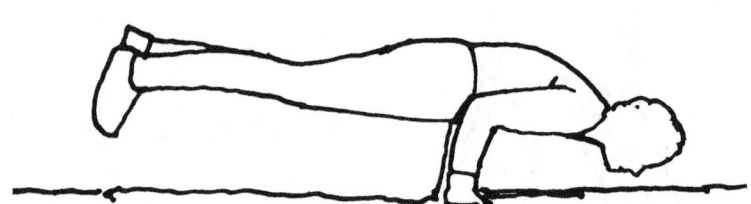

3. Body activities such as push-ups, chin-ups, sit-ups, lift-ups, leg-lifts, and body lifts incorporate two essential movements: one in the direction of the primary action of the event; the other in the return action. Be sensitive to the fact that the body ought to benefit from the return action perhaps a bit differently, but no less importantly than from the primary action. In both moves, relaxed energy and energetic relaxation are fully operative. So never rush through the return action in a hurry to get to what is generally presumed to be the more significant primary action. Both moves are true events in themselves.

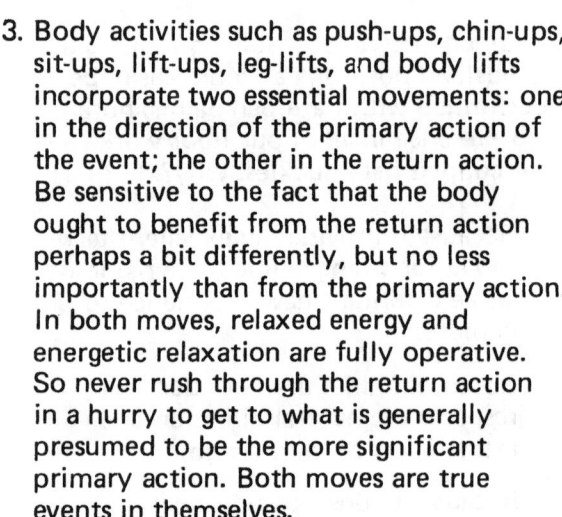

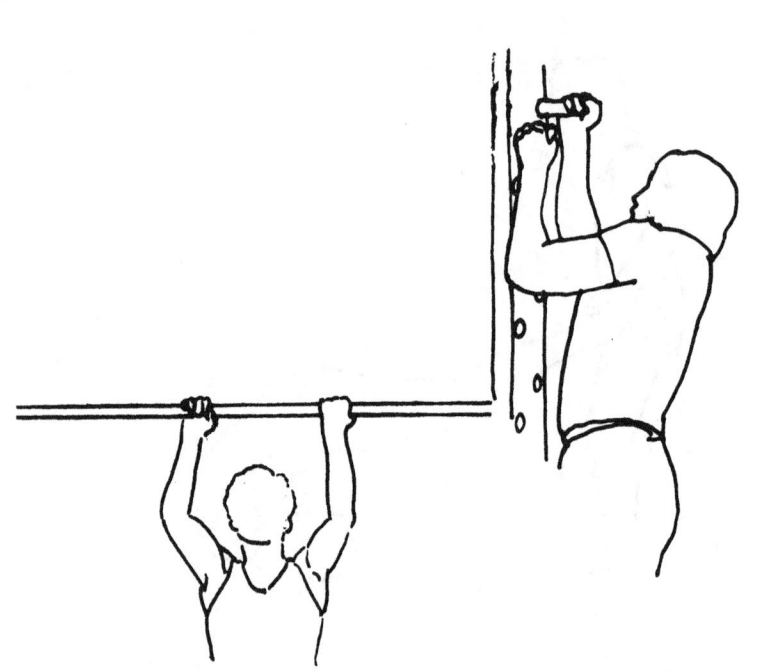

In a chin-up, for instance, lifting yourself above the bar is only half the exercise. The deliberate, slow-motion, settling-down buoyancy of the return action is equally significant and equally half of the task. This will become even more apparent when you advance, in later chapters, to running, springing, walking, and hopping **backwards** as separate, independent body experiences with the same importance as negotiating the action in forward direction.

The
Evolving
Body
Crescent

We are now ready to evolve the body crescent in vertical posture; to introduce wheels and loops into our experiments; to focus on the duality of body breathing and body posture in the upright; and to examine these inter-relationships as they determine the quality of physical, vocal, and emotional life. But now let us take a small break to review the conclusions of our work so far. Let us also image and discover additional creative applications, variations, and improvisations, particularly as they relate to "buddy explorations."

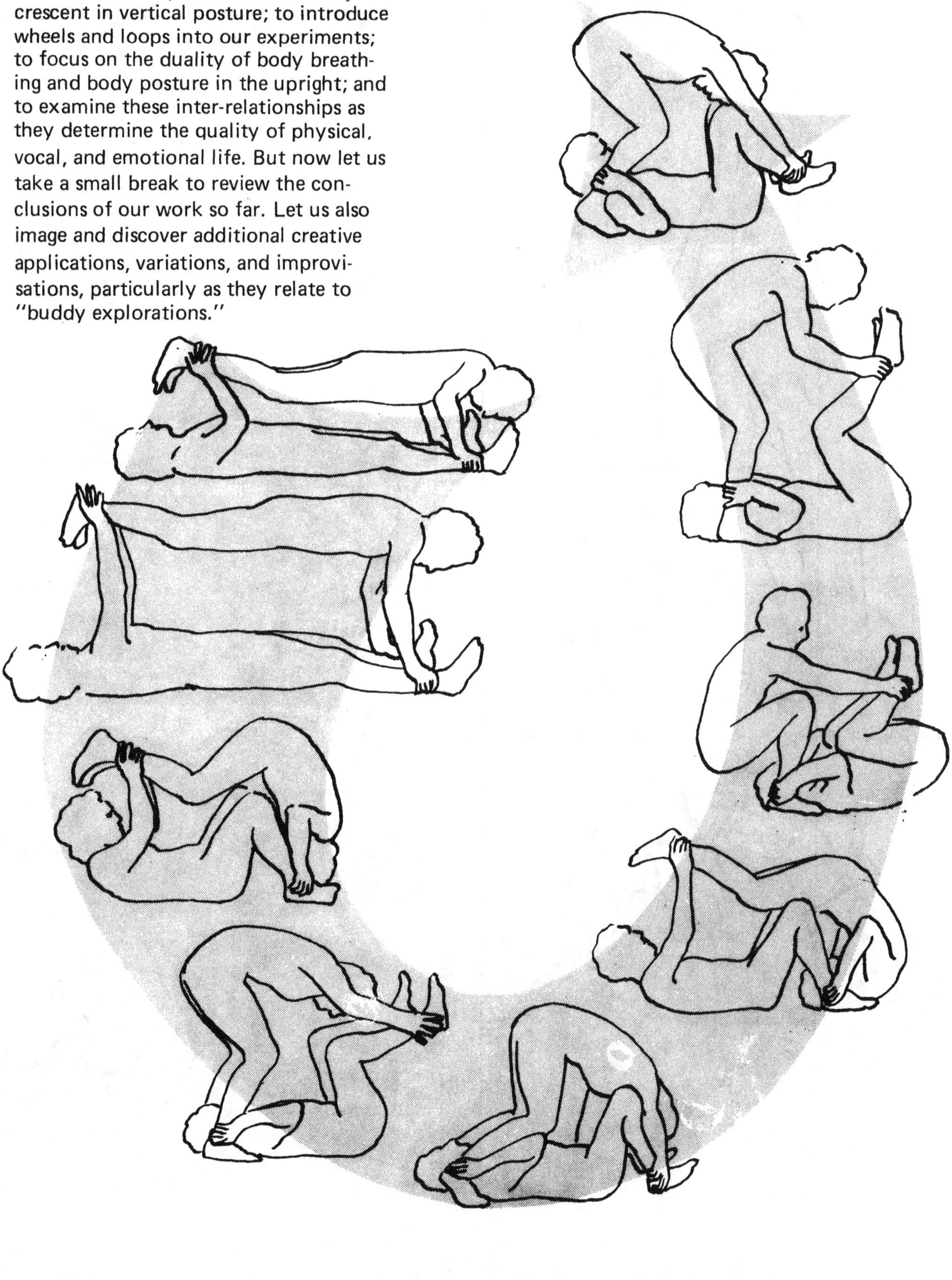

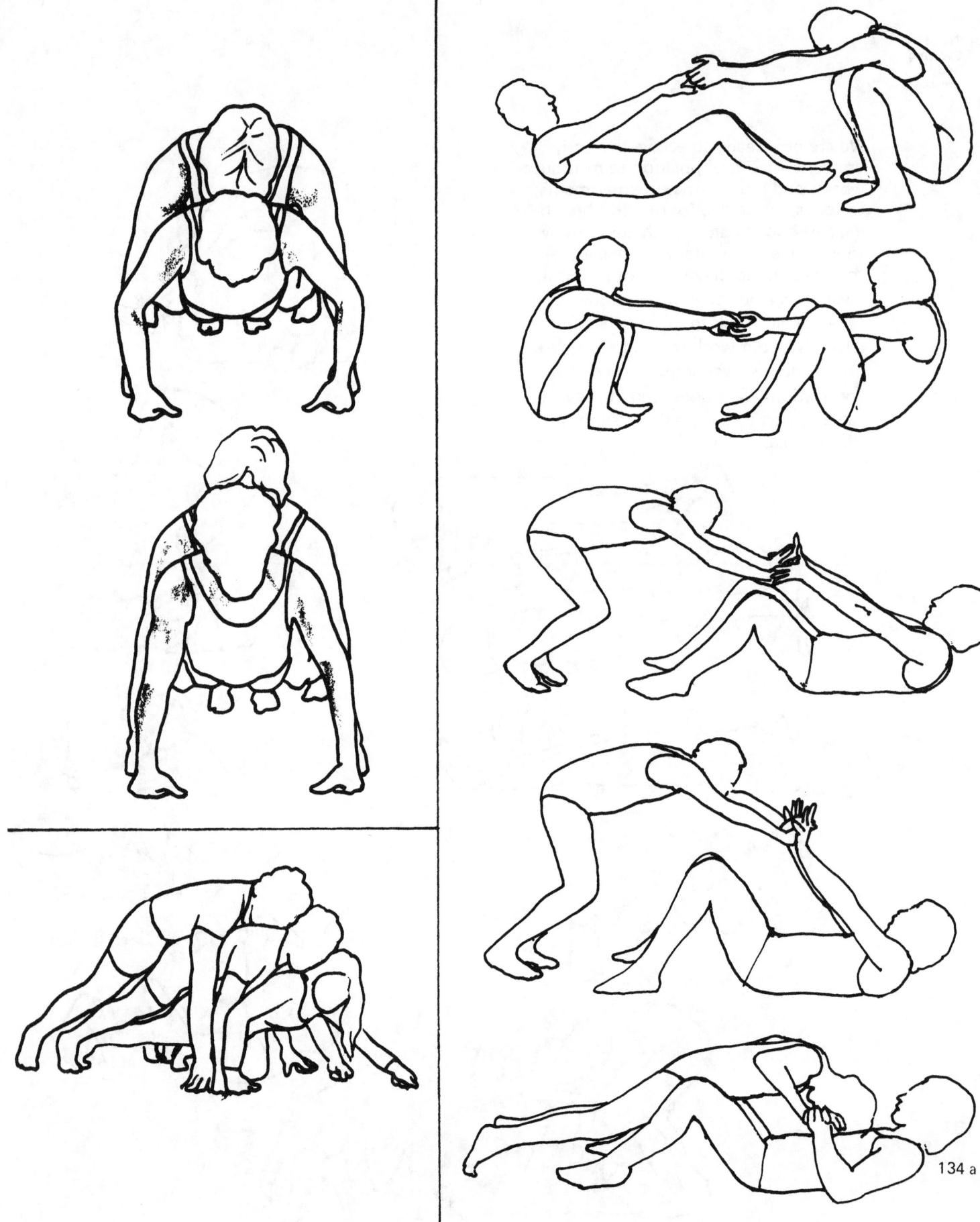

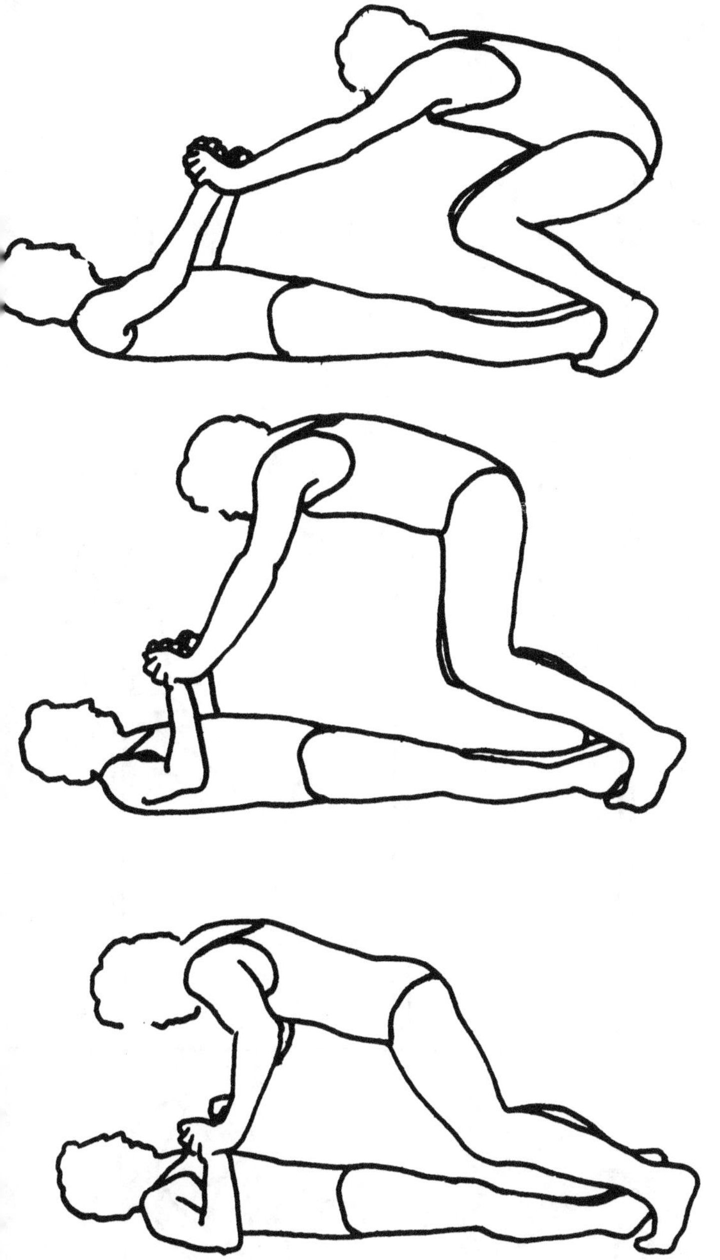

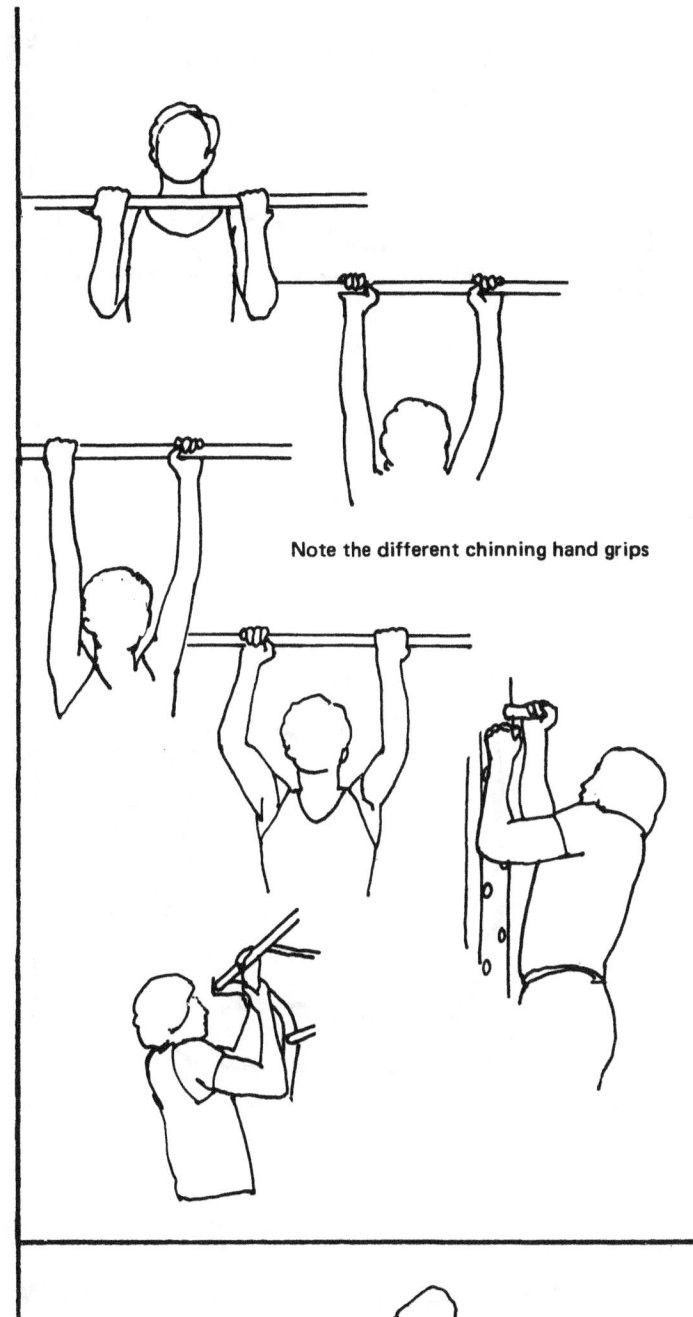

Note the different chinning hand grips

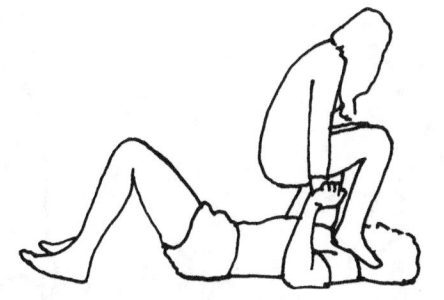

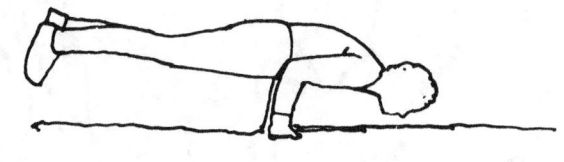

134 b

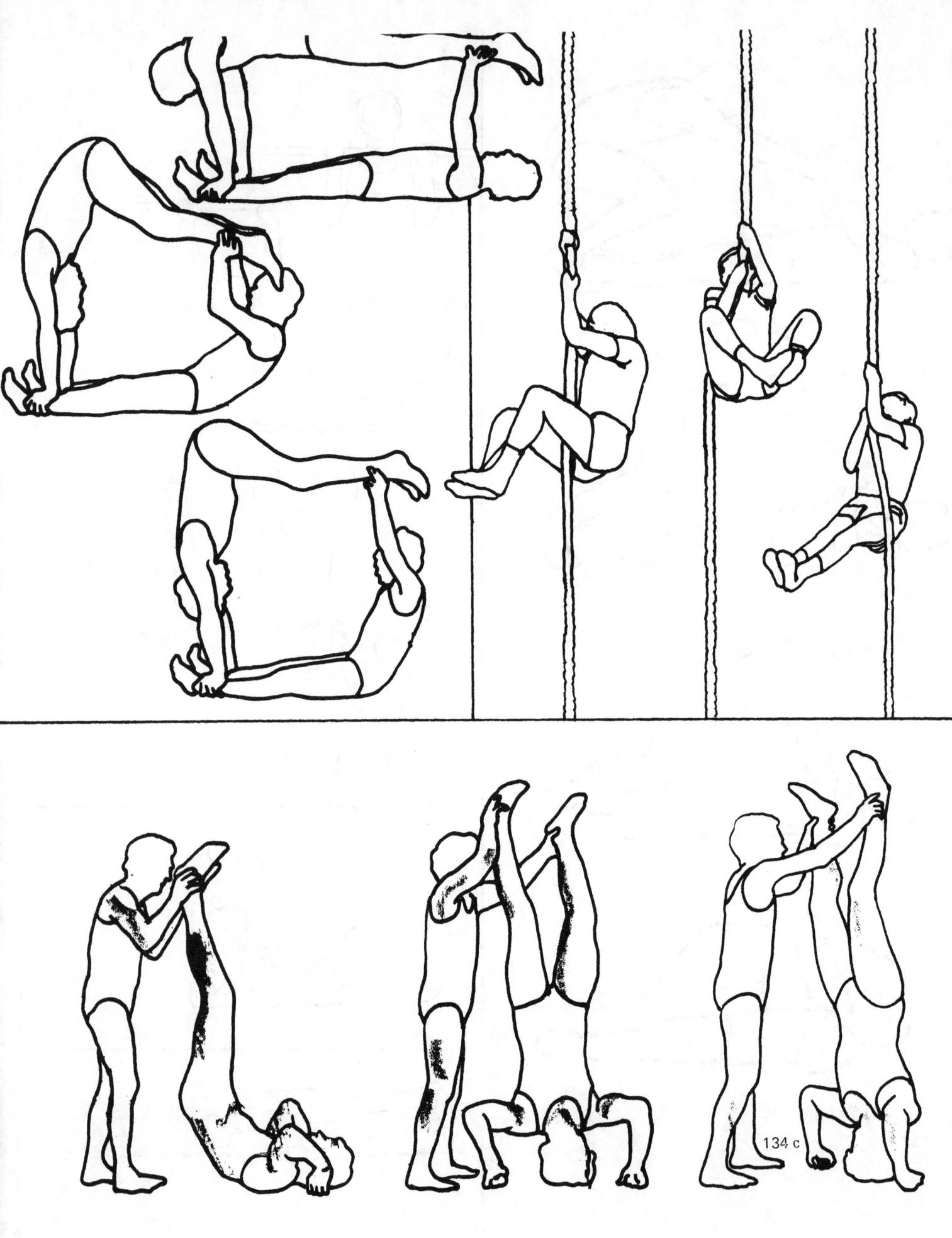

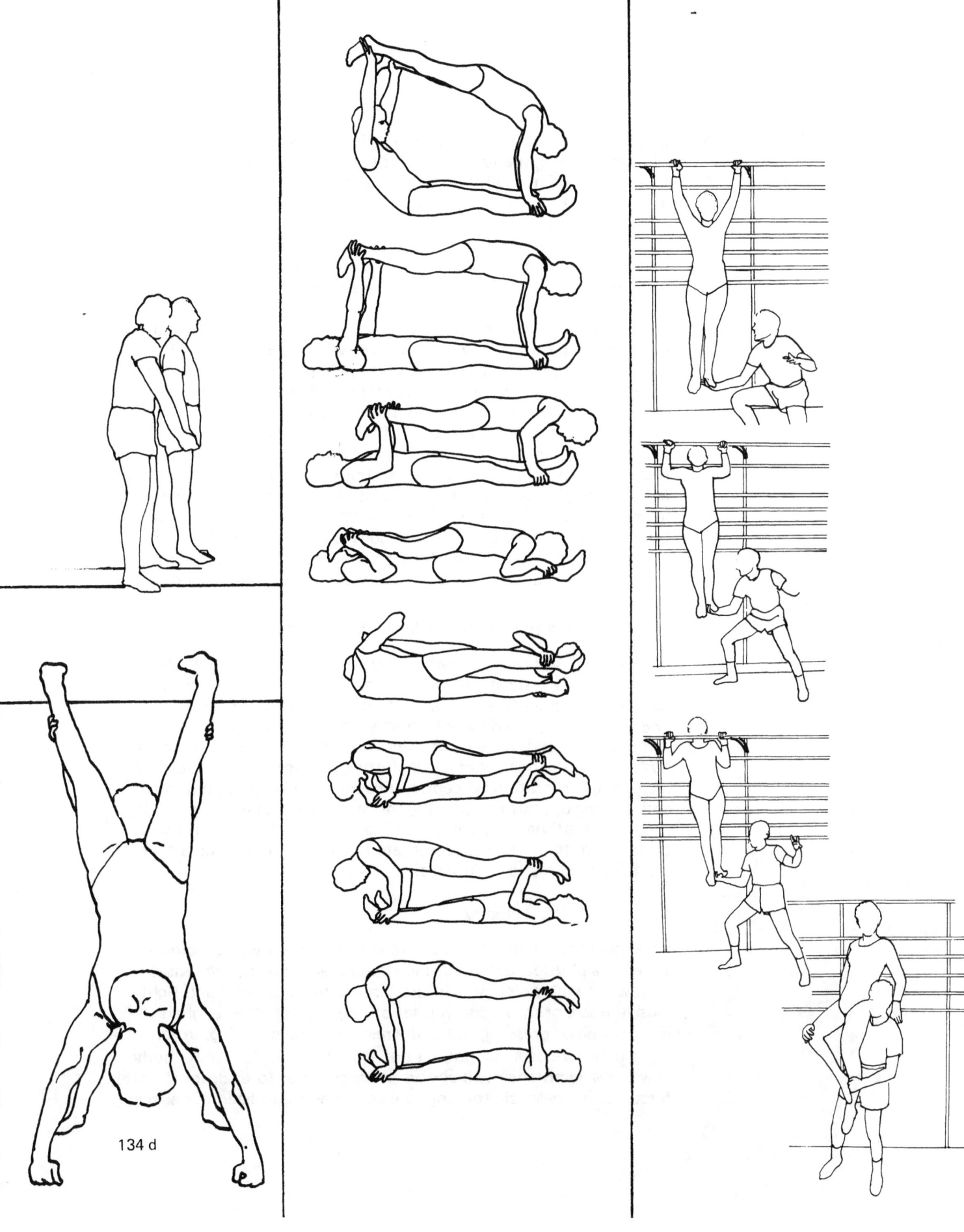

134 d

A MIDWORD BREAK

We are in the stage of kinesensic training increasingly concerned with body strength and body endurance. Rolling and tumbling accented an affinity with lightness, atom-to-atom discovery and contiguous continuity, vanishing contact point, finger-tip sensitivity, and just noticeable difference. Push-ups, lift-ups, chin-ups, pull-ups, and roll-ups concentrated more on strategies of balanced muscle tonicity, resting up and down at the same time, safety reserve cushion, and the feel of live weight versus dead weight.

All of these involved the concept of movement in the body and the body in motion. Each, in its own way, emphasized the basic curvo-linear, spherical contour of the body — its natural, biological inheritance. Throughout, we have employed and variously combined buoyancy, radiancy, potency, and inter-involvement energetics, not only to index the body wisdoms of balance, rhythm, esthetics, relaxer-energizers, image, play, safety-cushion, etc., but also in response to new cues and signals for body strength, body endurance, and the body's need for resilient flexibility. The result has been an increased range of sensations, perceptions, and awareness of the psycho-physical relationships that govern the body's self-to-self communication. Let us stop for a moment to examine some of the implications of these now active concepts for what lies ahead.

Resting Up and Resting Down at the Same Time

In resting up and resting down at the same time, we experience a double-edged alertness: the keen, sensitive energy fuel of rising buoyancy on the lift-off or take-off, on the chin-up or push-up; and the vibrant, yielding soft energy fuel of floating or settling-down buoyancy on the return from the lift, the pull, or the push, back to surface contact or starting posture. We must learn to identify this sensation-perception not only in lifting up, pulling up, and pushing up, but in climbing, throwing, weight carrying, leaping, running, wrestling, swimming, skating, skiing and striking (in golf, baseball, football, tennis, soccer, etc.) — in fact, in all events that call for strength and endurance.

Balanced Muscle Tonicity

We experience balanced muscle tonicity whenever we consciously apply to a physical act requiring strength and power, the sensation of yawn-stretch potency — infused into otherwise tense and tight muscle fibers or into a specific **set** of muscles. Whether applied to body-lifting or pressing, to hand-wrestling, rope-climbing, unscrewing a tight jar-cover, or pulling out a stubborn bottle cork, **body-yawn muscle potency will always prove superior to traditional brute force.** With kinesensic training, the strong-arm grip becomes a freer, energetically relaxed hold — just firm enough to exert a full, sustained body-yawn stretch that allows you to enjoy and tune into the rhythm and balance of the stretch, as well as to the muscle yawn itself — and more than firm enough to accept and accomplish the physical challenge.

Live Weight versus Dead Weight

Live weight versus dead weight helps, on the one hand, to clarify the image of "anti-gravitational energy feel" and on the other, to better understand the meaning of and our objection to the condition of body heaviness, passive-lethargic relaxation, body floppiness, and body imbalance — particularly as these anesthetics carry over to depression, fear of falling, and other anxieties that promote competitive conflicts within the body. In experiencing the feel of live weight versus dead weight, we can crystalize the "kinesensing" of body balance and body rhythm that directly result in aggressively counteracting "fatigue combat" — in an enduring warding off of extreme or collapsing body exhaustion.

Live weight versus dead weight is probably a matter of letting the body educate the mind when the mind suggests that limits have been reached. Adherence to the message — "You are at the end of the line, don't slow up...push harder, fella...Run faster to that old familiar home base" — would still have our runner-athletes doing the mile in just **over** four minutes. There is a difference between knowing your true limits, which means learning to live with healthy compromise based on sound, organic feedback, and taking the word of your mind which is not yet in sync with your body.

Until we recognize that there is more potential for relaxed energy and energetic relaxation in both everyday and special event activities, contrary to the mind's outer-conditioned message, we can never even dream of the body's full potential and inherent creativity that exists largely untapped within the organism. You will realize this for yourself when you dance and run on "leg wheels," put some rolling into your jogging, or "bow and wheel" your way up flights of stairs in upcoming chapters.

Safety Reserve Cushion

Directly related to the concept of live weight versus dead weight is the safety reserve cushion. The awareness of a reserve or safety cushion is established by developing those perceptions and images that serve to liquidate the tensions of fear, anxiety, and other energy-consuming body anesthetics. Conversely, these anesthetics, most often expressed through images suggesting fear of failure, can destroy any safety reserve cushion that has been built up by the body from intrinsic capabilities.

The safety reserve cushion is best understood as part of the body's complex feed-back system of internal cues, signals, and controls. It is a psycho-physical phenomenon with both psychosomatic cause and effect dimensions. Its cues and signals tell us that there is still a "reserve" of energy left. A singer or athlete or perservering pioneer, upon "feeling" the organic reserve cushion through body esthetics, knows it is safe to venture forth, to take chances, to invent, to innovate, to make the next extra move. The reserve cushion **creates** safety and **permits** a more exciting use of reserve energy, always available through an organic image such as the suggestion of buoyancy and radiancy in live weight versus dead weight.

When professional athletes, musicians, artists, and actors can teach themselves the meaning of, and the lambent feel of, body buoyancy and radiancy vitality, and orient their minds to the esthetic use of these body energy states, they (indeed anyone) will run, lift, jump, throw, dance, climb, play, sing, and act better; they will also sculpt, paint, design, or build more freely because their bodies will be **moving** in a different order of magnitude, on another level of creativity. Again, this is part of the body's safety-reserve-cushion feedback system.

Muscle-Sharing Responsibility

All our images have to do with the sharing or distributing of physical activity over the maximum amount of muscle substance, over a maximum number of muscle groups. This means minimal overloading or localizing of muscle-waste pile-up. And this, in turn, means easier collection of muscle waste, and more firing of muscle cells for production of chemical energy — resulting in minimal fatigue. This concept assumes even greater importance in the next two work chapters.

Relaxer-Energizers

We are based in a culture of "exercising" which demands that we hurt or overstress something in order to save, shelter or enhance it. There is no need for such a strategy. There is no virtue in learning of one's talent or creative skill **after** it has been temporarily harmed, crippled, or irretrievably destroyed. The proverbial story of the person who remarked, after a rugged workout, that he didn't know he had so many muscles in his body until they started to hurt, is not an especially amusing anecdote. No more than the oft-heard report, usually in a hoarse whisper: "Wow, what a workout! I didn't realize I had such a good voice and could sing so high and loud — if only I didn't lose the use of it I could have gone on forever!"

A
Midword
Break

But physical perception of relaxer-energizers can easily provide the necessary intelligence, without harmful side-effect, and readily inform what the body has to offer **before** any dangerous results develop. Such Body Wisdom can, indeed, communicate to the performer in many different ways, without hurting anything in order to preserve it. Using shivering, loosening, shaking, quivering, extension reaching to find out what is alive in the body is using natural relaxer-energizers to develop body awareness of sensations, perceptions, and muscle patterns that we usually ignore, or worse, **don't realize are right there in the body for experiment, exploration, and in the best sense of the term, exploitation.**

With the concepts discussed in this midword statement functioning as they should, we can look forward to satisfaction and exhilaration in the intense, initially challenging but highly rewarding work ahead. So, with radiancy-alert, let's move right on to the "body as a crescent — standing up" and "the perception of the upright."

11
THE BODY AS A CRESCENT
STANDING UP

Chapter 11

The Body as a Crescent - Standing Up

This chapter deals with the perception of being upright. Standing upright must be learned because, along with human speech, it is an overlaid rather than an immediately natural event. Both can either be learned well for optimal functioning or be learned so poorly as to adversely affect one's breathing, posture, and jointedness, one's communicating personality, and eventually one's emotional experiencing systems.

The perception of the upright, "how it feels to be human," should be preceded by the perception of **being** upright, "how it feels to stand up (and talk)." Our work so far — in the small ball, expanded sphere, and horizontal, elongated crescent-curve — has turned the body into a teacher of what instinctive functioning can be, under circumstances not subject to outer-environment conditioning. Now, we must teach ourselves, again through the body, how to apply that instinctive behavior to "being upright." We must teach ourselves, precisely because this is not an organically natural activity, though it is the final stage in our evolvement of the body curve, and in the ultimate instinctive potential of the body in motion.

For us, then, the evolving process continues. Being upright is a continuation of the small ball and the expanded sphere. It is a continuation of the open-curved crescent of the elongated body curve. It is the continuation of movement and the sense of extension, the continuation of the body's natural curves in breathing and posture. In this chapter, we will deal very specifically with breathing, posture, joints, and hinges — and their relationship to the emotional experiencing system as part of a psycho-physical instrumentality.

Your experience with breathing and posture has already shown you their cognate

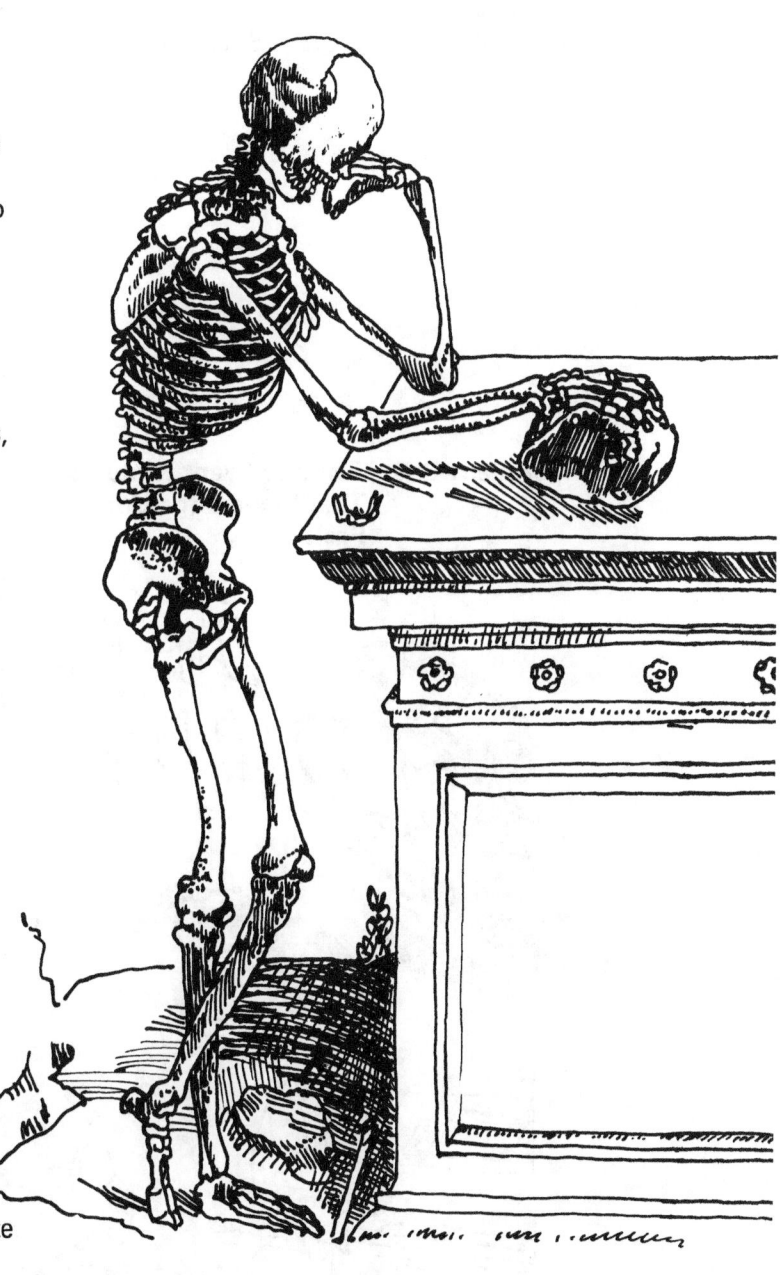

Energy and
Relaxation
in Movement

*"The function of breathing
determines the structure of posture,
at the very same time that
the function of posture
determines the structure of breathing!"*

character. Do one of them well and you have the positive benefit of both. Do either of them poorly, and you will destroy both — bringing discomfort and misalignment to the body. Stand poorly and you **must** breathe poorly. Breathe properly and you **must** stand properly.

You have sensed the natural breathing process in squat, crawl, and roll positions; in lying on your stomach, back, and side; in doing balance-stands on shoulders and head; in small ball, expanded sphere, cylinder and conical rolling; in body push-ups, lift-ups, roll-ups, and sit-ups. You are now ready to bring all this experience to upright position (to stand the crescent in vertical axis) and appreciate its new dynamics for everyday behavior and optimal functioning.

Experiment One: Familiar Event Postures That Prepare for Upright Position

The following are familiar event positions that bridge the semi-circle of the expanded sphere to the C-curve of the body in the upright. In other words, each of these comfortable and familiar positions carries the natural body curve that we will want to transfer to standing posture and exploit for more healthful and efficient walking, running, climbing, skiing, springing, etc. Do each exercise as indicated, becoming increasingly aware of the natural C-curve in each position. Use the illustrations as guides.

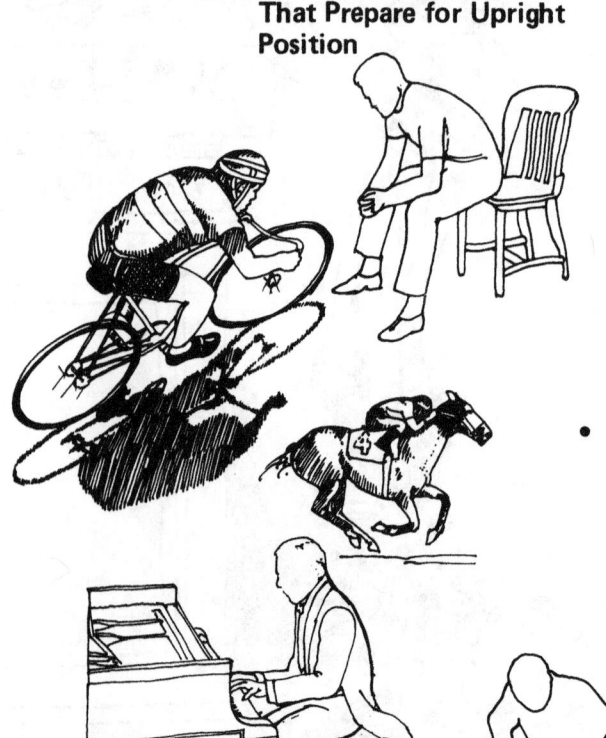

Illustrations above show
natural breathing postures

- Place yourself in sitting position as though you were:

    ◦ on the edge of a chair;

    ◦ bicycle pedaling;

    ◦ horseback riding;

    ◦ playing the piano;

    ◦ playing the drums;

140

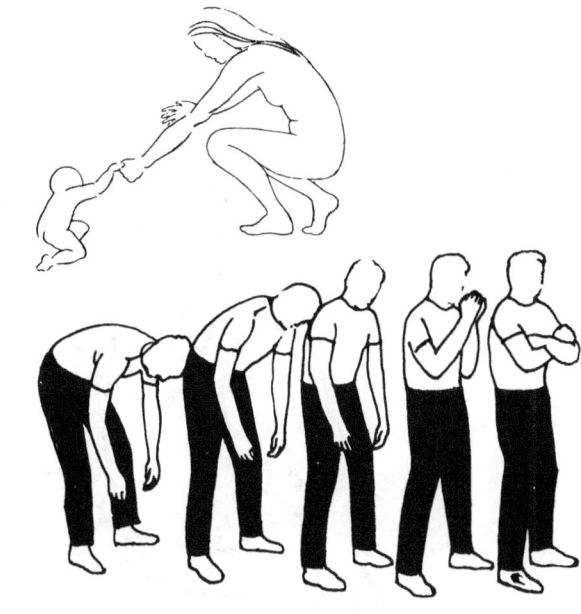

- beckoning a child into your arms.

Feel the natural breathing process in each of these characteristic postures.

- Bend over from the waist down. Breathe instinctively as you pretend to pick a flower, and continue inhaling and exhaling as, by degrees, you gradually bring the flower with you to upright. End by smelling the fragrant flower in the palm of your hand. Do this several times, each time adding more smoothness to the movement and feeling the flow and comfort of the C-curve.

- Check the illustrations and put yourself into each of these football positions. Breathe instinctively and naturally when experiencing them.

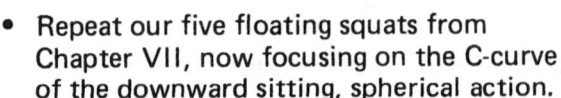

On the ready:
  one fist
  other fist
  both fists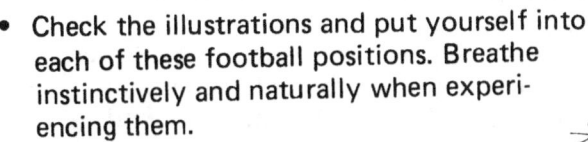

Set to go:
  one fist
  other fist
  both fists

- Repeat our five floating squats from Chapter VII, now focusing on the C-curve of the downward sitting, spherical action.

  - the flat-sole squat, heels on ground with toes apart;

  - the toe-stretch squat, on the balls of the feet;

  - the flat-sole squat, heels and soles on ground with toes pointing straight ahead;

  - the criss-cross squat;

  - the two-bladed squat, on the outside edges of the feet.

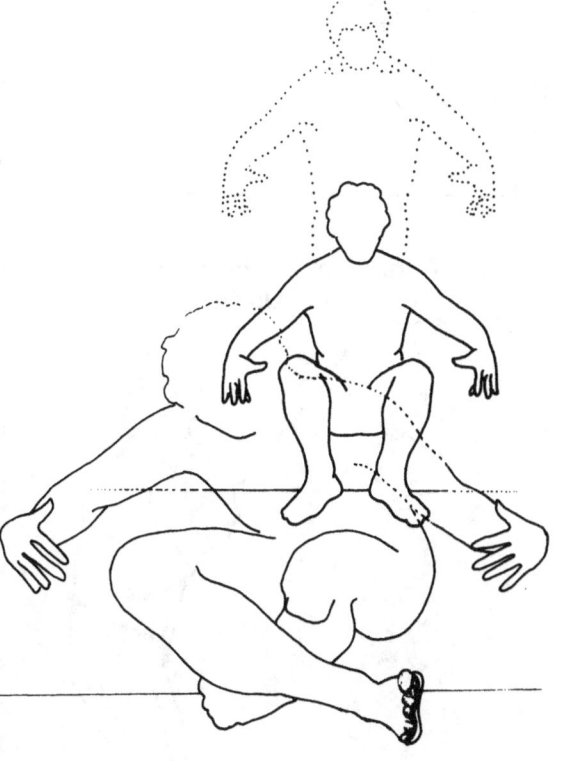

- The basketball dribble. As you recreate the feel of dribbling the ball over the court,

Energy and
Relaxation
in Movement

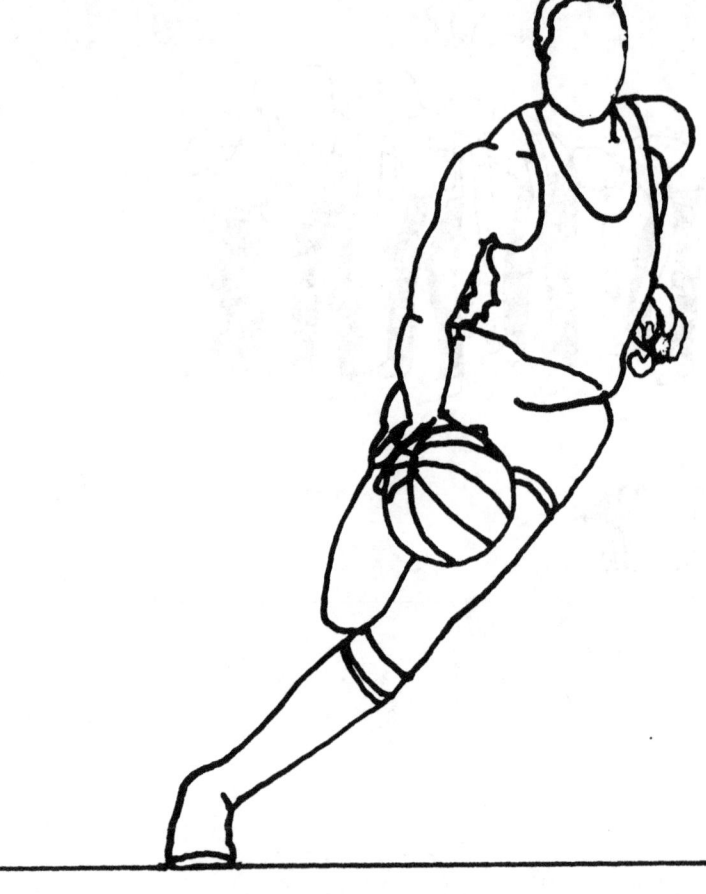

take note of your continuous C-curve movement, particularly its rhythm-feel and easy maneuverability; take note of your instinctive breathing action.

Transfer that same feel onto the low ball returns of an imagined, challenging tennis match.

In all of these exercises, you have no doubt registered the wave-like, combined action of instinctive breathing: a) the action begins in the lower abdomen, rolls gently toward the upper abdomen; and b) from there spreads the expansion to the sides; c) then to the relaxer-energizer center in the lower back; d) continuing to the large, broad back area; and e) finally waving around through the side and front expansion of the chest and rib-cage.

The familiar and comfortable "bridging activities" suggested below — and many more — are natural events that continue to induce the natural body curve with its instinctive breathing process. Feel that natural curve. Explore it and carry it over to the next set of bridging activities.

Experiment Two: Familiar Event Positions in the Upright

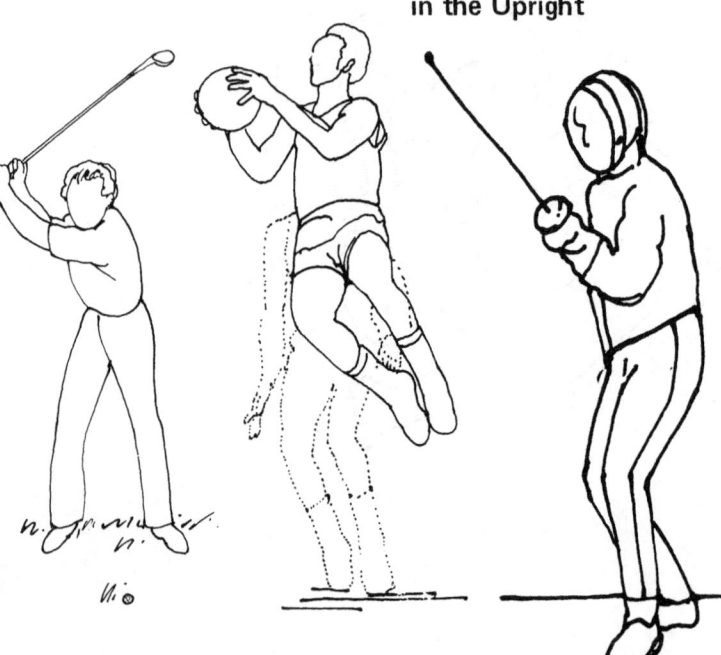

Recreate the position suggested by each cue and then check the illustrations for the different degrees of C-curves involved.

Breathe easily and comfortably in all of them.

- Golf:

- Basketball:

- Skiing:

- Fencing:

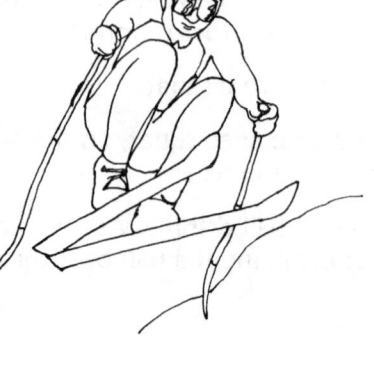

142

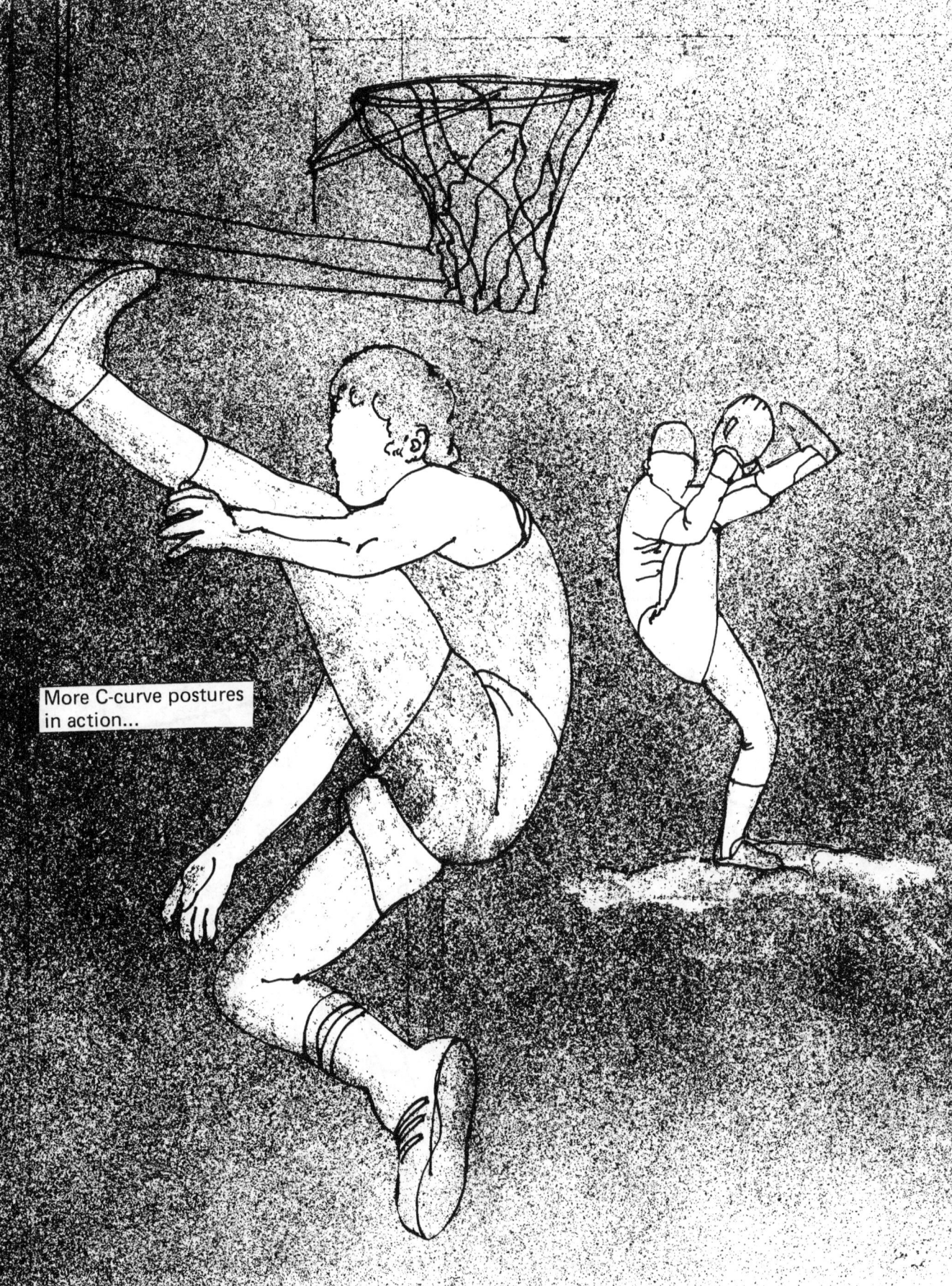

More C-curve postures in action...

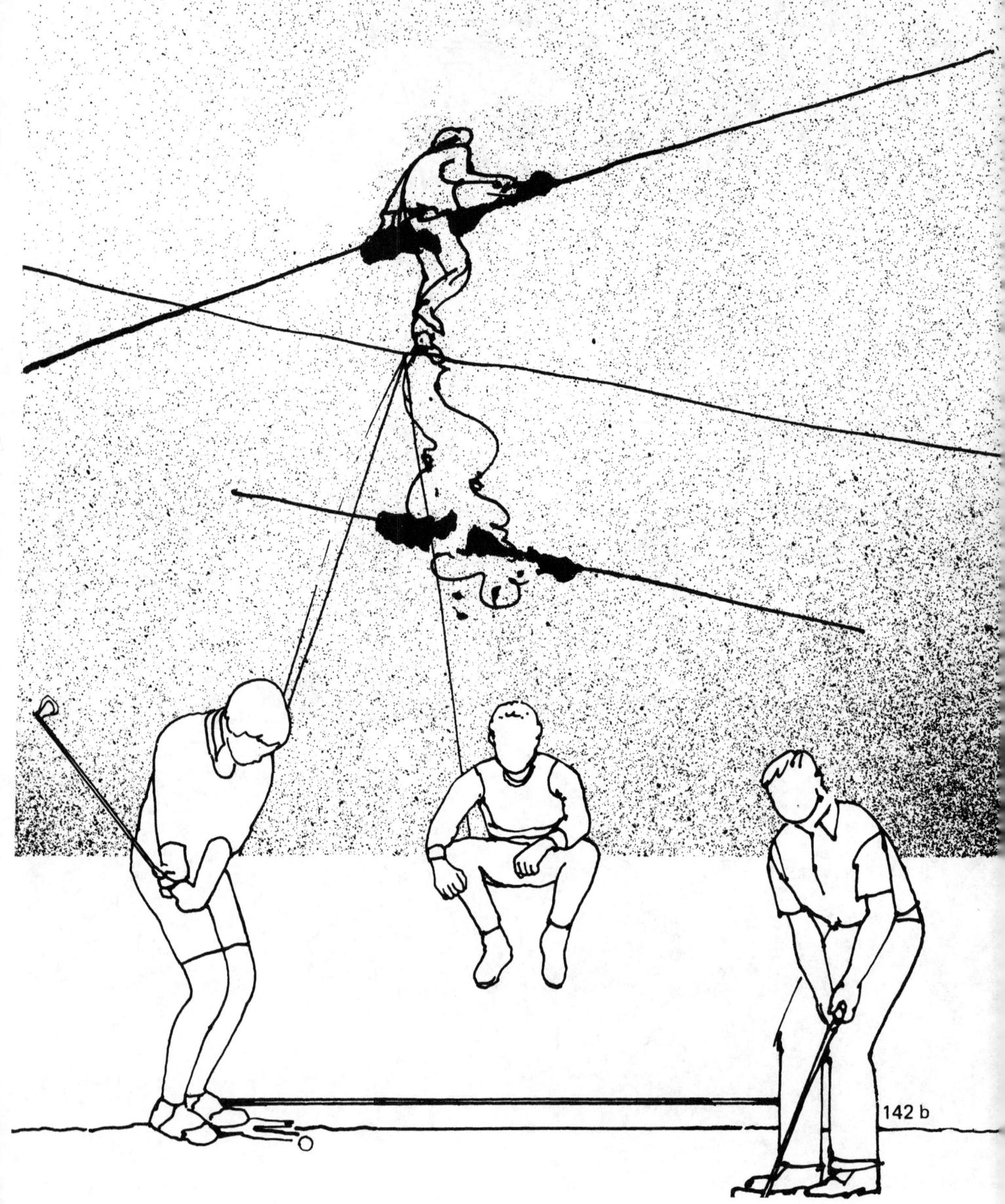

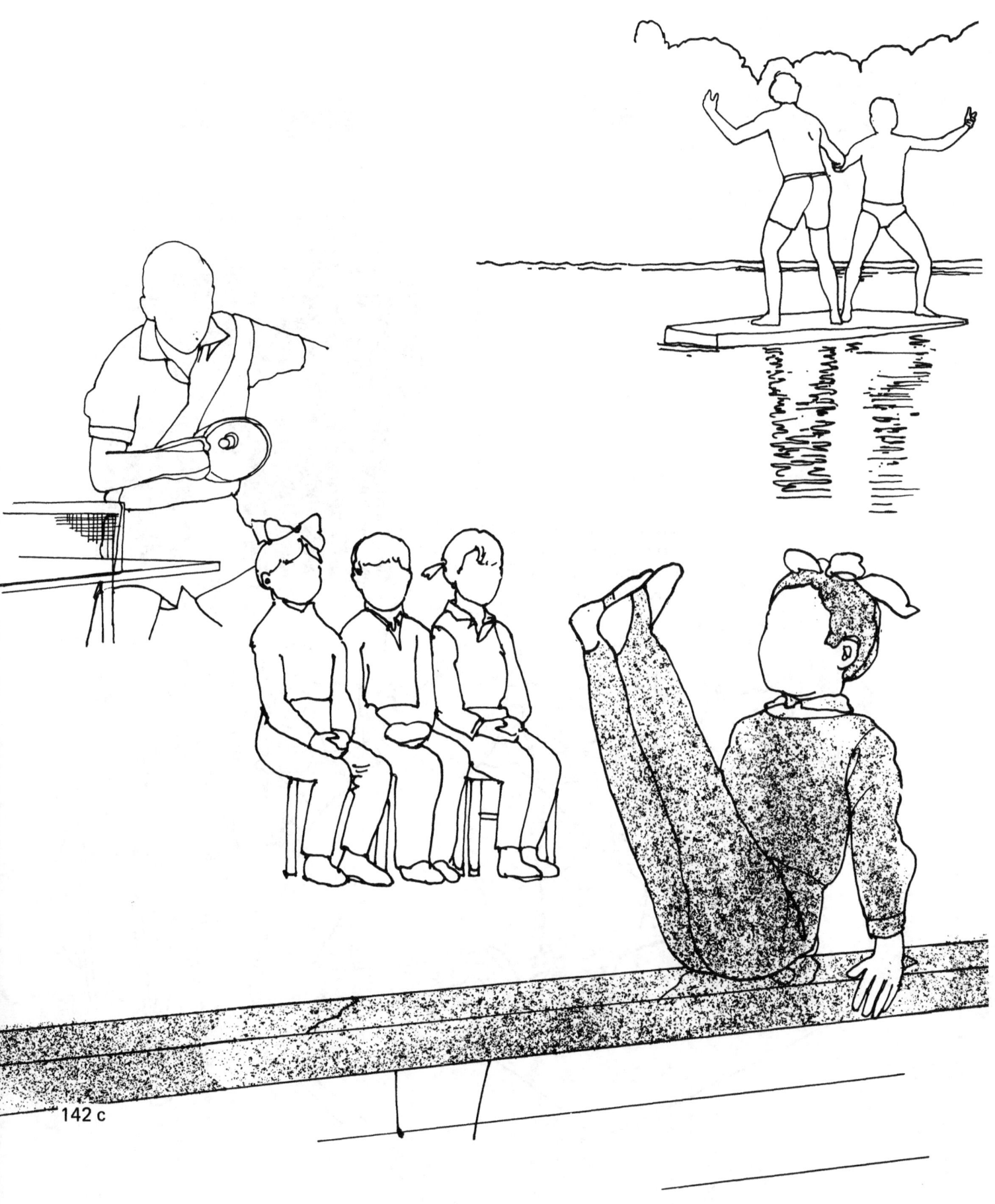
142 c

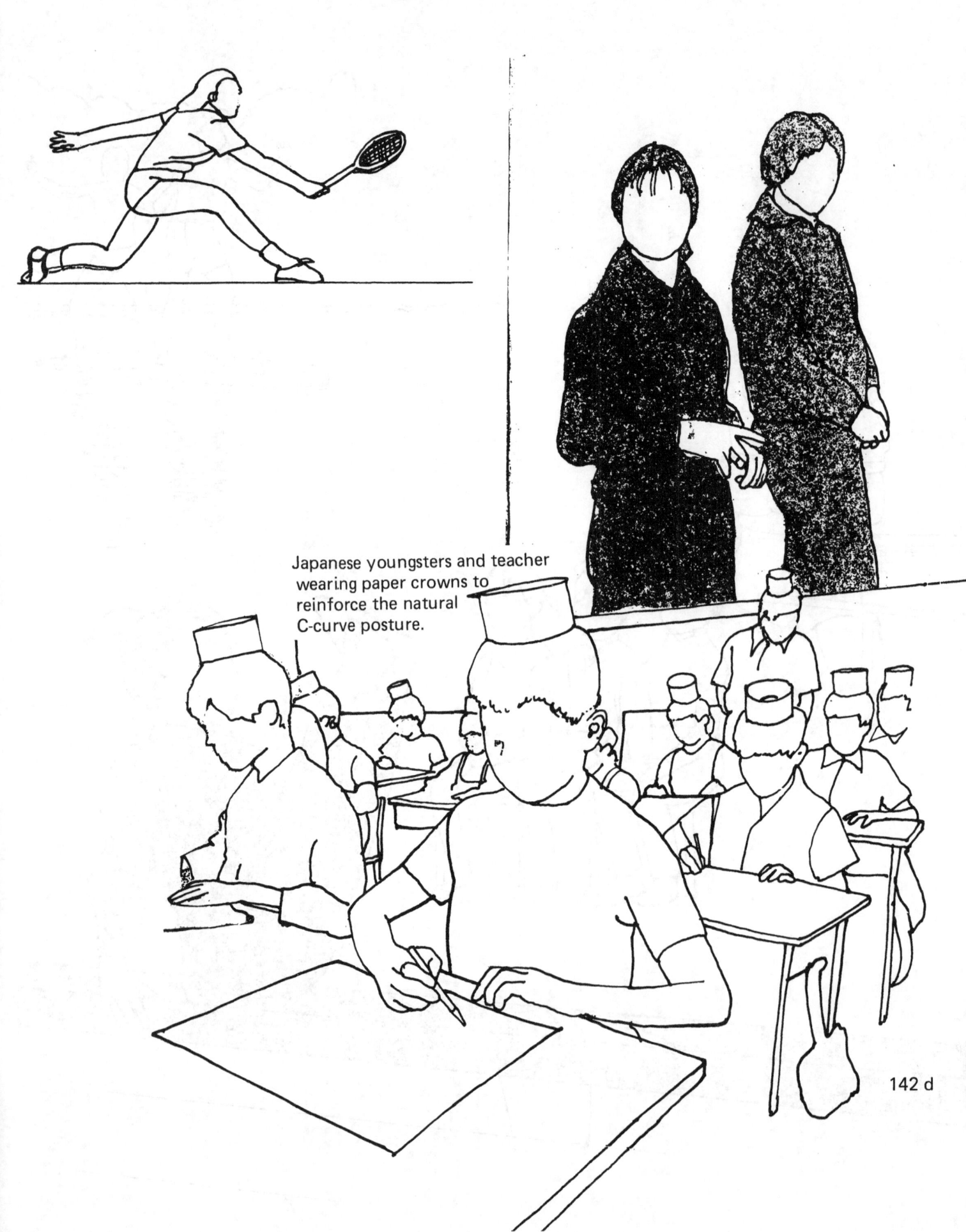

Japanese youngsters and teacher wearing paper crowns to reinforce the natural C-curve posture.

142 d

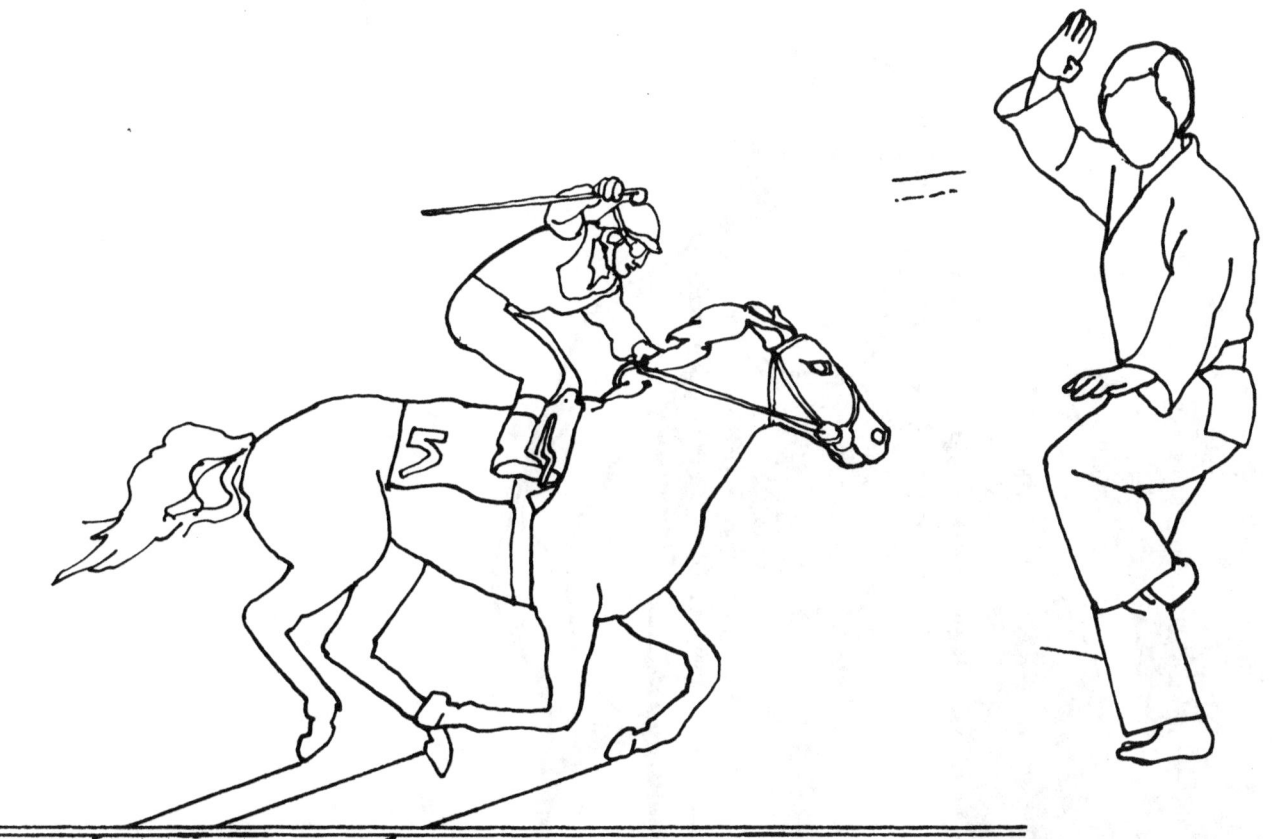
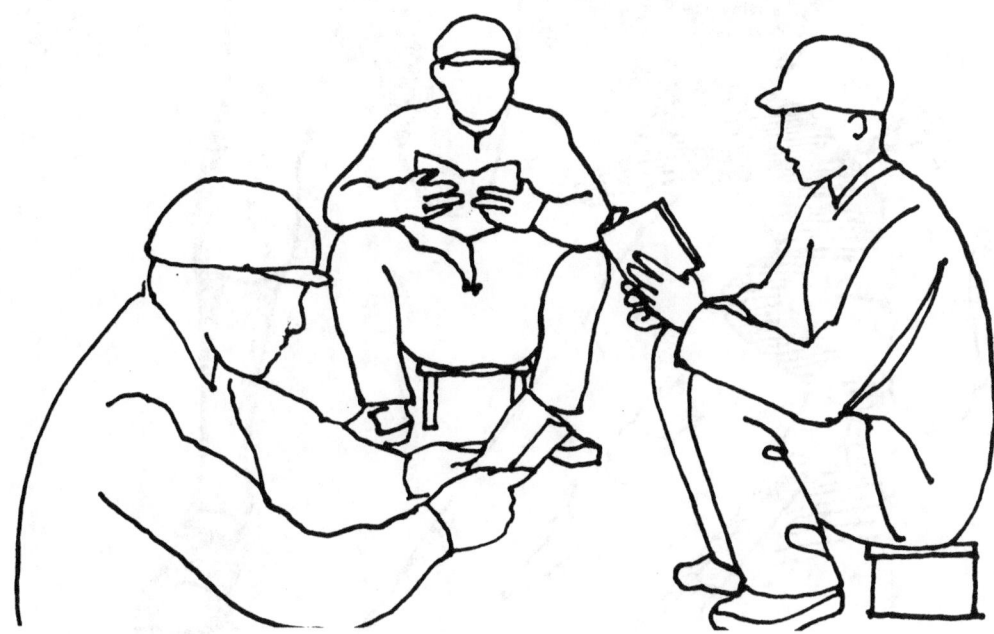

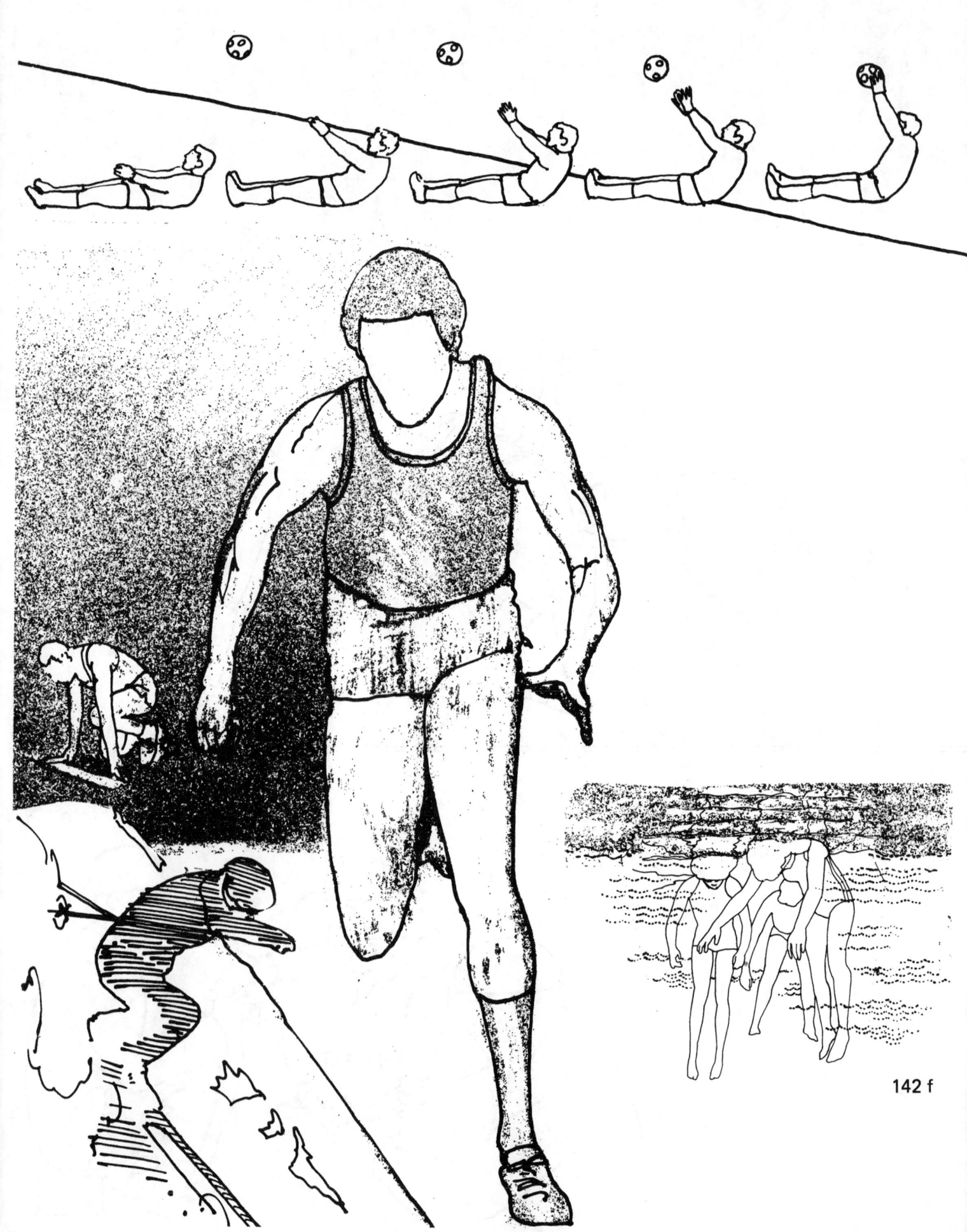
142 f

Body
Crescent
Standing Up

- Baseball:

- Tennis:

- Playing the violin

- Conducting an orchestra

- Sculpting

- Teaching or lecturing from a platform or in the classroom

   Sense and perceive the breathing experience in all these familiar events and transfer it to your own, consciously **normal** standing posture. Assess whether it feels precisely the same physically and esthetically as when you were hitting the baseball or leading the orchestra. Use your breathing process for **intentional** exploring.

Review the breathing associated with three of our primitive, non-derived energy states, but now put the breathing exploration into a three-part series and work through the series **standing up.** For most of our activities in the upright, buoyancy breathing is the preferred choice and closest to body esthetics.

Experiment Three: Breathing Related to Body Energy States

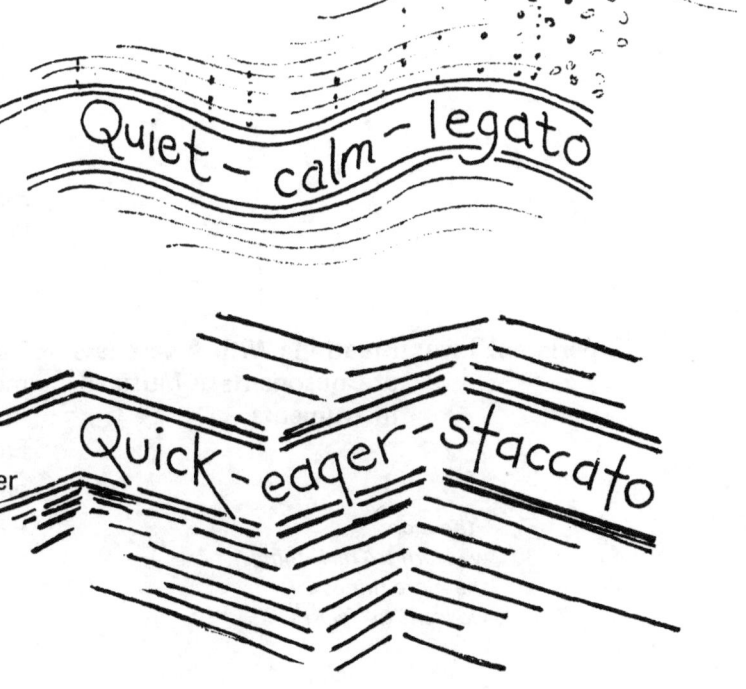

- Buoyancy: smooth, gradual legato and rhythmic breathing through the nose, with the tongue caressing the hard palate roof of the mouth and lips gently parted.

   ° inhale with rising buoyancy

   ° hold the breath with floating buoyancy

   ° exhale with settling-down buoyancy

- Radiancy: short, staccato, dart-like inhaling through the nose, with the front of the tongue running gently against the upper gum ridge, and lips comfortably parted.

Energy and
Relaxation
in Movement

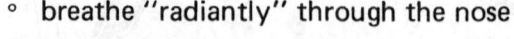

- breathe "radiantly" through the nose
- release the tongue from gums and/or palate and breathe lightly but "radiantly" through the mouth

• Potency: long, deliberate, inspired breaths.

- body-yawn muscle stretch with breathing through the nose
- face-mouth-throat-yawn with breathing through the mouth

Experiment Four: Breathing in Relation to Body Hygiene

A three-part exploration based on the concept that breathing through the nose warms and cleanses the air. The longer the passage of air, the warmer the air becomes with the hair cilia acting as natural cleansers.

*"discovering
additional energy-dynamics
is
an important process
of personal growth!"*

• Form an "M," with lips gently meeting while the upper and lower teeth are separated by approximately an eighth of an inch, and breathe delicately through the nose.

• Form an "NG" with the back of the tongue against the soft palate, lips apart, tongue-tip inclining gently downward, and breathe again through the nose.

• Form an "N" with the rim of the tongue, running it gently against the upper gum-ridge; breathe through the nose conveniently, and quietly, with lips and teeth apart.

How would you describe the different sensations?

Experiment Five: Breathing With Awareness of Consonants as Musical Instruments

Tasting the consonants as musical instruments and enjoying their music is a direct image that uses the device of metaphor. Satisfactory sensory perception of the taste and music of these instrumental consonants usually takes place on the exhalation.

*"the more
we learn to 'feel' things
the more things
we learn to 'feel'!"*

Body Crescent
Standing Up
(Breathing)

For purposes of breath training, bring each vocal sound as close to the associated sound of the orchestral instrument as you can. Sing melodies with it; play rhythms; create sound effects. The longer you feel the sensation on the inhalation and exhalation, the more practice you'll get in natural, instinctive breathing. For each vocal/orchestral sound listed below:

° breathe in quickly and exhale very slowly; then

° breathe in as quietly as you possibly can and at the same time, as slowly as possible; exhale the same way.

Listed below are the classifications in our instrumental "consonant orchestra."

First, the **Sound Effect Section** of the orchestra. These are all unvoiced breath sounds associated with wind-like and steam-like sound effects.

F as in snu**ff**, enou**gh**, **f**i**f**e, gra**ph**, hal**f**-way

S as in whi**s**per, a**s**k, ma**ss**, **c**ea**s**e, choi**c**e, voi**c**ed

SH as in wi**sh**, **sh**u**sh**, ba**sh**ful, bru**sh**ed

TH as in brea**th**, dea**th**ly, bir**th**day, ba**th**

H as in be**h**old, **wh**ipped, over**wh**elmed (pronounced: hw as in **h**wipped, over**h**welmed), and **h**ewn (pronounced: **h**yune)

Next, the **String Section**:

N (violin) as in incli**n**e, **n**oo**n**, e**n**ter, whe**n**, I**n**dian, e**n**d

M (viola) as in emba**lm**, e**m**pty, hu**m**dru**m**, di**mm**ed

"One develops the brain by finding new sources in the body for stimulating the senses!"

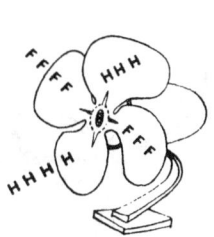
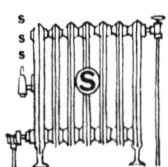

...make these sound effects soft yet keenly energetic; but no forcing of pressure — no escaping of breathiness!

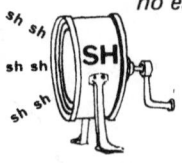

Image these as sound effects that add mystery to the orchestra!

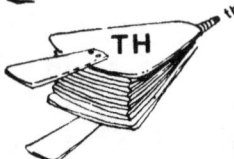

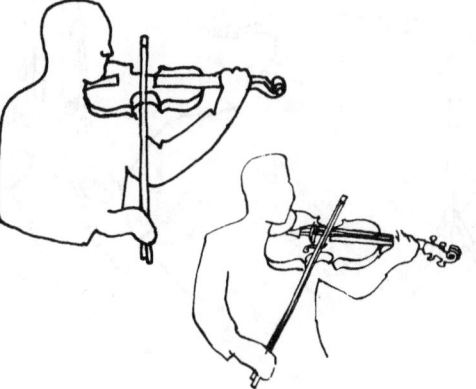

Energy and
Relaxation
in Movement

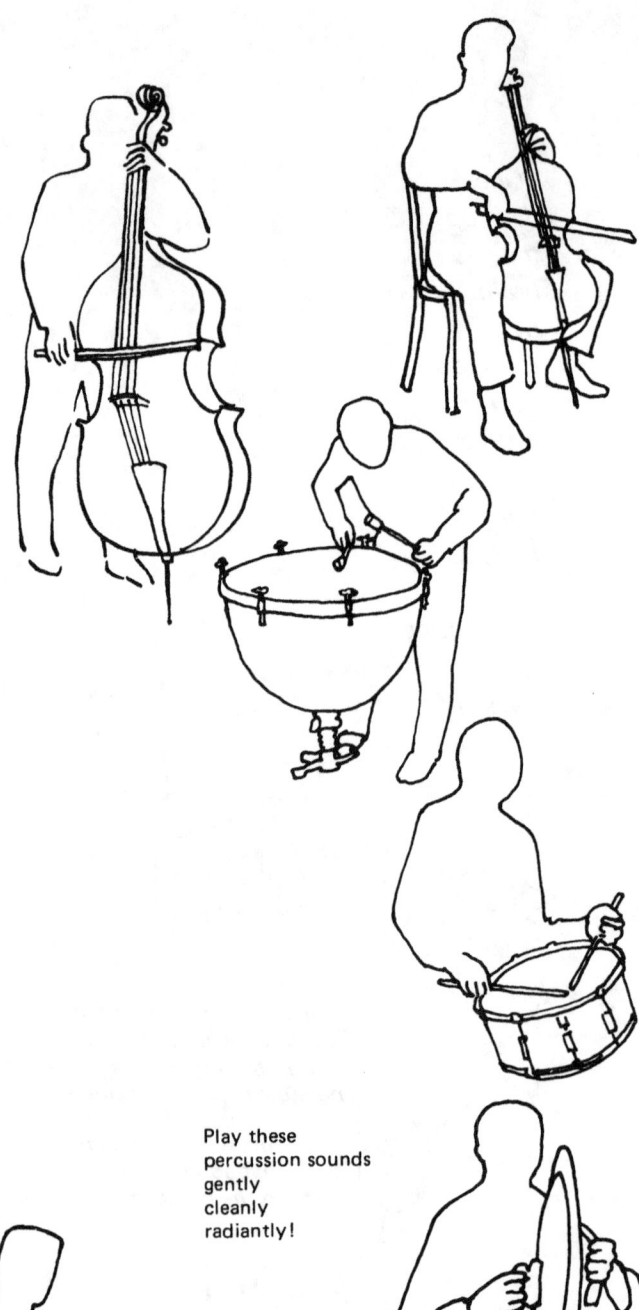

Play these percussion sounds gently cleanly radiantly!

V (cello) as in gi**v**e, themsel**v**es, lo**v**ely, positi**v**e

Z (bass fiddle) as in da**z**e, **z**ones, wi**s**dom, becau**s**e, Joe'**s**, hou**s**es

Taste the sound. Play it on the exhalation, sing a melody around it.

Now, the **Percussion Section** starting with

Tympani: (distinct, separated **voiced** drum-beat)

B as in jo**b**, o**b**vious, a**b**domen, co**b**web, a**b**horrence

D as in evolve**d**, a**d**vise, banne**d**, han**d**-made, hinte**d**

G as in lea**gu**e, su**gg**est, **z**i**g**-**z**a**g**, qua**g**mire

Drums (gentle, spring-away tap sounds):

P as in ro**p**e, ado**p**t, sto**p**, ti**p**-to**p**, clam**p**, ga**p**ed

T as in nea**t**, exci**t**emen**t**, reba**t**e, glance**d**, droppe**d**

K as in too**k**, atta**ck**ed, pla**que**, **c**o**ck**ney, **ch**e**ck**mate, monar**ch**, ti**c**, su**cc**ess

Cymbals (lightest tap-tap sounds):

DG (Chinese cymbals) as in fu**dge**, We**dg**wood, ra**ge**, encoura**ged**

CH (regular sized cymbals) as in ca**tch**, wi**tch**craft, ma**tch**ed, bewi**tch**, whi**ch**

TS (high-hat cymbals) as in ca**ts**, coa**s**t**s**, craf**ts**men, ha**t**e**s**, effe**cts**

DZ (tambourine) as in dee**ds**, husban**ds**, her**ds**man, buil**ds**, swor**d's**

Other Percussion (double clicks):

DL (woodblock) as in hur**dl**ing, cra**dle**, fon**dly**

146

Body Crescent
Standing Up
(Breathing)

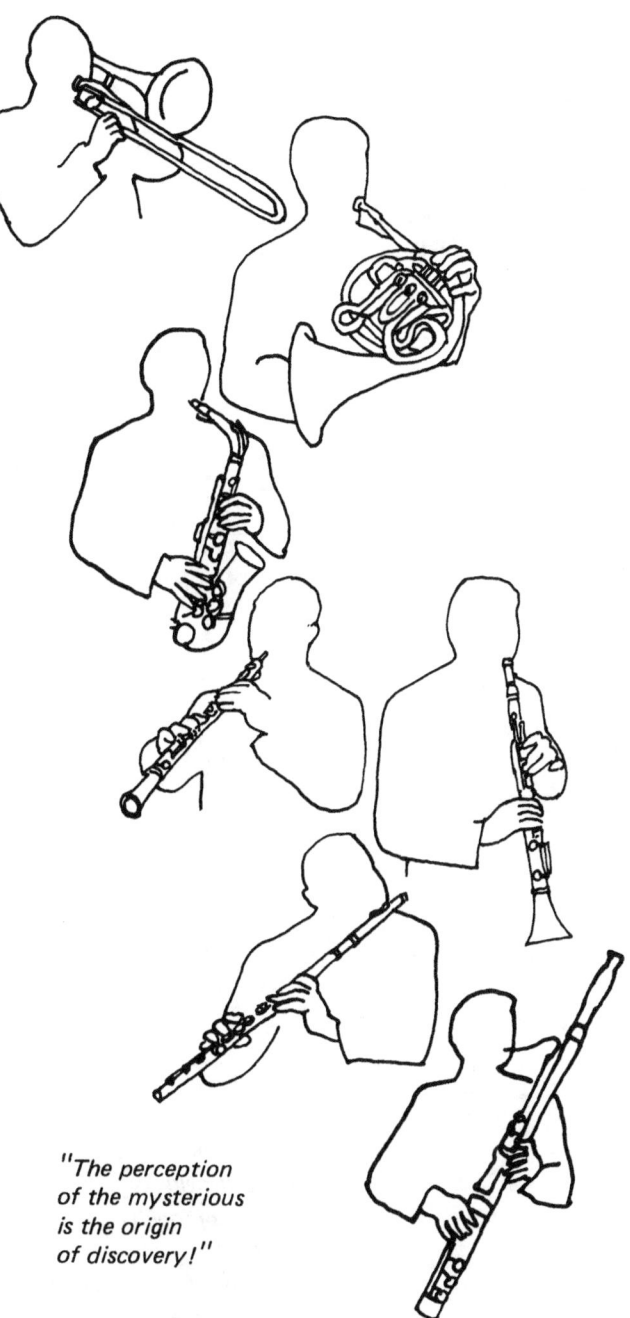

TL (woodblock) as in little, gentlest, exactly

The Brass Section:

R (trombone) as in roaring

Y (French horn) as in yesterday, beyond (Sustain a bit more to **feel the taste** of the French horn)

L (saxophone) as in old, level, kneel

And last, the **Woodwind Section:**

NG (oboe) as in tongue, seeing, things, swing and language

TH (clarinet) as in soothe, withdraw, breathe

W (flute) as in wigwam, away

ZH (bassoon) as in massage, beige, garaged, Taj Mahal, barrage (never played as a Chinese cymbal in these words)

Through the "consonant orchestra," you have been doing multiple variations on breathing, combined with vocal life; each a different experience, each a different sensation, a different musical esthetic, and a different breathing exercise. If the "consonant orchestra" holds special fascination for you, you can find more detailed explorations in *The Use and Training of the Human Voice* (PP. 132-171).

"The perception of the mysterious is the origin of discovery!"

These activities involve the physical experience of:

° a wide variety of emotions through the sense of smell;

° a range of different sighs;

Experiment Six: Breathing in Relation to Emotions

use these free marginal spaces for your own graphic designs that spontaneously tune you into these breathing-related emotions.

- gasps, yawns, sobs, and emotional panting;
- crying;
- laughing;
- trembling;
- shivering;
- sudden suprise, disappointment, and intense exhilaration.

All of these activities combine natural behavioral events with an awareness of that perfect equilibrium in the breathing process. When you learn to perceive and appreciate this, you expand your understanding and experience in sensing "breathing balance" as a generic component to be perceived in emotion-carrying behavior.

The **actor**, the **singer**, the **dancer** is in a general sense concerned with "emo-tivated breathing" every moment on the stage, but rarely understands it as an extension of a familiar event to a new and freshly unique situation, artfully integrated with movement, gesture, vocal life, characterization, "shadowing," subtext, etc. **The athlete** often goes through the gamut of emotions just before and during the application of highly tuned body skills to physical performance, but seldom, except for the great ones, turns these emotions to advantage through breathing designed to activate relaxer-energizers. All of us — at home, at work, at play — are incessantly involved with the by-play between our emotional and physical experiencing systems, but never stop to consider breathing as the transducer of positive energy from one to the other. That is why we are exploring here the **physicality of emotions** when there is nothing anxiety-provoking or disturbing to rattle our focus. The exercises that follow are meant to begin removing the self-consciousness, the

"the more
heuristic
the approach —
the more
holistic
the process!"

Energy and
Relaxation
in Movement

conditioned-impropriety, the fearful strangeness we have in dealing with such natural body esthetics as laughing, singing, dancing, yawning, etc. At the same time, we must begin to remove the conditioned fear reaction to sobbing, shivering, sighing, crying, trembling, and quivering — all of which have salutary effect upon the organism if we know how to exploit them with proper breathing. In other words, we need to provide instinctive breathing strategies for confronting the problem of the body's natural relaxer-energizers having been conditioned to function only in response to negative, threatening, or anxiety-producing situations.

...what different tempos, rhythms, flows, impulses, do you experience while exploring these breathing behaviors?

- **Emo-tivated Breathing Through The Sense of Smell**

To demonstrate exactly what we've been discussing, register the quality of breath produced by your instinctive reactions to the following situation: You are at home late at night and suddenly, you smell leaking gas. Your first thought is:

  ○ the house has been newly painted and all the windows are stuck tight;

  ○ you are all alone in the house;

  ○ your six-week old infant is fast asleep in your two-room apartment;

  ○ your invalid father is bed-ridden in the next room and can't be moved without professional help;

  ○ your parents are asleep; they're prone to hysteria and you **dare** not frighten them.

...do you find your breathing instinctively short, limited, economic and 'staccato'?

Your second thought is to seek out the leak without disturbing or frightening anyone in the house. In all probability, you will resort to a breathing rhythm that responds to the emergency with a quick, darting, staccato-like, 'smelling action' that relates to the

Energy and
Relaxation
in Movement

"Radiancy" energy state. In playing this role, you might even have felt the heaving and pounding of fear-induced breathing.

Now you wish to convert the situation. For purposes of control you change from "Radiancy" to "Buoyancy" breathing. You inhale slowly and deeply with rising buoyancy; exhale half-way and hold the breath for the feel of floating buoyancy which in this situation gives you a moment of calm pause to think through your options; then exhale fully and smoothly with settling-down buoyancy as you decide which option you'll take.

Now, compare the varying qualities of breathing (related through the sense of smell) experienced as you freely associate with the following, very different images.

— do you find that here you naturally breathe in long, inspired, and "legato" inhalations?

- It is a cool, lovely spring morning. You go to an open window and feel the fresh air coming right through the window and you are hungry for it. You want to get all of it into you because it makes you feel **so** good.

- It is summer, not cool but balmy. And you scent the fresh-cut grass and the trees swaying gently in the mid-summer breeze.

- You're moving through a crowded corridor and you get a strong whiff of exotic perfume that just passed by you.

- You now smell that same perfume on your wife — your mother — your secretary.

- You're doing the weekend shopping and as you go from store to store, you take in the aroma of rich, freshly ground coffee...a chocolate shop...a French bakery...a fast-food restaurant where

...hire yourself an image and draw yourself a graphic!

150

Body Crescent
Standing Up
(Breathing)

the frying oil is rancid. . .a fish and lobster market. . .

- You're traveling on a nearby turnpike or throughway and through the open windows of the car, you are bombarded with the odors of garbage, rotting food, industrial waste, and swampland smells.

- You're in a crowded elevator with no fan and you have to respond to "people odors."

- You are visiting a friend who has just undergone surgery and you are surrounded by hospital smells.

- You are in a garden and you smell a blooming rose-bush. . .or freshly turned soil.

...do you find yourself breathing 'stingily' and withholding your breath until the air clears?

The fact is: you respond differently to all of these "smells" or "aromas," with obvious bias even in the way you categorize or name them, depending upon how inhibited you are in their presence. We also tend to camouflage our responses when we don't want others to notice our reactions. Become aware of the different behavior rhythms, the contrasted reactions, and the varying qualities of breath that accompany emo-tivated response through the sense of smell.

- **Emo-tivated Breathing Through the Sigh**

A spontaneous sigh can be a most salutary, fulfilling breathing experience. It can also express contentment, deep disappointment, terrible tragedy, and considerable pleasure.

"if you really want to be responsive you must always find yourself in a 'moving state'!"

All are different. Discover these differences by practicing with a variety of sighs, each with its own expressive purpose, its own nuance and shading. Respond especially to the smooth, breath-rhythm of the easy, unintense sigh. You'll find that quiet, self-sustained, pleasurable sighs generally com-

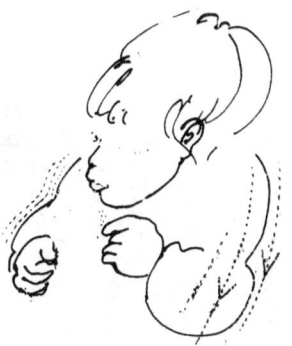

Energy and
Relaxation
in Movement

*...how do you
picture
your
'shivers'?*

bine an instinctively natural behavior-event with an awareness of healthful breathing, both activated in a state of perfect balance and equilibrium.

- **Emo-tivated Breathing Through Shivering**

   Experience the different breathing responses to different emotions that play into, and express themselves through, shivering. Situational contexts for emo-tivated shivering may include the following:

   ◦ You are out in the freezing cold fairly bundled up, but it is too cold to stay out very long...and you begin to shiver while breathing.

   ◦ You are out in the same cold, but underdressed for the weather and you start almost immediately to "shiver-breathe."

   ◦ You have just come out of the water, after a bracing, refreshing swim. The air is a bit breezy and just cool enough to induce mild shivering.

   ◦ You have just come out of a dry-hot, wood-scented sauna and you plunge into the cool clear waters of a mountain lake, and feel a tingling shiver go through your completely relaxed body.

   ◦ Practice shivering and breathing through the lips, letting your teeth chatter.

   ◦ Now shiver and breathe while your lips-teeth-tongue make the sounds: F — S — H.

- **Emo-Tivated Breathing Through Trembling**

*compose
your own
anatomy
of a
'tremble'!*

   Whereas shivering is associatively "weather-oriented," trembling, a basically similar physical activity, tends to be "fear-oriented." One trembles from fear, guilt, nervousness, unanticipated calamity, unsettling results, uncontrolled excitement, trepidation, etc. One can tremble from a weakened body

Body Crescent
Standing Up
(Breathing)

condition or from temporary disorder or imbalance of the nervous systems; and most interesting of all, one can tremble with no apparent physical cause.

- ° Recreate your own image-serving situations (as I presented here in the earlier emo-tivated breathing sections above) and respond with your varying "tremble-breath" behaviors and actions.

- ° Try trembling on different consonants with different sounds, i.e. F — V — N — NG — S — SH — H — L — etc., registering the feel of each.

- ° Improvise trembling situations that help you re-orient to it as a **positive** vibration or shake activity. Learn how to help its salutary action rather than hinder it through fear, anxiety, and apprehension.

- **Emo-tivated Breathing From Crying (Sobbing) and Laughing**

  Crying and laughing are truly "breath-emotive" activities. They can be loud or quiet, controlled or uncontrolled. They both involve panting, gasping, residual breathing, shaking, and quivering. As best you can, as though you were an actor, explore the breathing experience by experimenting with the following actor's explorations: (see page 101)

  - ° Explore crying and laughing by trying **not** to cry or laugh — by holding back the action.

  - ° Explore crying and laughing audibly, but gently.

  - ° Try to cry and laugh in full voice.

  - ° Now cry and laugh without apparent control.

  - ° Cry out of joy, then out of gratitude.

Explore!
    Taste!
Perceive!
    Discover!

    Do not pretend
or presume
    to play-act!

Energy and
Relaxation
in Movement

*...borrow
an image
from your
inner screen-
and
ride with it!*

- Try to laugh "with tears in your eyes."
- Try to belly laugh "till your belly hurts."
- Try to cry out of rage.
- Finally, explore crying and laughing on consonants in the order indicated below. Always start this last exploration quietly, privately, and imperceptibly, as though avoiding the action of crying or laughing publicly and noticeably.

The action always starts with a slight shiver or tremble for the "crying" improvisations, and with a vibrating smile or gentle shake in the "laughing" improvisations. Initiate this with each series of consonants:

S → Z → N → NG (NG as in sing)

F → L → L and NG together → G

N → S → V

SH → Y (Y sound as in be-yond)

Do not invite pain or hurtful stress in these explorations. Avoid heavy panting as it is an incorrect use of the body that can only be tolerated once we teach ourselves to do it correctly. On the other hand, the activities such as crying, laughing, sighing and the others suggested here are truly **explorations in learning how to aid in some of the body's natural healing process**. As such, they are more than just acting exercises, though in fact they serve the actor well. Likewise every athlete ought to have a full range of possibilities in the breathing process. Indeed, every one of us ought to have that range to exploit in our own personal repertoire of physical activities.

It should be clear by now that the sigh, tremble, shiver, laugh, and yes, also the cry, are really relaxer-energizers for the body. Even stressful panting can be converted into an esthetic — into a relaxer-energizer. Whenever the body's cardio-vascular system

*...between the "fundamentals"
of inhaling and exhaling,
lie the "harmonic overtones"
of:
..crying & laughing
..fear & joy
...anticipation & astonishment
..sobbing and panting!*

Body Crescent
Standing Up
(Breathing)

has been pushed too far (overburdened) and needs the "pant" for self-protection, one must immediately turn the heavy panting behavior into a firm sighing behavior, and the breathing process converts itself forthwith, into a comfortable, pleasurable activity.

- Through the nose (tongue in N position, lips and teeth parted) quietly, and aided by a gentle sigh.

  ◦ Breathing through the nose brings cleaner, warmer air to the lungs. The gentle contact of "front-of-tongue" to "front-of-hard palate" is the most comfortable way to breathe through the nose.

  ◦ Quiet and smooth breathing, in and out, is the body's most hygienic and energy-gathering way to breathe. The resulting feel, as you know well by now, is that of rising buoyancy on the inhalation and floating buoyancy on the slight pause before returning to settling-down buoyancy on the exhalation. It is the very essence of comfortable "sigh-breathing."

  ◦ Breathing must feel good, fulfilling, and vitalizing. The quiet, gentle rhythmic sigh of satisfactory appreciation is the best and most esthetic way to inspire and accommodate breathing energy.

- In comfortable, natural breathing:

  ◦ There is little noticeable body action — no push-pull-lift action of the belly, chest, sides, or shoulders. Instead, one feels only the soft billowing of gentle back inflation.

  ◦ There is the feeling, as in Experiment One, of a combined, complete breath experience. This is so whether the

Experiment Seven: The Best Way to Breathe for Psychosomatic Health

". . . that which produces 'peace of mind' is good maintenance —

that which disturbs it is poor maintenance;

your BODY is your mind's 'maintenance man'!"

expansion travels only to the lower-back energy center through a "complete small breath" (so-called "shallow breath"); whether it continues to travel to mid-back through a "complete half-breath;" or whether it extends its action through the upper-back energy center and around the chest/rib cage to a "complete full breath."

- All that is necessary to replenish your breath supply is a flick of the tongue back to the "N" position with lips and teeth parted. The complete small breath, half-breath, or full breath which combine the same body responses only in different degrees of back expansion, is sufficient to provide you with a refill of "instant breath."

We have spoken at length about the salutary effects of breathing through the nose. The fact is that while talking and maintaining smooth utterance, we have little recourse but to breathe through the mouth as well. Clearly, during normal speech, there is insufficient time to stop and breathe through the nasal tract; this would only pre-occupy the tongue, lips, etc. from their proper business of comfortable everyday speech (involving both consonants and vowels).

Also, communication becomes ineffectual when phrasing, inflection, intonation, and rhythm are interrupted or disturbed by open-gap breath hiatuses. In addition, the spontaneous tempo and involvement of conversation often prevents the quiet, controlled equilibrated breathing through the nose. This explains why, particularly on stage, the noise and character of forced "nose-breathing" is not esthetic and negatively affects the actor's performance or the communicating personality in general.

Body Crescent
Standing Up
(Breathing)

So while mouth-breathing is not the most hygienic, salutary, or esthetic practice, there is small choice during the stream of involved talking. Vocal life **does**, however, appreciate all the help it can get. During pauses or breaks or listening moments, you can and should return reflexively to nose breathing. Otherwise, the mouth breathing can become labored, turn to panting, and forcibly (psychophysically) impose an unintended change in the emotional climate.

Some of you may want to explore breathing through single nostrils. Any such additional variations are welcome and you ought to explore them, as long as you stay clear of noise, force, push, pull, strain, or pressure. We will suggest additional breathing activities when we come to our posture, running, and lifting work. For now, it is important to approach the "perception of being upright" with eight basic conclusions about breathing energy.

1. There exists a strong relationship between breathing and internal exercising of body organs and inner structure.

2. Breathing is a distributing agent that cleanses the body and picks up muscle waste.

3. Buoyant "sigh" breathing returns you quickly to relaxed respiration and body comfort, even after a strenuous, rugged workout (or after an unnerving emergency).

4. Because fear limits and inhibits easy, regular breathing, our physicalization of the breathing experience helps reduce anxiety, dispel fear, and liberate inhibition.

5. Breathing can be "felt" as a vital, distributing force throughout the entire body that you can learn to respond to, and follow psychophysically with your blood circulation,

radiating heart beat, kinesthetic energy, and nervous energy.

6. There is a close relationship between respiration and perception, between physicalized breathing and the exploration of emotions.

7. Whatever your current reaction, you can teach yourself to respond to these relationships consciously, as well as subtextually, with more spontaneous awareness, greater integrity, and more realistic application.

8. Proper and instinctive breathing behavior is an important therapy instrument in clinical conditions such as: stuttering, cleft-palate, hysterical aphonia, chronic throat conditions, and other articulatory disorders.

POSTURE and ALIGNMENT

Having explored breathing activities rather intensively, let us consider just as intensively the other half of the Breathing/Posture cognate: **the perception of being upright!**

"Being upright" presents new vistas of seeing, hearing, and reaching out. Anxieties laid low during our evolving process are perhaps now fanned anew. Concerns and questions regarding one's communicating personality, body personality, and emotional personality rear their little heads again and whisper incitingly: "How do I look? — How do I sound? — Am I making a fool of myself? — Do they believe me? — Do they like me? — Do I walk funny? — Do I stand up straight? — How am I projecting? — How do I feel?"

Once in the upright, our relationship to the outside world, counterweighted against the sensing, understanding, and imagining of our emotional experiencing system, be-

Body Crescent
Standing Up
(Posture)

gins again to impinge upon us. If these inevitable impingements are not to become fixations, we must learn to perceive ourselves in the upright in such a way, with such integrity, that we can avoid measuring ourselves exclusively or primarily against the outer environment.

So let us return to the body for instruction. Let us continue the evolving process by unfolding the body curve into upright structure; and responding to at least five levels of perception that will help to safeguard the body, especially in the upright, from further deterioration or imitative behavior.

"Being upright" includes:

1. The perception that breathing and body alignment depend, relate, and respond each to the other. If outer-environment influences induce or condition us to "blow out the chest" and "accordianize" the spine's vertebrae, we shall destroy or inhibit natural healthy respiration and sound cardio-vascular condition. If, on the other hand outer conditioning encourages shallow, depressed breathing, such suppression will produce, among other things, a caved-in chest and over-rounded shoulders that adversely affect the neck line and head position.

2. The perception that body joints, hinges, weight distribution, anatomical relationships, and body balance must now enter a new phase of consideration and awareness regarding the body in movement.

3. The perception that body "jointedness" is pivotal to that fundamental curve as it progresses and evolves into wheels, circles, and loops.

4. The perception that "standing still" involves the sensation of "posture as a form

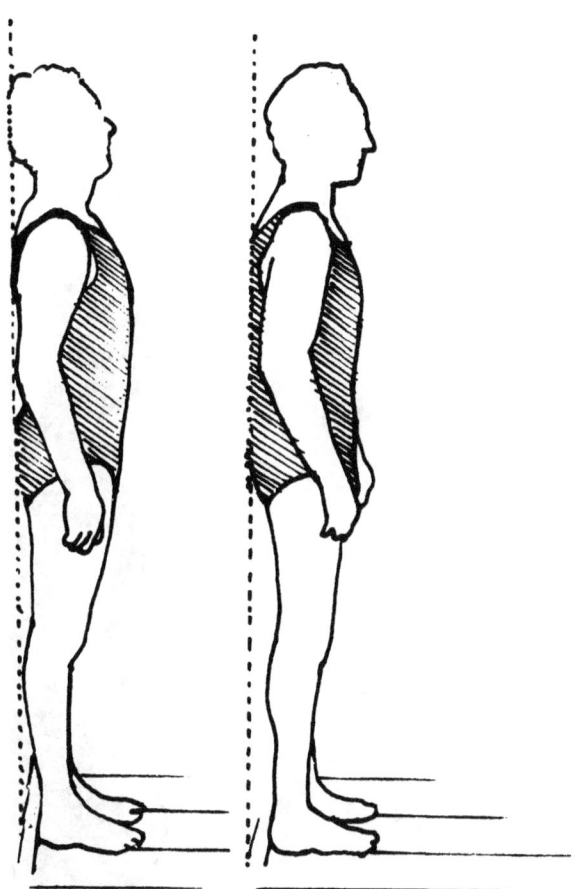

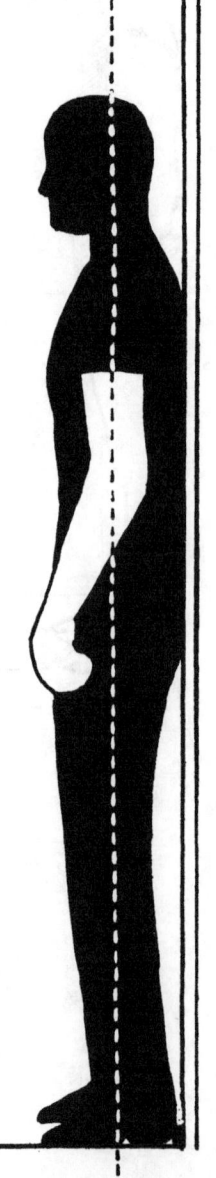

of **movement.**" We don't really stand **still,** do we? What we really do is **experience the feeling of movement while standing** — as an activity in balance, rhythm, and energy; as a new experience in rising buoyancy, resting up and resting down, and live weight versus dead weight. Not only is upright posture a **form** of movement — it can be sensed as the **continuation of movement,** and the continued extension and expansion of the elongated body curve.

5. The perception of every seeming straight line in the body as curved or bent, and therefore not really straight at all. This key perception allows us to respond to **the body in the upright as a curvo-linear structure** and not, as is widely held, as a rectilinear one. Thus, the joints and hinges become intrinsic parts of the curve itself, rather than merely angular connectives between two straight lines.

This last perception warrants closer attention. The only straight line we can admit, in regard to upright posture, is an imaginary one that runs along an internal axis from the top of the head to the soles of the feet, through the precise center or inner core of the body. A graphic visualization of this theoretical inner axis is represented in the illustration.

Otherwise, our experience suggests that the gentle parenthesis curve of the spinal back is the organic image-instruction that best conveys the most natural and optimal body line and structure. Our investigations further indicate that the more the dorsal curve progressively elongates along a single, convex line, the closer the body comes to a perfect integration of alignment and balance. Hence, the single convex curve of the outer spinal axis equals the single straight line of

Body Crescent
Standing Up
(Posture)

the body's inner core. And it would seem that an axiomatic, architectural principle also applies to the functional model of the human body: that whereas curves are strong and resilient, straight lines tend to be comparatively weak and brittle.

We are discussing here **viable posture**. Anything viable must continue to be capable of growth, development, movement. Applied to upright posture, viability necessarily implies "natural" body articulations, alignment, and energy states. But by "natural," I mean neither habit-patterned functioning nor the way most anatomy texts illustrate "normal" human posture. In fact, the standard anatomical charts reveal only the outer-conditioned behavioral pattern and structural **deformity** of body posture.

For only a very brief period in infancy do we maintain a truly natural, unconditioned and of course, very pliable spine line and posture. Though the body potential is there to sustain this organically natural condition into adulthood, it is almost immediately conditioned away by imitation and improper early guidance toward **un**natural, distorted misuse of the body. What results is a "distorted norm" that is passed on to us as "normal" in the anatomical texts, which deal only with what **is** rather than what is meant to be.

If posture pairs up with alignment, weight distribution, balance, lightness, rhythm, and movement, along with breathing, it should follow that each of these energetic-esthetics strengthens the other and influences the other qualitatively and creatively. However, this occurs only when we perceive upright posture as conforming to an interdependent, curvo-linear structure.

The bone structure of the spine consists of vertabrae which I regard as "ellipsoid-type"

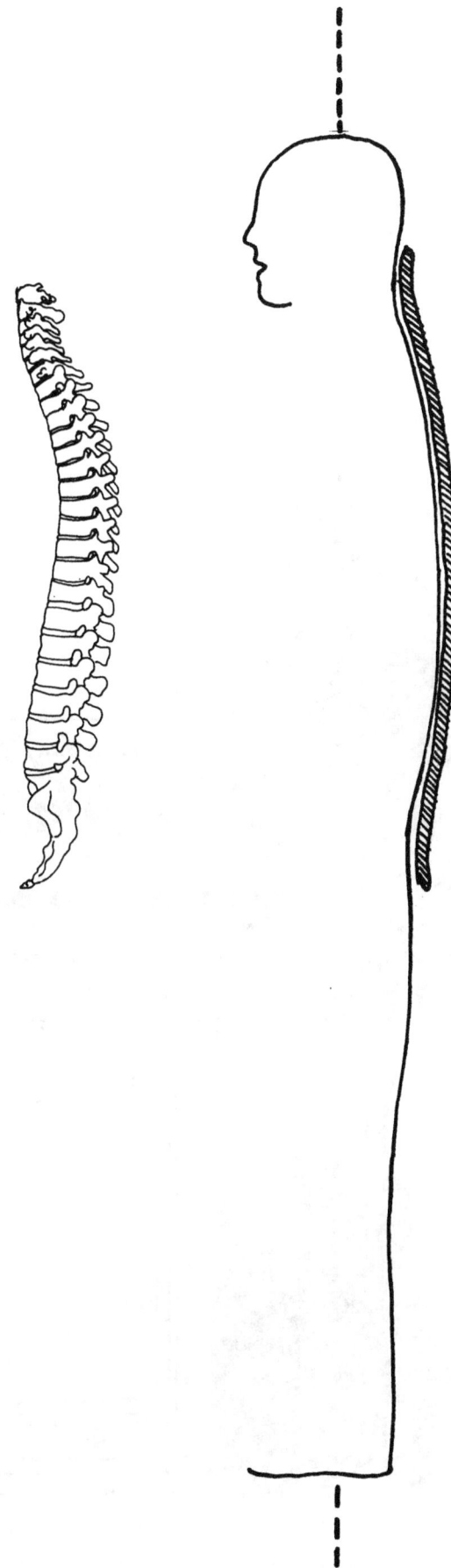

Energy and
Relaxation
in Movement

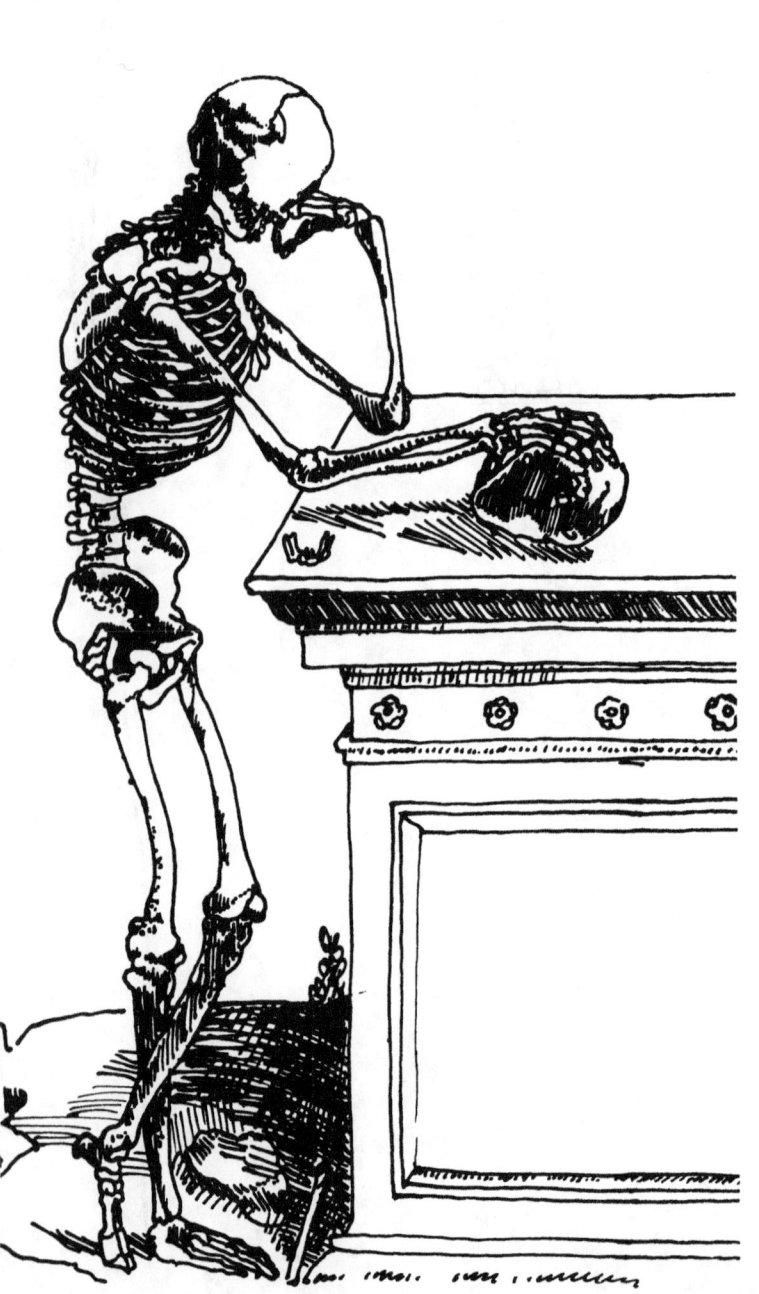

hinge-joints. Check the illustrations and note that when the joints of the spine swing to a forward "bend," a natural articulation of the spine joints results. Conversely, when they swing to a backward "bend," there is imposed a spinal articulation that can easily lead to fracture or pain. Within the gamut of the human spine's **natural** articulation, it bends, curves, and stretches with relative impunity.

The parenthesis curve of the spinal column should be viewed on your inner "screen" as starting from the top of the head with a continuing flow right down to the pelvis-coccyx. It then branches off into the thighs and legs, forming a progressively graduated C-curve from the top of the head into the hollow of the knees. It is in such a graduated C-curve that the back and spine contribute so much, and so mightily, to body leaping, springing, running, climbing, walking, and sitting.

Another image to keep flashing onto your mental screen, as part of organic instruction, is the interplay between the shape of the back spine and the form of the front body surface. Specifically, when the dorsal body surface is extended in convex shape, the front body surface takes on a complementary, concave form. When, on the other hand, the back spine is formed into one or more concave shapes, the front surface, in complementary response assumes an awkward, belly-protruding (convex) character.

Notwithstanding opinion to the contrary, it is clear to us that the adult spine and back, multi-curved into an "S" form and other deformities, does not enjoy natural, structured alignment; and in almost any physical activity, such distortion could do real bodily harm. Only when we have taught ourselves the perfectly natural articulations and alignment, and only

162

Body Crescent
Standing Up
(Posture)

in emergency situations or in required professional use, should we tolerate the radical concave back-stretching or back-bending; and then, only if we have also taught ourselves, viscerally and cortically, **how to do the incorrect correctly!**

As indicated above, the vertebrae of the spine are actually hinge-like joints that move in more or less oval manner. The vertebrae, along with joints of other types and movement — knee joints, pelvic hip joints, shoulder, ankle, toe, finger, wrist and elbow joints, as well as jaw-bone joints and hinges — are for us, absolutely central to body health and function.

Joints and "jointedness" maintain the body's curvo-linear construction and bear a direct, structural relationship to its manifold curves. Abrasive treatment to any of the body's joints not only distorts one's appearance, but does serious injury to one's psychosomatic health.

For most of us, body jointedness remains one of the least understood, and routinely misunderstood, areas of human physiology. The experiments of this second part of "The Body as a Crescent — Standing Up" provide objective evidence of the intimate relationship between jointedness and the perception of being upright. Specifically, they offer self-teaching strategies for developing:

1. awareness of the natural and unnatural articulations of body joints;

2. sensation and awareness of ever-present looseness and living space within the joints; and

3. perpetual avoidance of pressure-weight "feel" in or upon the joints during

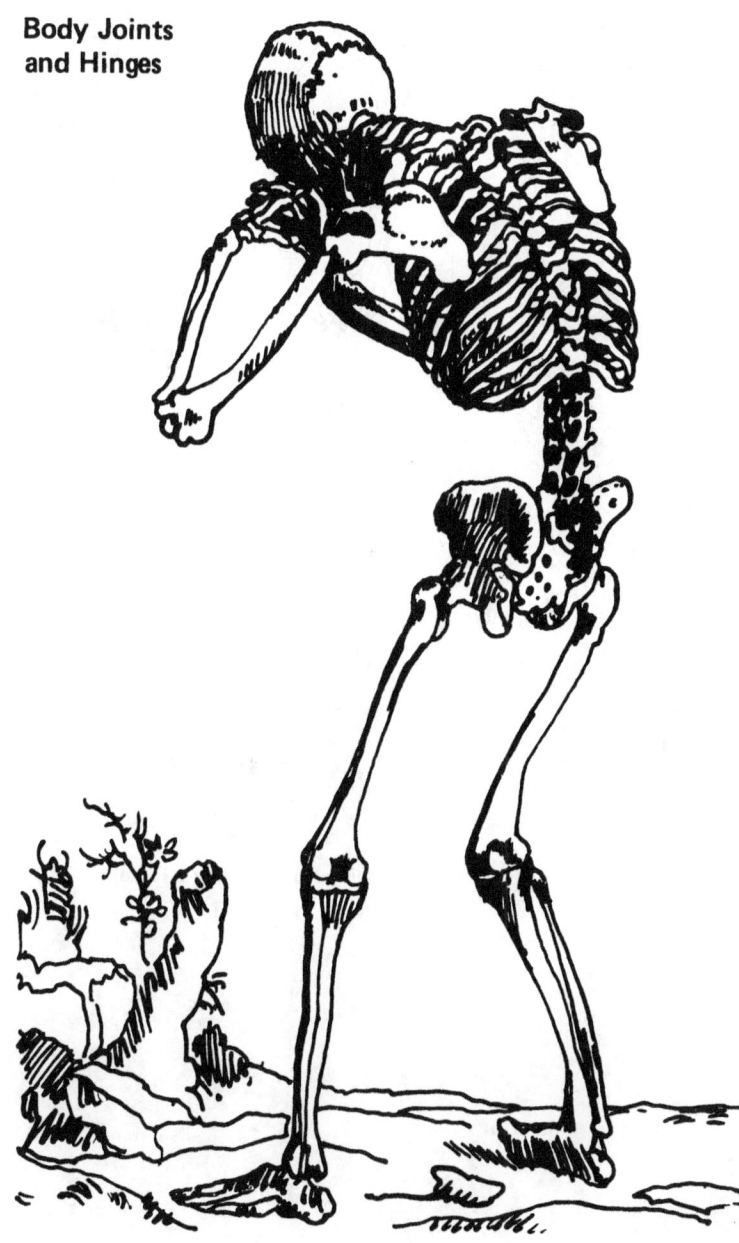

Body Joints
and Hinges

Energy and
Relaxation
in Movement

physical activity, be it dancing, gymnastics, running, or carrying heavy groceries.

A pressured joint forces a pressured overcrowding **within** the body environment. If you want to "stay loose-jointed," while still enjoying the body's different energy states, then you will also want to avoid "tennis elbow," "housemaid's knee," weak wrists or ankles, lower back pains, neck tension, and tight "rusty jaw."

Since every joint has its own natural articulation and direction, consistent with its individual structure and protective device, each accommodates its own optimal latitude for movement — whether that movement is one-way, two-way, criss-cross, or circular. By "latitude," we mean to suggest a bit of scope and range in the movement of the joint; a freedom from confinement, an "emergency shoulder" alongside the highway for the driver in trouble. One purpose of the joint is to maintain this latitude as a subtle, physical "safety cushion" to reinforce body balance, flexibility, agility, and special awareness. Thus, any joint, with whatever is connected to it, can articulate maximal motion without ever feeling tight, locked, or forced. Only pressure brought to bear from the outside, that disrespects this natural latitude and articulation, will lock the joint into a rigid jaw, a tennis elbow, a locked knee, a lower back pain, a stiff neck, etc.

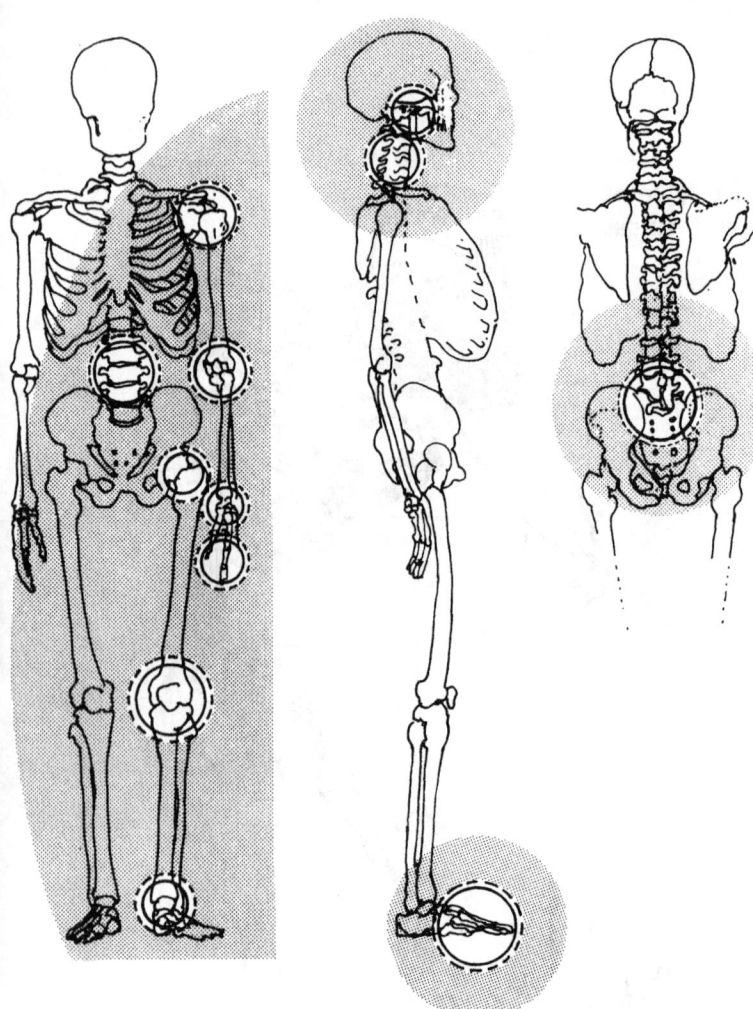

Joints and hinges in the body structure

Primary training activities for developing movement and flexibility in body joints fall into radiancy, shaking, swinging, rowing, and rope-skipping classifications. However, almost every physical action involves "joint participation," as the body in movement is controlled by many more joints than one generally considers.

Body Crescent
Standing Up
(Posture and
Alignment)

- Follow the graphic instructions. Dotted lines indicate body expansion resulting from breathing action.

- Breathe in each gradation of posture change, as illustrated, and elongate the C-curve according to the degree of body expansion produced by inhaling and exhaling.

- When you reach a comfortable, but still casual upright posture, complete the breathing experience by pretending to smell a fresh flower in the palms of your cupped hands.

- **The Head**
    - Your head should be as high as possible at the crown point. If the crown is the tallest part of the body, then the head is level and can swivel from side to side without tilting. Also, the chin will neither protrude nor stick into the neck; the head is neither held up nor held down.
    - Send a rising-buoyancy feel up through the back of the neck and cervical spine joints first into the crown of the head, and then forward from there toward the forehead and face.
    - The back top of the crown will feel as though it is attached to invisible helium bags constantly urging it skyward.
    - The measurement of the back of the neckline will be at least two inches longer in the parenthesis posture than in the usual, rigid S-curve.

- **The Neck**
    - As indicated earlier, the cervical area of the spine must be as elongated and extended as possible.
    - It should feel like a continuation and part of the shoulder and back muscles.

Experiment One: Breathing Yourself into Upright Posture — From the Large C-Curve to the Longest "Parenthesis" Curve

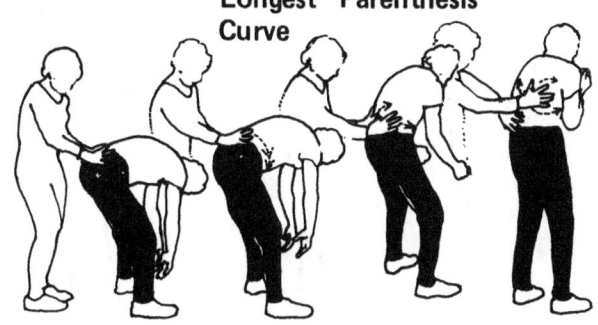

Experiment Two: Survey Your Own Perception of Being Upright

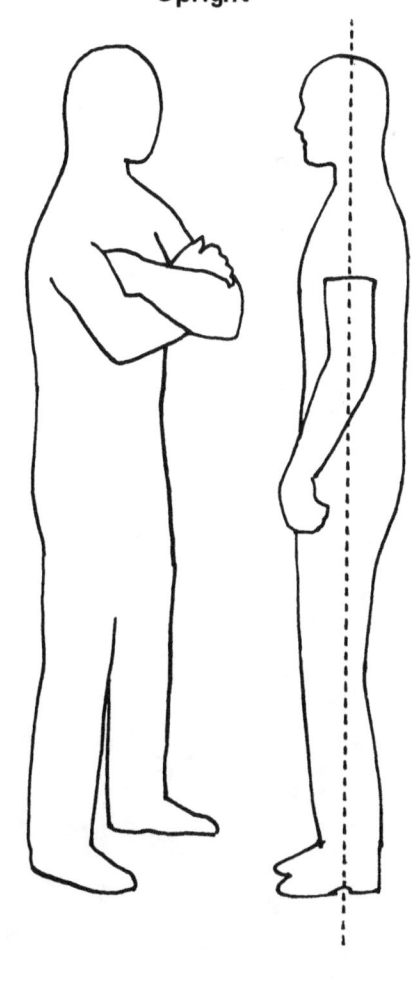

Energy and
Relaxation
in Movement

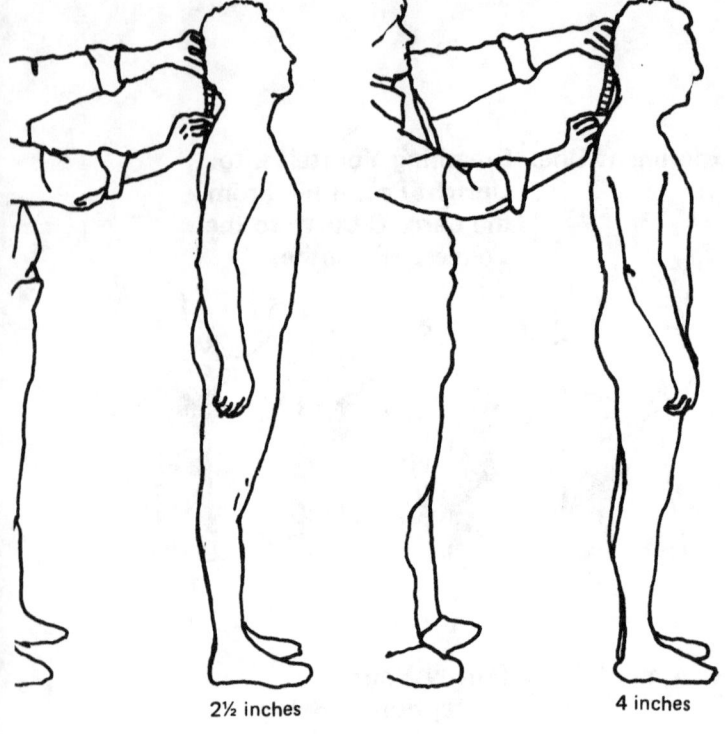

2½ inches   4 inches

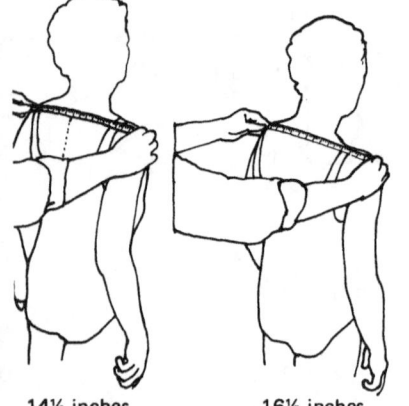

14½ inches   16½ inches

We're actually dealing here with the "trapezius muscle" which is distributed over most of the back, most of the shoulders, and the back of the neck.

° You should feel that the neck is being extended by this muscle, rather than contracted by it. Remember: the contraction in the back of the neck is responsible for a good deal of tension. As mentioned elsewhere, this part of the body contains more nerve tissue than any other part except the brain itself; and when misused or abused, becomes susceptible to tension headaches, "rigid jaw," tense neck, and tightened throat muscles.

- **The Shoulders**

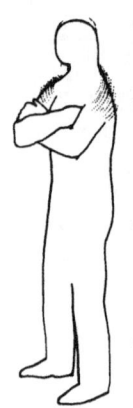

° The shoulders should enjoy maximum muscle looseness and extension.

° The shoulder joints should feel as though they gently slope around in forward direction.

° With good, relaxed, really normal posture, the arms appear to rest slightly in front of the thighs.

° Compared to shoulder measurement with poor posture, the shoulder line will be at least two to three inches longer with the proper posture.

- **The Upper Back**

° The back should feel broad and extended, as though attempting to fit a snug garment.

° A radial flow of lambent energy appears to move out from the relaxer-energizer center in the upper back.

° The pleasant sensation of an extended fit around the upper back area will remind you very much of an incipient, muscle-yawn feel.

166

Body Crescent
Standing Up
(Posture and
Alignment)

- **The Middle and Lower Back**

  ○ The mid- and lower-back area must feel as though it continues the convex spine line, not permitting even a mild concave curve. The convex sensation continues into the pelvic area and on into the hollow of the knees.

  ○ The torso will have the energy feel of curving into the pelvis...around through the under-pelvis...and up into the groin, abdomen and stomach area.

  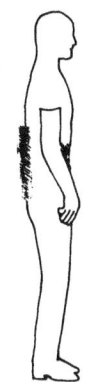

  ○ The line of the stomach and abdomen and the line of the small-of-the-back relate to one another through a kind of "call and response." If the small-of-the-back line is convexly curved, then the front groin, abdomen, and stomach areas have a slightly concave curve

  ○ It is this posture that permits a waistline anywhere from one to two-and-one-half inches **smaller** than that which attends incorrect posture.

  ○ With this bow-shaped body curve, the full spinal measurement increases correspondingly from one to four inches.

  ○ **The broad, rounded, expanded back is the strongest, most powerful back.**

  ○ **The most elongated, parenthesis-curved spine is the strongest, most flexible spine.**

  ○ **Because the rounded back and full chest expansion inflates naturally and curvingly, around the complete thoracic area, neither the C-curved nor the parenthesis-curved body postures will ever appear round-shouldered or chest caved-in.**

- **The Chest**

  We can measure three different chest dimensions:

  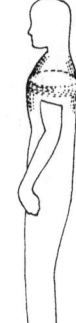

Energy and
Relaxation
in Movement

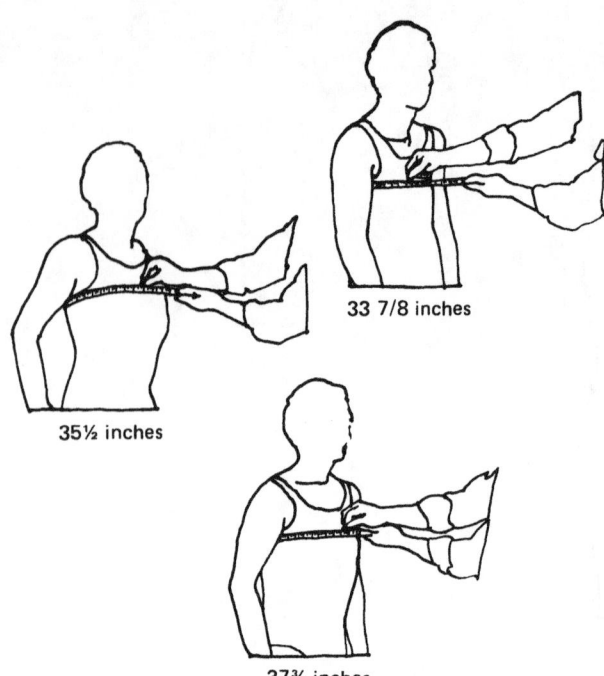

33 7/8 inches

35½ inches

37¾ inches

○ the shallow chest;

○ the conventional chest expansion with rigidly "straight" posture; and

○ the natural, instinctive expansion that arises from the properly C-curved breathing-posture experience.

Expansion in the third posture exceeds that of the second by two to three inches. Yet this maximum expansion looks casual, normal, relaxed, and entirely comfortable — not inflated, military, or "posture-posing" as does the second. Compare illustrations.

• **The Thighs**

In the C-curve posture, the thighs seem loose, relaxed, and slightly forward.

• **The Knees**

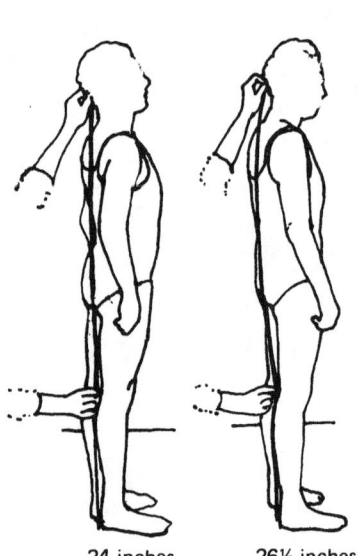

24 inches   26½ inches

○ In the C-curve posture, the knees are always loose and flexible.

○ These most important joints have as much as two inches of movement latitude without falling into either a bent knee or a rigidly locked position.

○ The line extending from the crown of the head to the inside hollows of the knee is one continual parenthesis curve; and this curve measures at least two to four inches longer than the rigid "straight line" of conventional S-shaped posture.

• **The Feet**

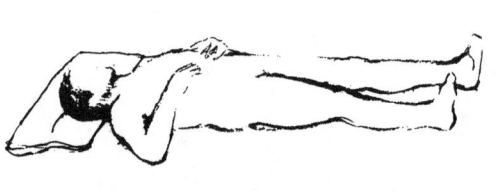
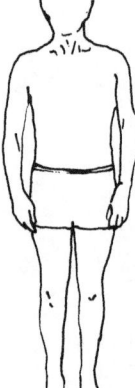

○ Whether on your back or in upright posture, your feet should not point diagonally outward; that is, the toes should really not be any farther apart than the heels during walking, and just barely farther apart while standing.

168

Body Crescent
Standing Up
(Posture and
Alignment)

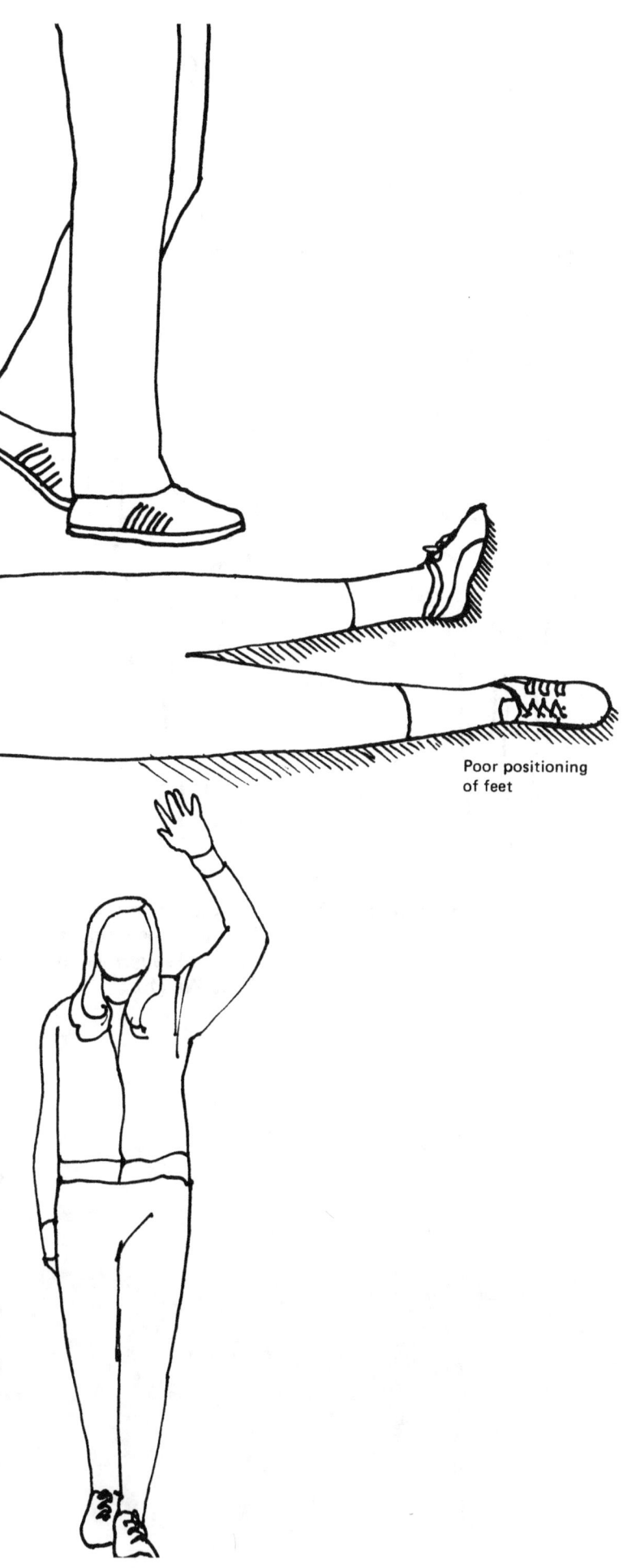

Poor positioning of feet

- The thigh, knee, calf, ankle, foot, and toes should follow one another rather precisely along the same body line.

- In natural, healthy body behavior, the ankle joints should no more be misused by being radically turned out than should the knee joint or even the thigh joint.

- A real test of the leg and foot posture occurs as you lie on your back. If you submit to the "path of least resistance" and the feeling of dead weight, then the knees, calves, feet, and thighs will most certainly turn out. The weight of the feet being pulled down will be felt on the **outside** of the calf muscle, and this amounts to dead weight. You may think you are relaxing, but in reality you are harming and distorting your body, particularly in the knee and foot areas.

- Instead, try to find a new balance for the legs by resting on the **inside** of the calf muscle. This will help to balance the feet and the toes, as they maintain a comfortable, straight-upward position.

- Whether standing, lying, walking, or running, the feet normally ought never point outward or inward. These are both defective postures, although outward pointing is the more harmful to the knees, to body alignment, and to body balance.

- Standing with your toes pointing out, regardless of the position of your heels, can be justified only as an intentional posture for achieving a particular characterization or dance position, or a special "sports-event" requirement. It is not conducive to normal, healthy, esthetic stance.

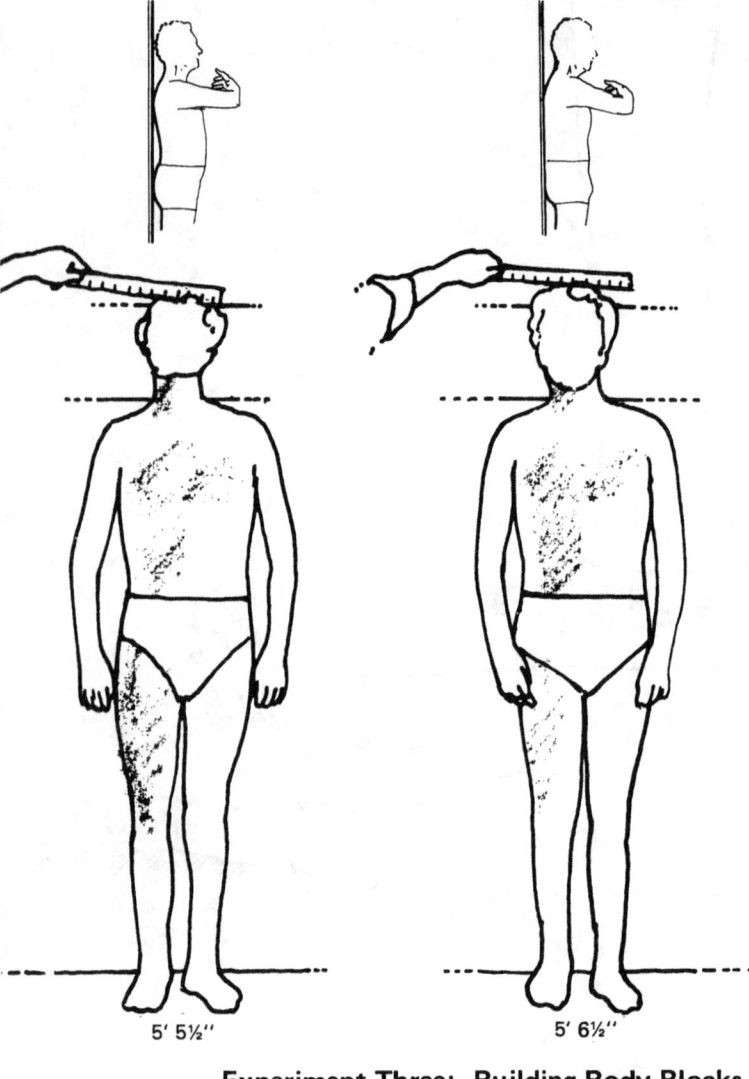

Experiment Three: Building Body Blocks Through the Concept of Live Weight versus Dead Weight

Energy and Relaxation in Movement

- **Body Height**
  - The formal "physical education" or "military" stance is at least one-half to three-quarters of an inch shorter than the natural, instinctively correct posture.
  - The rigid, conventional posture makes it difficult for the back to come into full contact with a vertical column or wall surface (as in illustration). However, the natural posture achieves complete contact with the wall from the pelvis to the top of the back, and looks easy and relaxed.
  - A rigid, straight, upright posture makes a tall person seem inaccessible and defensive; the parenthesis-curved posture makes that same person seem friendly, natural, and pleasantly reaching out.
  - A rigid, straight, upright posture makes a short person shorter; the single parenthesis posture actually makes that same person taller.

Once we understand and appreciate the interdependence between the body's joints, hinges, and curves, we are prepared to perceive the body in the upright as a series of building blocks constituting and fortifying the whole. Central to this image is the support provided by live weight versus dead weight — by the feeling of anti-gravitational urges that buoy up the body as opposed to the feeling of heaviness or compression within the body that incline it to falling, collapse, floppiness, or gravitational pull.

The following exercise in building a column of body blocks does not originate with me. But its application directly and potently relates to our **Body Wisdom** principles and concepts.

170

**Body Crescent
Standing Up
(posture and
alignment)**

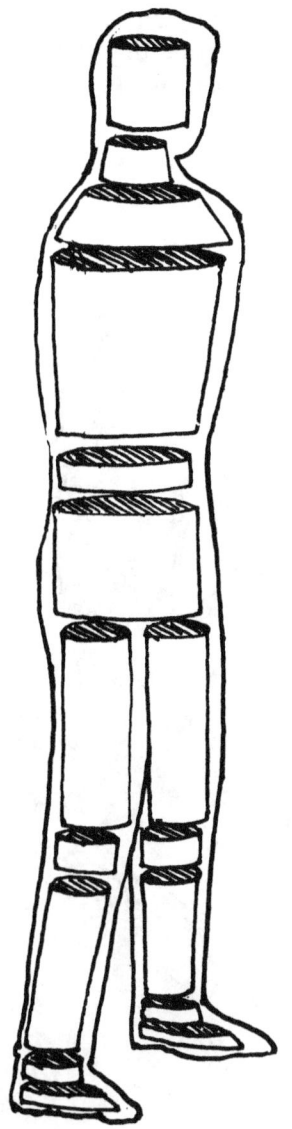

- Check the illustration for a graphic representation of thirteen, specific body blocks: head — neck — shoulders — back — waist — pelvis — thighs — knees — calves — ankles — feet — arms — hands.

- Assume that each block, starting with the feet, will "rest down" lightly on its bottom surface while it simultaneously "rests up" to its top surface, gently reaching for and receiving the next block. Once received, both surfaces rest up and down simultaneously. Each block is fully centered as it rests with the others, with no overhanging edges. Thus the body column, when completely assembled, appears to the eye as a perfectly balanced "straight column," creating a vertical version of contiguous continuity.

- Now transfer this image to your own body of building blocks. Walk your body column around and let the upward energy flow make you feel your tallness. Remember: any rag-doll limpness is heaviness and heaviness is the feeling of weightedness, the feeling of dead weight that induces muscle fatigue. In this connection, you might review the "body-block" exploration in Chapter 10, Experiment One: Coordinated Breathing with the Body as a Crescent Lying Down (pp. 126, 127).

- If you should feel dead weight pulling down the body column, stop for a moment to realize that the feeling of dead weight anywhere in the body generalizes throughout the entire body. And if it generalizes to all parts of the body, it weighs down the brain and psyche as well! Thus buoyancy has not only been deserted by the intellect, but it has vanished totally from the body!

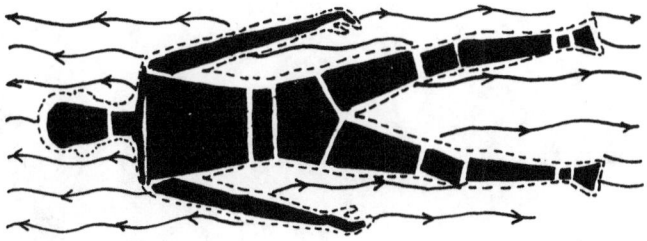

Obviously, these concepts imply both realistic and imaginary self-suggestions used as body instructions. They involve a **combined** bio-physical, bio-neural, and bio-psychic intelligence and experience.

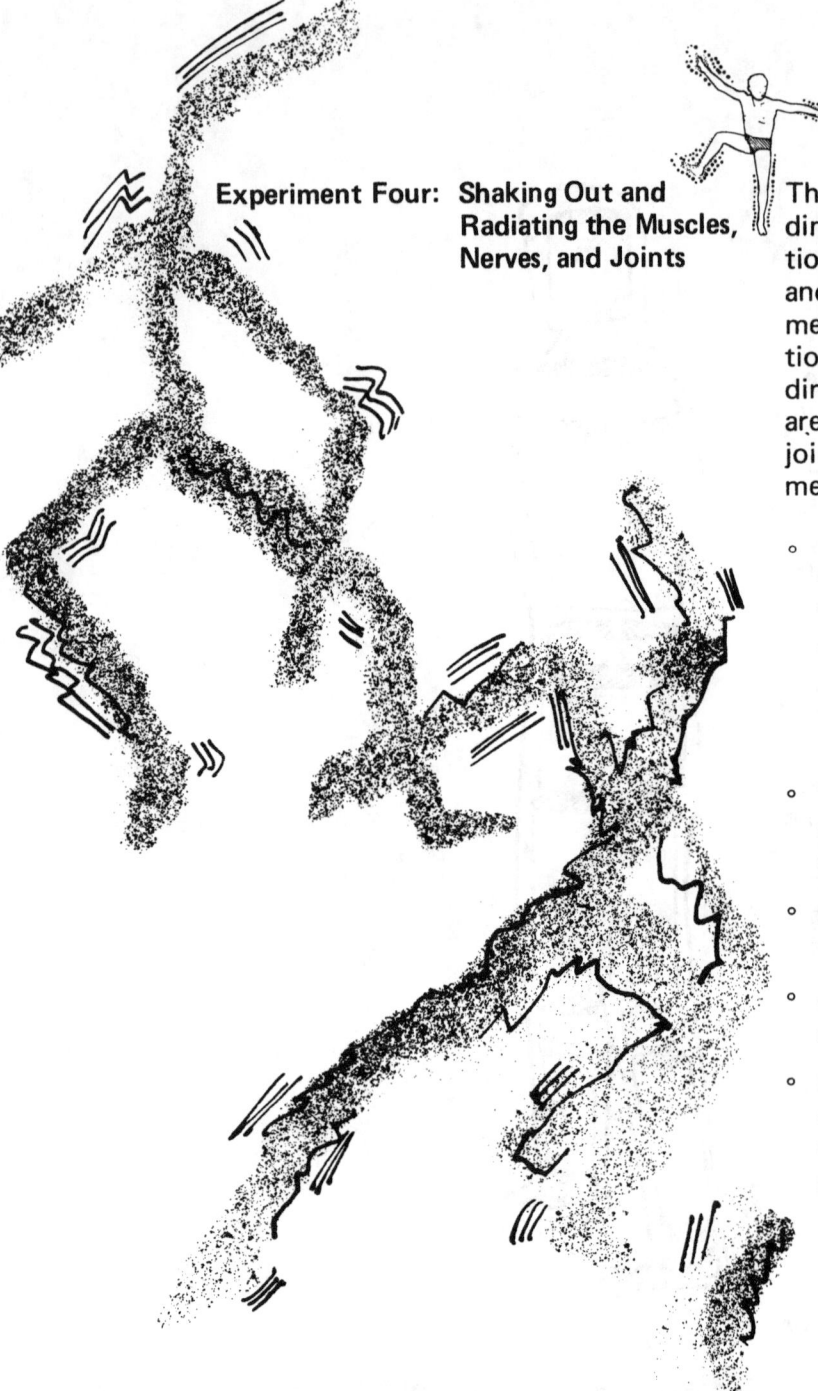

Energy and Relaxation in Movement

Experiment Four: Shaking Out and Radiating the Muscles, Nerves, and Joints

These Shaking and Radiancy activities diminish impingments, loosen up fixations and reduce internal over-crowding and pressing of the organism. Body alignment, posture, breathing, weight distribution, and body energy state sensations are directly affected. Also directly affected are the visceral organs, muscles, nerves, joints, and the circulatory, respiratory, metabolic, and digestive systems.

° Refresh your memory by reviewing "Radiancy Energy" in Chapter 4; "Shaking" in Chapter 5; and the section on "Emo-tivated Breathing" through sobbing, crying, laughing, trembling, shivering, presented in the first part of this chapter, pages 152, 153, 154.

° Then invent shake activities of your own; explore them as a "would-be" actor or dancer might do;

° develop variations on any of the "shaking" themes presented so far in this work;

° devise a series of short "Radiancy" dances as a personal form of art-exercise;

° improvise with the three Radiancy activities — for the fun of it — for good strong workouts — for the creative ideas you may get.

172

Body Crescent
Standing Up
(Rope Dancing)

Experiment Five: Rope-Dancing and Skipping

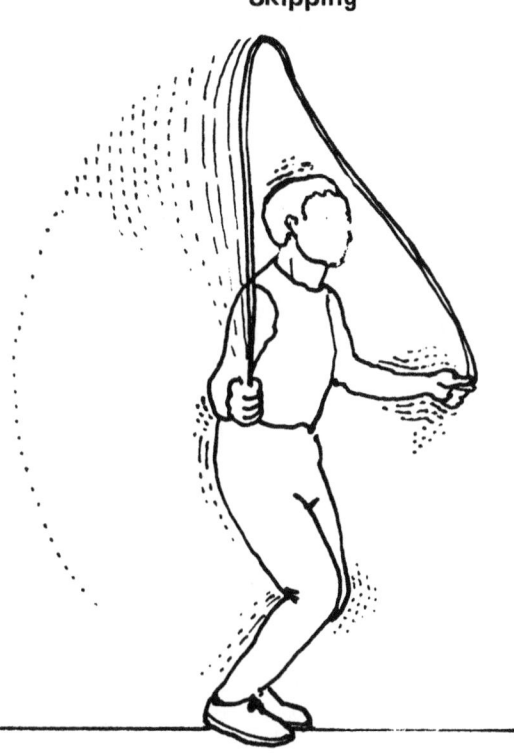

Rope-skipping is one of the few total "art-skill" exercises that particularly affects the building and developing of: body strength, endurance, flexibility, agility, balance and rhythm in the upright. It also contributes to cardio-vascular improvement, bi-lateral body development, and complex, combined body team work.

It should be started early in life, but only as "play." The adult should consider rope-skipping simple, pre-dance training; rope-skipping itself as dancing; and dancing, in this case, as a pleasant, familiar event.

While I introduce "rope-dance-skipping" here, the subject is specifically discussed and illustrated in Chapter 12, Experiment Twelve, on pages 198 - 202.

- Select the simplest hop-skip step that feels good and just enjoy its light, tip-toe, coil-spring quality, first on both feet, then on one, then on the other. Dance — don't jump!

- Now use the rope and coordinate your arms with the rhythm-feel. Don't focus on the rope or its successful clearing under your feet — only on the dancing and the rhythm!

- After you've enjoyed the activities above, pause and ask yourself four questions:

  ◦ How much lighter can I be?

    How much longer can I maintain the action before stopping?

  ◦ To what extent can I smoothly increase the speed and then return to the slower rhythm, while still observing the lightness and length of the action?

  ◦ How can I accompany the rope-skipping with comfortable breathing while controlling the lightness, length, and smooth rhythm-speed of the action?

Energy and
Relaxation
in Movement

The major theme of rope-skipping must be play and dance; activities that are simultaneously and spontaneously esthetic, exhilarating, and invigorating. Variations on the theme will evolve later. Also, it is very important that the rope be of proper size and weight, not just any rope. It must be a **live** rope that feels as though it is swinging on its own, rather than through your effort.

We are now ready to advance our perception of being upright into the specific activities of running, walking, springing, climbing, swinging, etc. In the next chapters, we will therefore treat the body curve as it evolves into wheels, circles, loops, and rocker-rims — and from these, into what we call "personal space spheres."

12
THE PERCEPTION OF THE UPRIGHT

So far, our work has placed primary emphasis on the back and spine. In the last chapter we began our explorations with the body crescent in vertical position — using it as a fulcrum for breathing and posture; understanding its hinge-jointedness, as interrelated with our structural bodyblocks; supporting it with the work/play therapy of shaking and rope-skip-dancing esthetics. We have reinterpreted the traditional tension centers at either end of the spine as relaxer-energizer centers that permit organic instructions and body energy circuits to positively affect body alignment balance, strength, flexibility, and overall vitality. **The spine and the back have, together, become the "umbrella" of the bodywhole; and the back has become the most effective, participating image for the body in movement.**

Graphically represented (see illustration), the body's natural loops, wheels, circles, and rocker-rims encircle to form a double figure-eight. The major objective of this chapter will be to unfold the evolving process of that double figure-eight and apply it to our body training. In the structured activities that follow, we continue to roll. Only now, we roll not as spheres or hemispheres but rather on "leg wheels" and "foot-rocker loops," as a way of reorienting the body to natural, instinctive running, walking, climbing, dancing, jogging, sprinting, springing, leaping, and jumping — all functions of good breathing and proper posture in the upright.

The double figure-eight of the body in motion (see illustration top of 176) invites the image of five kinesensic energy circuits:

1. neck-head-face to neck circuit; (Head Loop)

Chapter 12

The Perception of the Upright

C-Curve, Leg Wheels, Arm Circles, and Body Loops in Motion

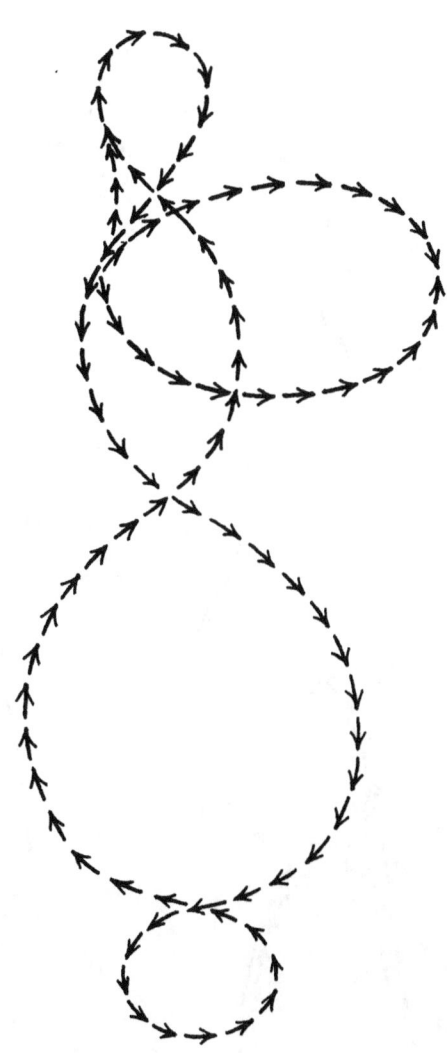

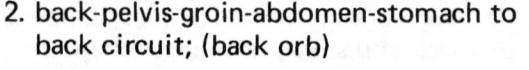

Energy and Relaxation in Movement

2. back-pelvis-groin-abdomen-stomach to back circuit; (back orb)

3. back-pelvis-thigh-leg to back circuit; (leg wheel)

4. foot-heel to foot circuit; (foot rocker)

5. plus shoulders-arms-hands-fingers circuit. (arm circle)

Experiment One: Feeling the Relatedness of the Parenthesis Curve and the C-Curve

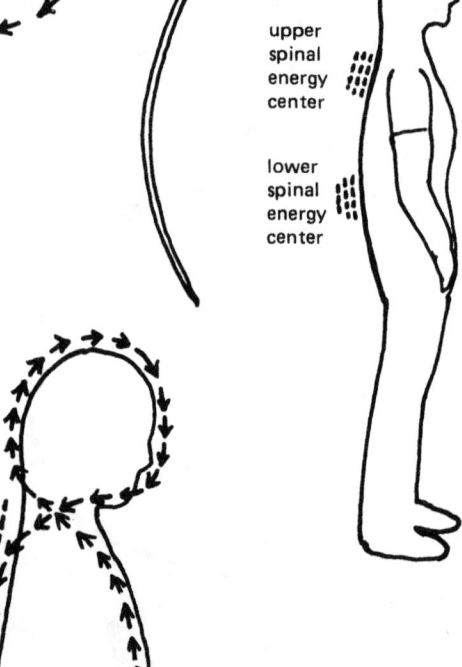

Starting with the parenthesis curve in upright posture, follow the graphically illustrated steps. For the first series of illustrations, consider the crescent bow as your spine. You should be keying into a number of sensations and perceptions of your body in the upright. Among these:

- The lower and upper energy centers create the image of two separate "cruxes" for body movement.

- The upper energy center urges an "upward and around" flow, while the lower center urges a "downward and around" energy flow.

- **The upper spine center** "motors" alignment through expansion of the upper back into the expanded chest; extension of the shoulders and shoulder girdle into an expanded arm circle; extension of the back-of-the-neck into a forward-rotated head and reflexively relaxed jaw. It energizes upper body posture and relates to breathing.

- **The lower spine center** "motors" alignment and relates to breathing and posture through expansion of the lower back into the rotating pelvis and upward-extended energy of the abdomen and stomach; as well as through the vital circular movement of thighs and knees.

Perception of the Upright

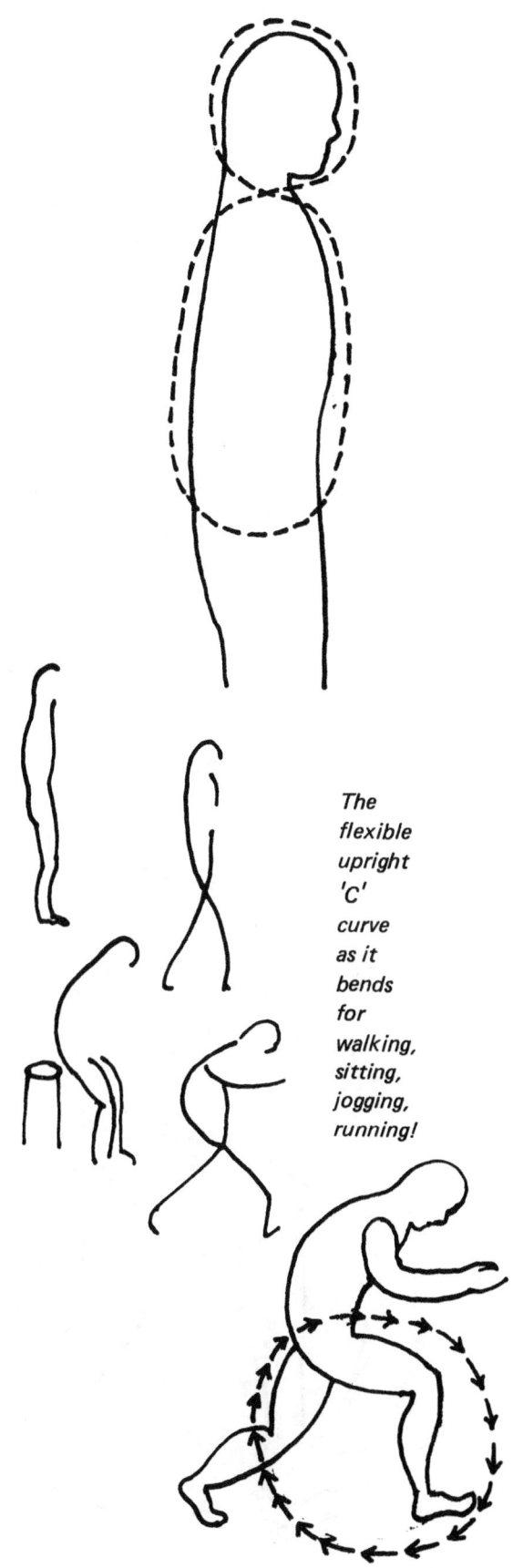

The flexible upright 'C' curve as it bends for walking, sitting, jogging, running!

- ○ The two-way energy flow converts the two traditional spine-tension areas into two new relaxer-energizer centers, particularly in terms of breathing and posture.

- ○ When you incite buoyancy energy, stimulating combined feeling of rising buoyancy in the upper energy center and gentle but firm floating plus settling-down buoyancy in the lower center, you achieve a reinforcing feel of dynamic buoyancy in "still body movement." The three body buoyancies in motion also tend to raise the arms into level circles as well as balanced arm and hand gestures.

- ○ When you put these opposite buoyancy-flows together in unified action, producing a third-force familiar event in posture and an organic instruction for breathing, you develop an energy circuit that assumes the image of our first upper figure-eight.

- As though sailing with the active current, walk buoyantly as you gracefully move the upper figure-eight around your outside space.

- Notice that as the crescent bow bends, it becomes a C-curve. As the bow becomes a C-curve, the body walks, sits, jogs, and runs, but always maintains its spherical contour and curvo-linear style. As the crescent bow progresses into a more mature and longer curve (to the knee-hollows), it incorporates the thighs and knees, and motors the "leg wheels." (See illustrations)

- Note that when the back is instinctively curved, the convex crescent or C-curve guarantees retention of the spinal centers as relaxer-energizer centers. You may think of the back as a shield, an umbrella, a parachute, or an envelope. Whichever image you select should accommodate the notion of the back as a prime fulcrum, coordinating and assisting the centering,

Energy and
Relaxation
in Movement

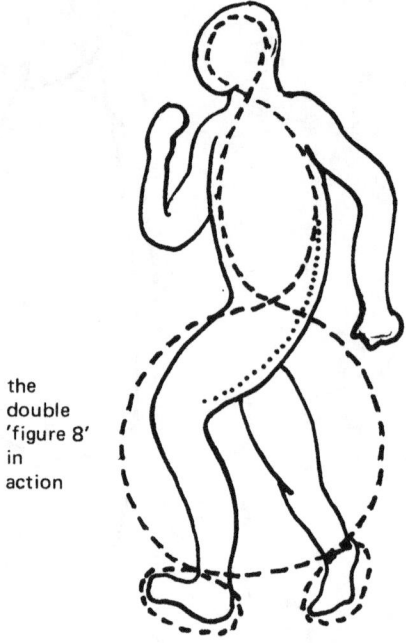

the double 'figure 8' in action

balancing, and freeing of the body for physical action. As you explore, increase the dominance of the back as a fulcrum, so that the front area can accept the pleasant, kinesthetic responsibility of responding causatively, and in complementary concave (in-curved) manner, to the convex (outcurved) back.

- Note again, how your posture and breathing will follow the same circular energy flow, the same wave-like body contour; moving from the lower energy center into the pelvis and sides, around into the groin, abdomen, and stomach which, firm and relatively flat, continues its "elastic" extension to meet the expanded upper back and chest cavity.

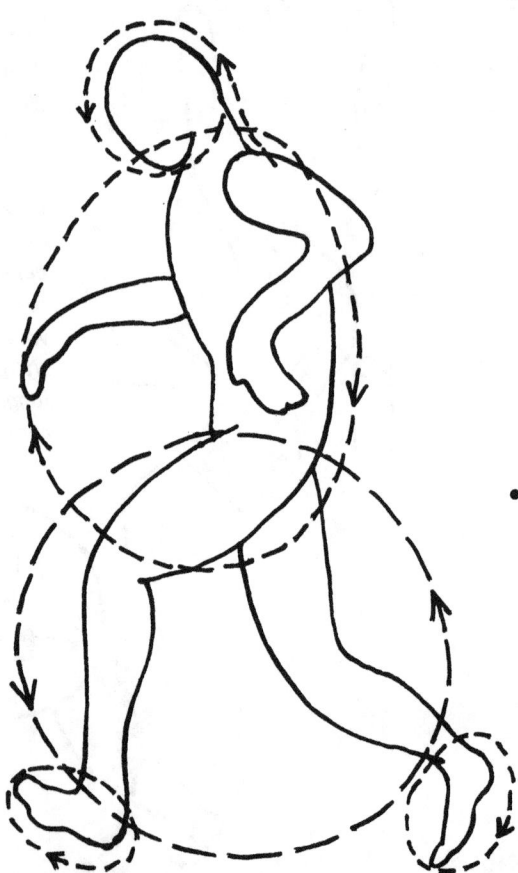

- The two energy centers, by sending kinesthetic energy flow in opposite directions, meet and intermingle. They appear to unite: the "kidney bean" torso-loop posturally with the head-loop above and the leg wheel below (under the thighs); the leg wheels with the foot "rocker-rim" loops. At the same time, the breath flow, itself, seems to unify within the "kidney bean" torso-loop; radiating in the opposite direction to create an unceasing, cause-effect relationship between the torso's front and back action. **All of this creates the sense of being centered.**

- Recall that, in upright posture and upright movement, the crescent back curve branches off downward, like two giant roots, joined through the pelvic muscles with the underpart of the thighs. The accompanying image is that of the lower back lifting the under-thighs to form a leg wheel, with the energy flow sent right through the bottom of the C-curve into the hollow of the knees. It is this energy flow that creates a motor-sensory "lift and roll" action in the thighs, leg, and foot.

Perception of the Upright

A similar motor-sensory lift action radiates from the mid- and upper-back into the shoulder muscles, resulting in the arms being raised into cooperating circles or loops. Here, the kinesthetic sensation travels from the back to the shoulders, from the shoulders to the arms, from the arms to the hands and fingers. Observe this action in the illustrations of the skier, the surfer, the runner, the jumper, etc.

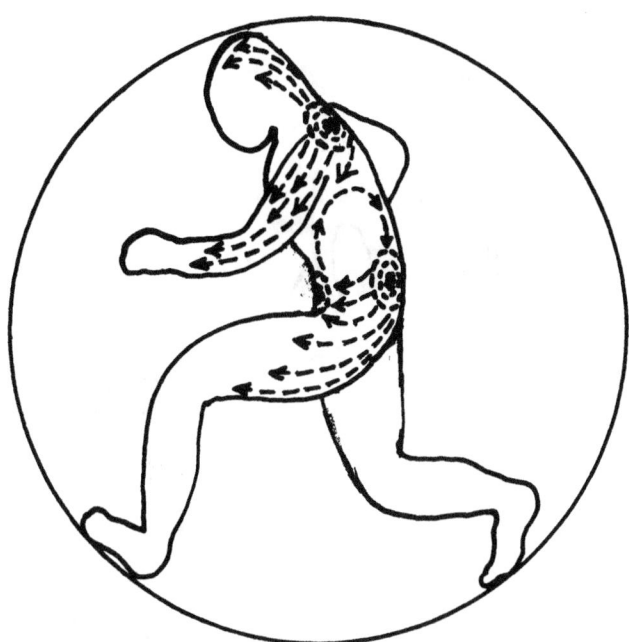

Experiment Two: Walking, Running, Climbing, and Dancing on Wheels

The five energy circuits of the double figure-eight are maximally involved in running, walking, and climbing. Walking — running — climbing are not actions of the feet and legs alone. Particularly as regards the legs and arms, they have nothing in common with piston-like foot thrusting, with forced pumping and kicking actions, or with jolting, jerky stop and start actions. They involve no push-pull propulsion; no shock-landing bounce to the ground; no drag-heavy dead weight, either in movement or at rest.

Rather, the image to hire for these upright actions is that of your energized lower back center pedaling a bicycle over a smooth level, as well as an up-hill road surface. Kinesensically, walking, running, and climbing are best imaged through graceful body circles, C-curve back, leg wheels, and foot rocker-rim loops — all in coordinated, continuous, circular motion.

Circular motion implies multi-directional movement. This seemed natural when we were rolling and rocking as small, compact balls and expanded hemispheres. But how, without eyes in the back of our head, do we run backwards, climb downward, walk sideways? The notion of body intelligence that can accommodate multi-directional movement, without fear of falling, is not new — not, at least, to the consummate

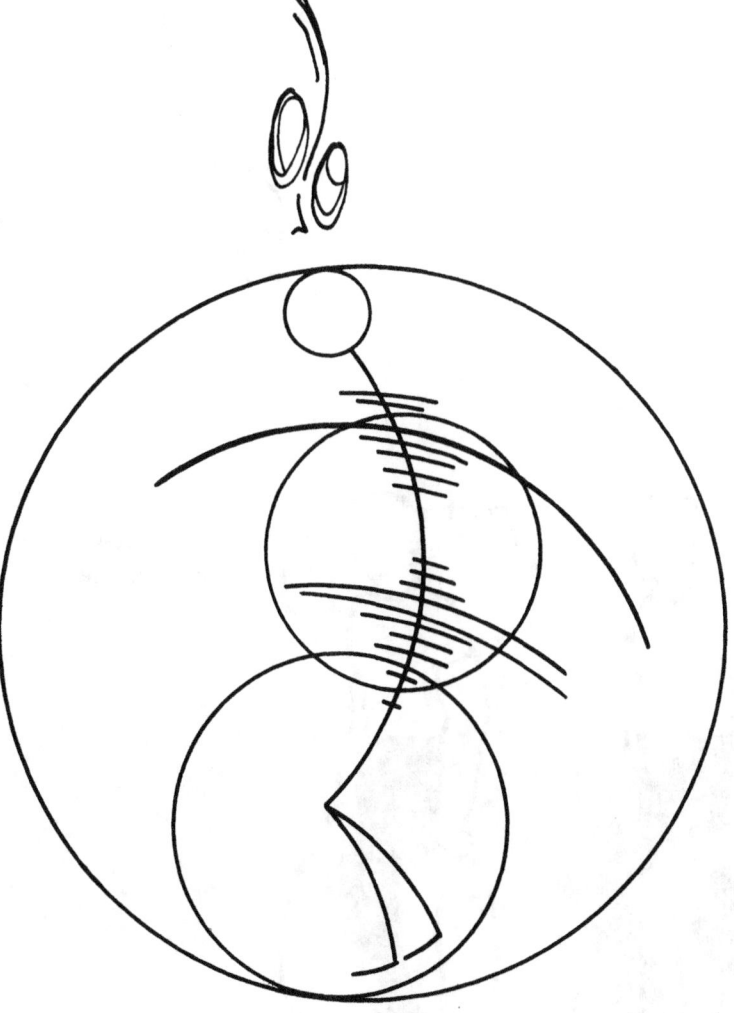

Images for hire

Energy and
Relaxation
in Movement

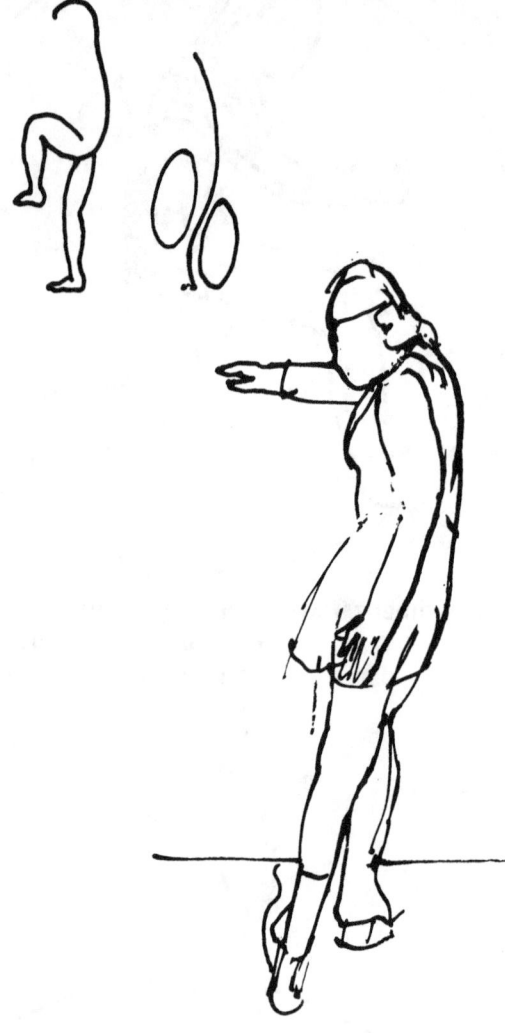

skater, gymnast, diver, football and basketball athlete, or dancer. For these and other "body artists," the body **does** roll, slide, tumble, or dance backward, sideways, and upward as well as forward and downward. All these moves are equally creative and accessible as potential body skills and talents.

Furthermore, they often embody an important "countering" or counterbalancing action. The body is meant to move and balance itself so there can exist a maximum freedom for moving backward as **defensive or offensive action,** without harm to the organism. Perhaps the best example of countering action is the intense sharpening of outer senses and alternate modalities by the blind and deaf, in order to maintain the body in movement and balance and enjoy an equilibrium and sense of physical esthetics most of us would envy.

This is not to suggest that we need to lose our vital, outside senses in order to achieve circular, multi-directional motion with full retention of balance. **Quite the contrary, we need to gain inside harmonic senses that put eyes, ears, touch, and taste in our back and spine, thereby sharpening our outside senses, reducing fear, and developing the use of greater portions of the brain.**

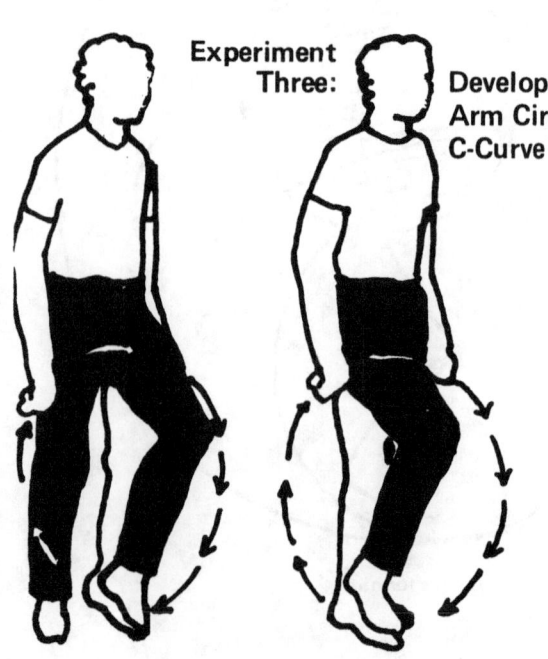

Experiment Three: Developing Leg Wheels, Arm Circles, and the C-Curve

- This is an exploration of the "Bow and Wheel" activity. It consists of extending the **crescent line** on one side; and motoring the **leg-wheel** (along with arm loops) on the other.

  · From the waist up, induce radiancy and some potency energy;

  ° From the waist down, induce a buoyant "resting down" that continues the curve of the extended crescent into one leg;

180

Perception of the Upright

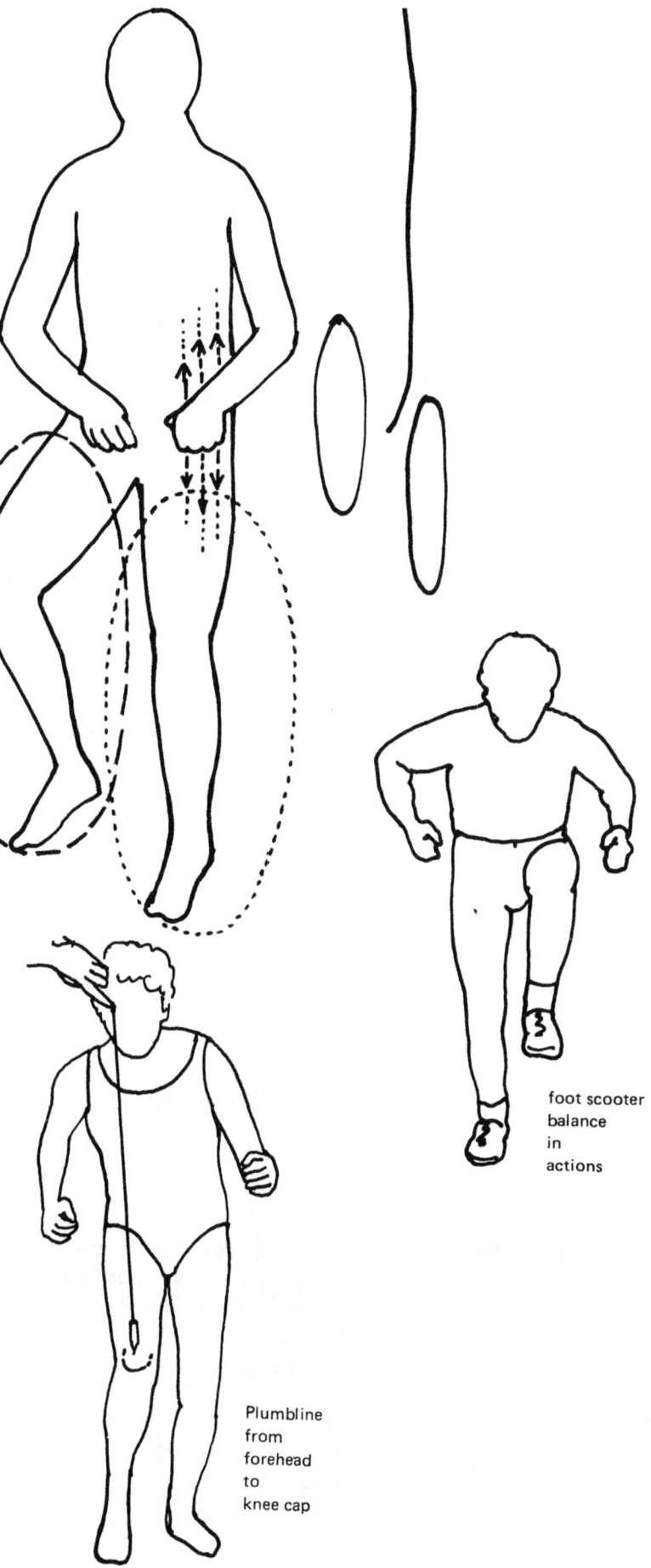

○ Note how the other leg, as part of a countering or counter-balancing action, floats up in rising buoyancy to form a wheel; and how the arms, fed by the extended crescent and expanded back, buoyantly rise to form an arm circle.

This is the feel of 'one-legged' bicycle pedaling we referred to above. Or perhaps, we should imagine this activity as a "foot-scooter" exploration.

• Repeat the experiment, moving into it quickly from either standing or walking position. Feel how the balance esthetic is fed by activating all the body energy circuits of the double figure-eight within the buoyancy, radiancy, and potency states.

• With the same activity, explore turning the leg wheel and arm circle while standing in place, as illustrated.

As previously mentioned, posture derives from movement, not from a standard of shape! Whatever the body action — from casual walking to vital sprinting, from easy sitting to knee-bend springing — the balance image must be a "plumb line" from the forehead to the knee-cap (see illustration).

If, in terms of organic image support, the face is far ahead or far behind the knee position, the body will be out of balance, and will not roll, move, glide, or float with proper control, pleasure, and inner harmonic rhythm. "Plumb-line balance" works most effectively and creatively when the body most fully enjoys the longest C-curve extension and radical expansion flow.

The body is always being sensed as exclusively curvo-linear, whether in the

foot scooter balance in actions

Plumbline from forehead to knee cap

Energy and
Relaxation
in Movement

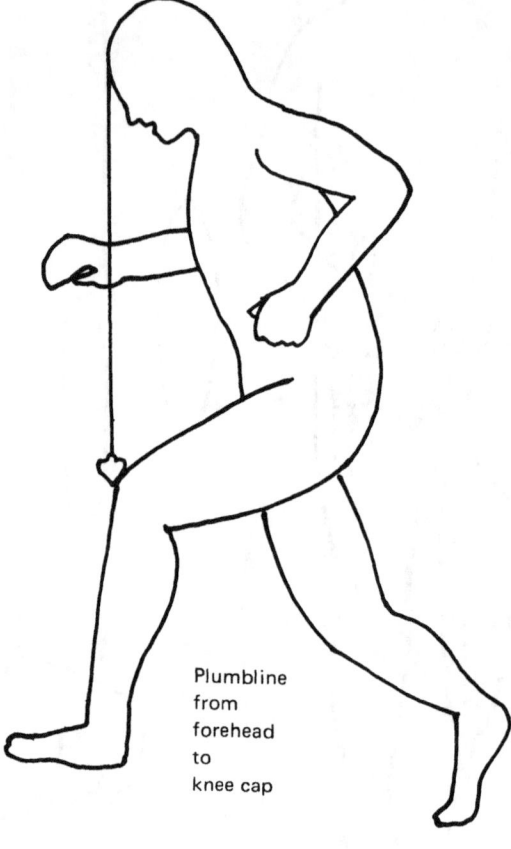

Plumbline from forehead to knee cap

Standing foot scooter balance

Experiment Four: **From the "Standing Foot-Scooter" to the Walk Series**

shape of a ball, orb, rocker-rim, crescent, circle, or wheel. If you maintain this perception, you may count on experiencing body movement with solid equilibrium and a center of balance. In fact, any point of surface contact, where the body **feels** the curving surface, is a centered point of contact! Equilibrium is lost only when that curving surface becomes a straight line; when the rigid, straight line causes "disproportionate" concern with balance; and when as a result, the fear of falling follows quickly head over heels.

- As you explore each variation of the experiment, look for

    ◦ the start of energy flow at the waist, fed by the lower spine center;

    ◦ the extended crescent-bow;

    ◦ the expanded C-curve in sit/run position;

    ◦ the rocker-rim sole of the foot;

    ◦ the leg-wheel action in a standing "bow and wheel" exploration;

    ◦ the arm-circle action coordinating with leg-wheel movement;

    ◦ the weightless quality of the **leg wheel** as it counter-balances the axle-like **crescent-bow** in rising buoyancy; and

    ◦ the "plumb-line" balance center in running, walking, climbing, and sitting.

Having attended to the body in alignment, the following walk-series provides a working guide for dealing with the body in movement. It is part of the developing perception of curves, and as such, it prepares our kinesthetic senses for further progression into running, climbing, and springing.

Perception of the Upright

The "Bow and Wheel" Walk:

- Begin the walk-series by walking in place with an easy foot-scooter, or bicycle pedal action. Then take light, gentle, short steps using the same "bow and wheel" movement.

- Now adapt this movement to a "penguin walk," using your arms and hands to fill out the image. The smoother, more rhythmic and expressive the movement, the more like a penguin-walk it will feel. Note how the "rolling" steps roll **downward** rather than **forward**, and that the downward rolling heel is never ahead of the other foot (or toe). It is an extremely small, and almost dance-like leg-wheel action.

- Accelerate the small wheel "penguin-walk" and vary the action further by turning the alternating "bow and wheel" movement into an approximation of a "racing walk." Much to your surprise, you'll find that this is easily achieved without the usual, exaggerated hip-swivel and jutting out of lower spine and pelvis from side to side. The bicycle or scooter is beginning to course quickly over smooth roadway.

As you work through the series, note:

- the alternating counter-actions of crescent bow and leg wheel.

- the alternate foot action of rocker-rim heel-to-toe contact with the floor.

- the **downward** roll of the leg wheel which by rolling down, rather than forward or ahead, covers surface distance more fluidly, gracefully and efficiently.

- the **gliding** rhythms of the marking walk (in place), the penguin walk, and the racing walk.

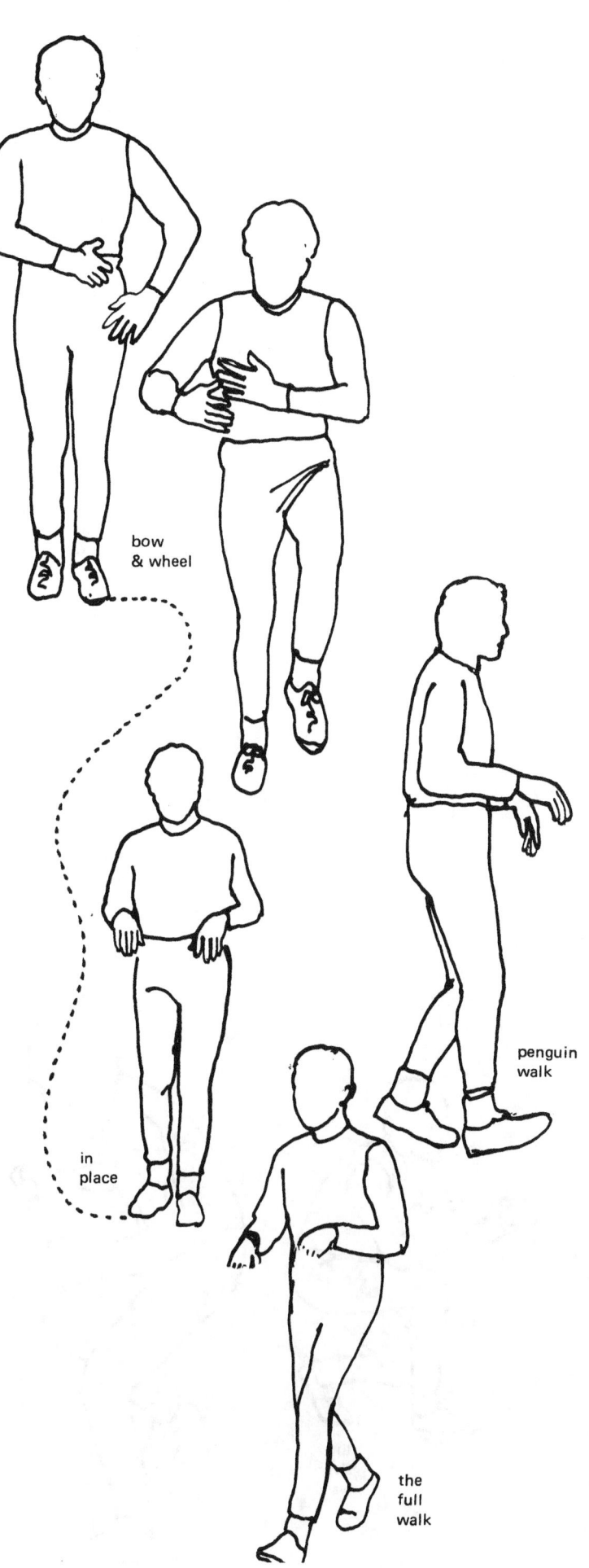

Energy and Relaxation in Movement

- the ease with which variations can be effected once the rhythm and movement of the basic "bow and wheel" are controlled.

To aid your exploring of the walk-series, as new familiar and unique events, at home, at work, and at play, a few general rules and gentle reminders are offered.

1. When shifting from one leg wheel to the other, avoid transferring your weight from one side of the body to the other. Your crescent torso, neck, and head-curve should remain perfectly level as floor contact to one wheel after the other is achieved, without the slightest disturbance to body balance. Success depends upon how lightly one wheel floats up while the other alights on the ground, and how conscious you are of walking on an "air cushion" rather than a hard surface.

2. To change the degree of the C-curve from a mild to a deeper bend, pretend you're skiing and use your arms as though holding onto ropes or ski-poles.

3. Remember: when one wheel is up, the other is down. The revolving leg wheels, like pedals on a bicycle, follow and precede each other. Recall that they are not rod-like pistons being thrust forward and pulled from the back, but "riding wheels" with rolling action. If you think of the leg wheels as simply rolling, rather than rolling forward, you'll find that they naturally roll downward toward the ground, not ahead of you.

The Sitting Walk:

- Start either with the "bow and wheel" walk, or penguin walk, and gradually allow the C-curve to bend and lower itself into

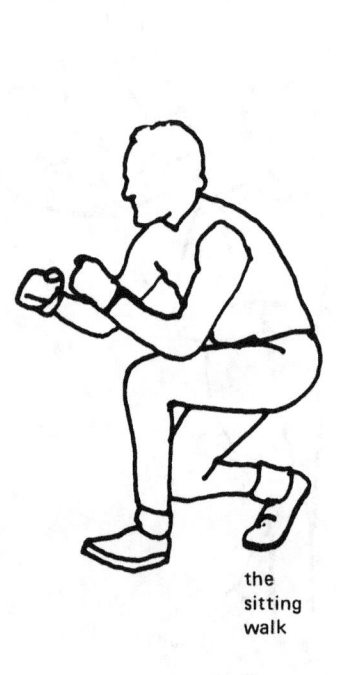
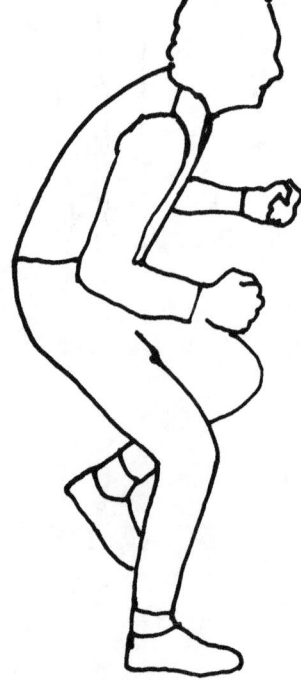

the sitting walk

Perception of the Upright

a comfortable sitting position, as close to the ground as possible. Keeping the same easy rhythm, initiate your walk in the sitting position. Then, by degrees, work your way back up, returning to the mild crescent curve of the original "bow and wheel" walk.

- Practice a comfortable one-quarter sit-walk; increase it to one-half, then to three-quarters. As you master your own movement in these modulated sit-walk positions, you are also adjusting the degree of the C-curve bend.

- When your seat is very low to the ground, let your arms and hands, particularly in the elbow area, assist the leg and foot rolling. Use your arms to help make the body feel lighter and prevent wobbling from side to side. Hire the image of a goose walking or a duck swimming.

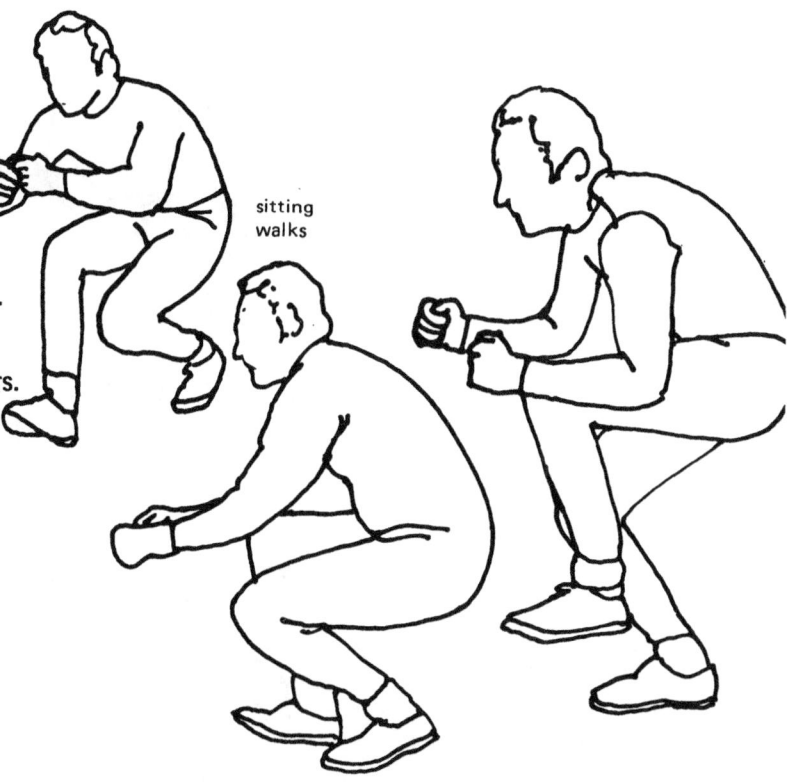

sitting walks

Experiment Five: Small Wheel Dance-Walk

The dance walk is a bridging experience between walking and running. You will feel your walk becoming more like a dance whenever inner rhythm becomes the dominent modality.

- Use a small leg-wheel, but with liberal arm and hand motion, to lead you into the dance feel and perceive its rhythm. Explore dance-walking to different types of music with distinctive beats or, better yet, to the melody and beat of your own "inner-felt" body rhythm.

- Bring the dance feel into your arms, hands, legs, lower energy center, upper back, knees, thighs — into the entire crescent! These spontaneous, improvised dance walks will plant the seed-feel that walking is a creative, artistic activity with all the esthetics of dancing.

- After you've practiced several dance walks and gotten into the "swing of it," ask yourself: Is walking fun? Is it like radiant

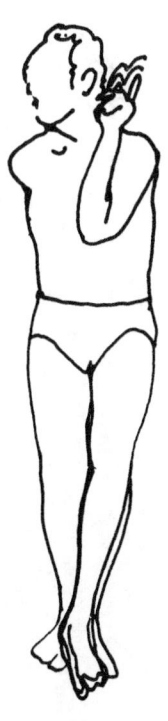

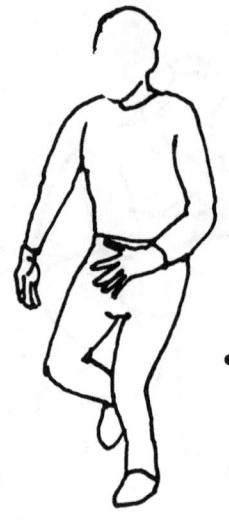

dancing? Is it like buoyant dancing? Does it feel physically as well as psychologically satisfying, relaxing, energizing, reinforcing? Expect to be pleasantly surprised by your self-to-self responses.

- Finally, use your plumb-line balance center as a realistic and safe image to keep the body in equilibrium, while experiencing the radiant spontaneity of dance-walking to outer and inner rhythms.

Experiment Six: A New Approach to "Jogging"

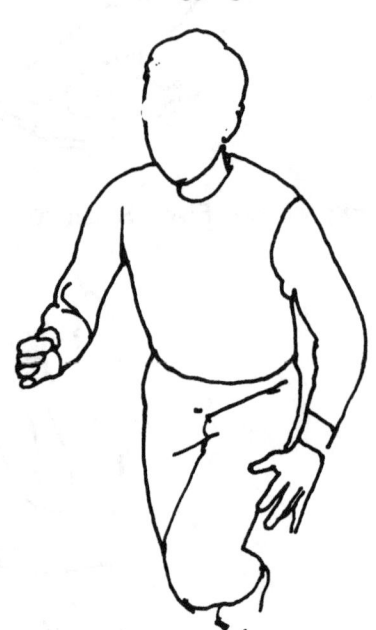

Strictly from the viewpoint of exercise, jogging is an in-between activity — half-way between a fast walking pace and an easy loping gait. True, jogging has become, especially in America, a cultural phenomenon unto itself, largely appropriated by faddists and marketed like instant broth to the weary, the over-worked, the impatient. Yet despite its current consumer orientation, jogging has served to awaken people to the need for more energy-gathering exercise and relaxing recreation.

Jogging should do both, but in fact, in its regularly practiced form, it does neither. For most, even among the zealous, jogging becomes an uneventful, humdrum way of perpetuating a desultory, purposeless pretense to body training. Joggers may momentarily experience the ecstasy of running and the joy of walking, but from all appearances, despite television commercials to the contrary, they do not in the least understand the esthetics of jogging. If we are trained to look, all that we see is a monotonous and repetitious series of shock-bouncing, body flopping, and push-pull-jerk-jolting movements — about as interesting and salutary as a loaf of pasty, white supermarket bread.

It therefore seems timely to offer an alternate approach to jogging. Such

Perception of the Upright

an approach, kinesensically reconsidered, embraces the following techniques and objectives:

1. To "dance" from a walking gait into a smooth-sailing running gait, on small leg wheels;

2. To "roll" on the full sole-bottoms of the feet rather than rely upon "toe-landing;"

3. To reinforce the movement of jogging with a specific regime of breathing;

4. To vary both the jogging posture and the body energy states used in jogging, as a way to vary one's responses and thus improve body balance, rhythm, and endurance;

5. To consider jogging as non-exertive, full-fledged running; and

6. To understand that the only distinction between jogging and racing (far from a question of style) is the size and rhythm-feel of the leg wheels and arm circles.

There is more than one way to experience the dance feel in walking, running, and jogging. The idea is to combine the attributes of body lightness, personal pleasure, internal rhythm, and physical enjoyment with, quite literally, a "sensing" of humor.

You can start with radiancy energy and your sense of humor will tune into the nimble prancing steps of an imp, a Puck, or a Charlie Chaplin. You can begin with buoyancy energy and take personal, physical pleasure in the feel of a seagull skimming the water's surface or an eagle soaring through air. You can connect with the flow of breathing energy or the vibrato of nervous energy — or just **think dance** (Look, Ma, I'm dancing!) and take off with your sense of humor on a million

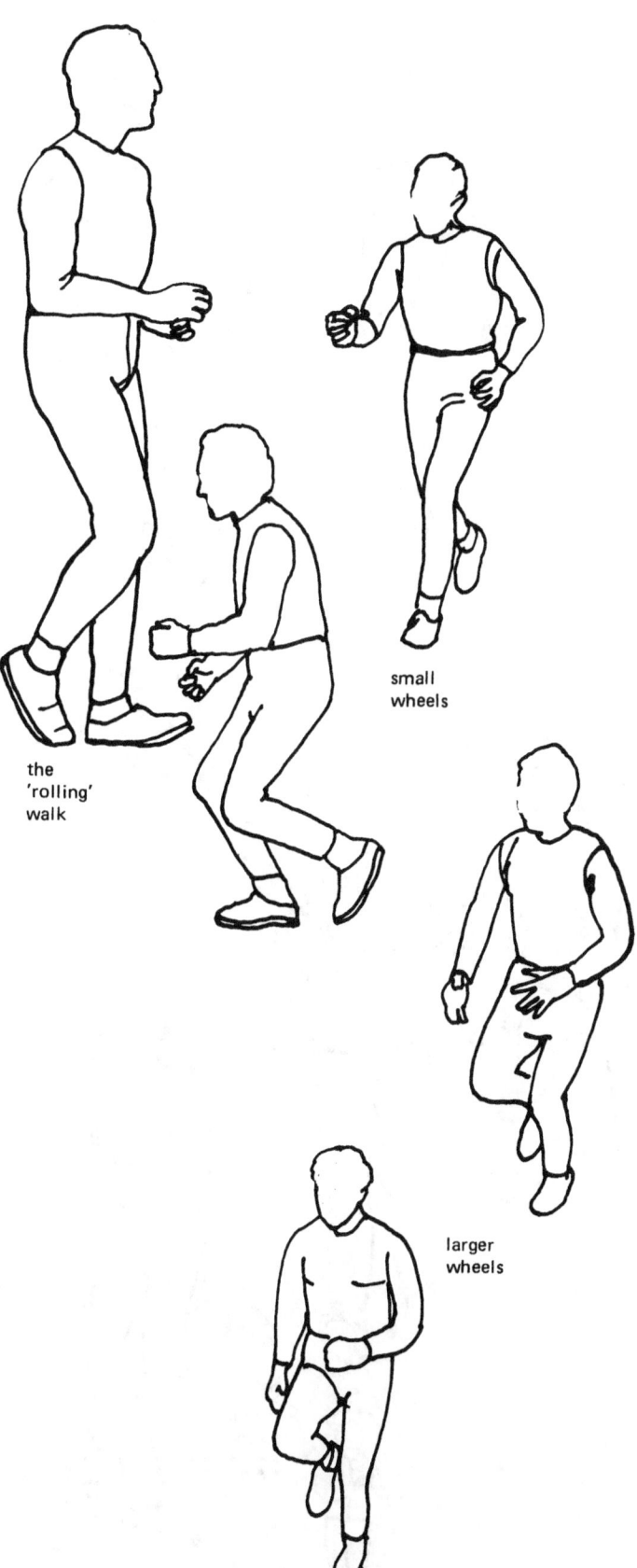

the 'rolling' walk

small wheels

larger wheels

Energy and
Relaxation
in Movement

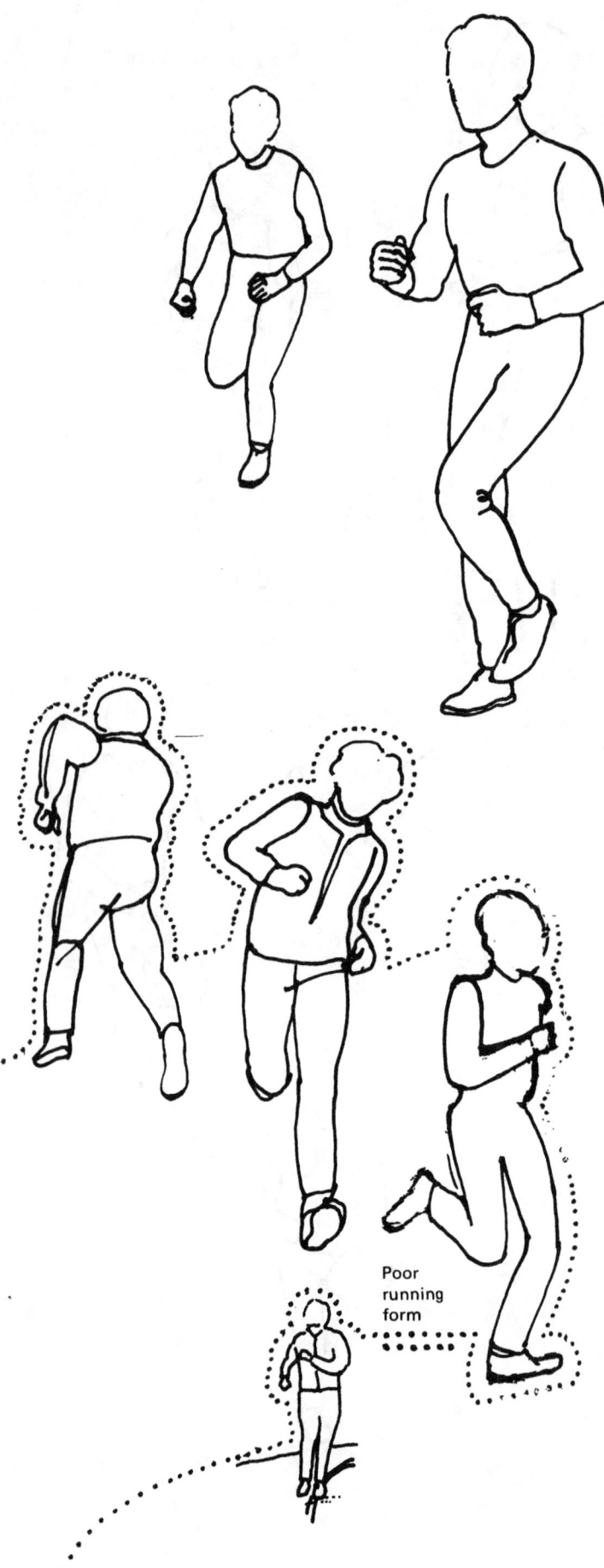

Poor running form

little helium bags and begin to know what it's like to "rest upward." This is what we mean, in kinesensic training, by the duality of "play" and work.

As we noted at the outset, the difference between walking, jogging, and running is not one of quality, but of degree. The penguin walk leaves no space between the heel of one foot and the toe of the other, whereas the rolling walk leaves a distance of nearly eight inches between heel and toe. It is this distance, expanding the periphery of the leg wheel, that matures a rolling "walk" into a "jog," a "jog" into a "run," a "run" into a "sprint." The distance between **front heel** and **back toe** in the jog is approximately twelve to fifteen inches.

But it is the rhythm feel that gives the sense of the body in movement, of "wheel rolling" back and forth between walking and sprinting. It is the rhythm feel that produces feather-weight rolling without swaying, bouncing, jutting, jerking, or heavy landing on the feet. It is the rhythm-feel that instructs you organically on the distinction between the "rolling walk" (faster walk) and the small wheel running (jogging).

With dance-walking and feather-weight rolling, your C-curve for jogging will not lean from side to side; your shoulders will no longer jut forward and backward, or up and down as you move at a clip. Instead, you should feel the body in equal balance with the drawn bow of your spine remaining perfectly vertical as your leg wheels along with the arm circles turning freely in coordinated action. Because all the joints in the body are loose, the body-curve bends freely in this vertical posture while maintaining the plumb-line center from eye-bone to kneecap.

And remember: You don't have to concentrate on lifting your legs and knees.

188

Your spine, branching into each under-thigh, "bend-lifts" them for you — weightlessly; without transfer of weight from one side of the body to the other; and with no disturbance to body balance as each foot rocker-rim continues the curve line of the previous leg wheel in making light contact with the ground.

Experiment Seven: Breathing Regime While Running or Jogging

- As you run or jog, experiment simultaneously with the number of strides you can easily take while holding your breath. (The term **stride** refers to the action and distance covered by a single leg; thus, the action of both left and right leg constitutes two strides). Check the number of strides on one breath three or four times to feel sure that the average count is a reasonably standard guage.

- Let us assume you are in pretty good shape and in three succeeding breaths you can conveniently do: 53 strides the 1st time
  58 strides the 2nd time
  48 strides the 3rd time;

  Now divide the approximate numbers in half and you might accept a norm of about 25 strides per breath for the purpose of this exploration.

- Having accepted half your computed measure as your norm, start the following series of steps:

  Step 1:
  a. Start running or jogging comfortably;
  b. while doing so inhale easily as though in a gentle sigh (the inhalation may require a duration of 2, 3, 4, or 5 strides);
  c. while holding your breath run or jog your 25-stride norm;
  d. then, while still running or jogging exhale smoothly and freely, which may again require a duration of 2 to 5 strides (or seconds); then,
  e. inhale (without interrupting your running or jogging) and repeat the 25-stride norm; exhale and prepare for step 2;

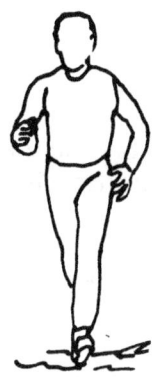

Step 2:
Repeat step 1, from 'a' through 'd', except that in 'c' you run only 20 strides.

Step 3:
Repeat the same activity, only now in 'c' you run or jog only 15 strides;

Step 4:
Repeat the same activity, only now in 'c' you run or jog only 10 strides;

Step 5:
Repeat the same activity, only now in 'c' you run or jog only 5 strides;

Step 6:
When you reach the "5 stride" complement, repeat it about five to ten times, always preceded by a fresh, easy, new breath. This "5 stride" sequence will become so comfortable and efficient that you will find yourself reinforcing an optimal inhale/exhale breathing rhythm, which will almost instinctively serve as a flexible time/rhythm clocking device. You may require from 2 to 5 strides to do the inhaling and maybe 2 to 6 strides to do the exhaling, and you will surely enjoy running or jogging from 5 to 10 strides while holding your breath. Thus, your breathing and running 'time-rhythms' might be considered a form of inhale/running/exhale "key signature" that works well for you.

The breath/rhythm "key signature" is flexible and variable to serve the runner's needs (just as is the musical "key signature" to serve the composer's needs). The runner's "key signature" responds to the grace, tempo, power, — to the very "rhythm and melody and harmony" desired (and/or required) in your running activity. The "key signature" assists in equilibrating the time, speed, endurance **and esthetics** relevant to any running situation. After effective exploration, one gets the **feel** of the necessary time/rhythm/body music to be generated for optimal results.

The object is to build a resilient endurance while simultaneously developing a challenging but managable speed, and at the same time **experiencing the esthetics** of running. Keep reminding yourself **to not push yourself stubbornly,** and that the esthetics of running (or jogging) begins with the sensing and perceiving your body as a "sphere" rolling on "wheels" rather than as an "upright structure" push-pulling and propelling itself through the pressure-pumping of arm and leg "pistons".

Note: a) When you research this inhale-run-exhale "key signature", explore it whenever possible, without resting between breaths, and turn it into a short but complete activity (or workout) that is measured in comfortable though challenging time/rhythm/balance relatedness to "breathing while running". The problem is that most people forget all about their breathing while running or rope-skipping and the result is disorganization and body chaos. As your body rolls along on your "leg wheels" you will become accustomed to inhale your breath, hold your breath, and exhale your breath smoothly and instinctively -- yet always with the optimal number of strides in each action -- depending only on how you feel and on the specific objective of your running activity. Please note that while the "key signature" intelligence is helpful in **feeling** the time, rhythm, balance, and reserve energy in your running, after a time one tends to forget about specific "key signatures", and is only **habitually aware** that the **feel** of a "key signature" exists. Particularly is this true in **sprinting.**

b) On occasions you may desire some extra relief and require more than one breath between the "six steps of the breathing while running" regime just described. **Do not hesitate** to avail yourself of the comfort of a few additional breaths whenever you deem it necessary or desirable. Also, for variation and relaxation, alternate your running with a slow jog or a rolling walk for forty or fifty strides and then resume your running or fast jogging.

A good rule to remember is that the breathing process simply must not be permitted to break down or be neglected. If during the running explorations you do tire (or feel truly 'out of breath') you ought not stop altogether to rest, but instead, introduce another relaxer-energizer or "body esthetic" by shaking, or skipping, or dancing, or dance-walking, or pleasant sighing for about 30 seconds or so, and then resume your running to complete your workout.

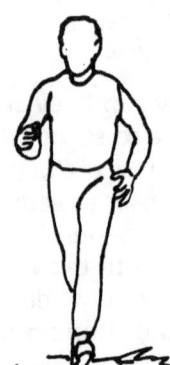

Experiment Eight: Medium Wheel Rolling and the Loping Run

"Loping" should be considered enjoyable, full-fledged running — something short of sprint racing or maximum effort. Essentially, loping embodies the consistency and gait of long distance running with a rhythm feel that, without extreme exertion, accommodates speed changes relative to the size of the leg-wheel.

Perception of the Upright

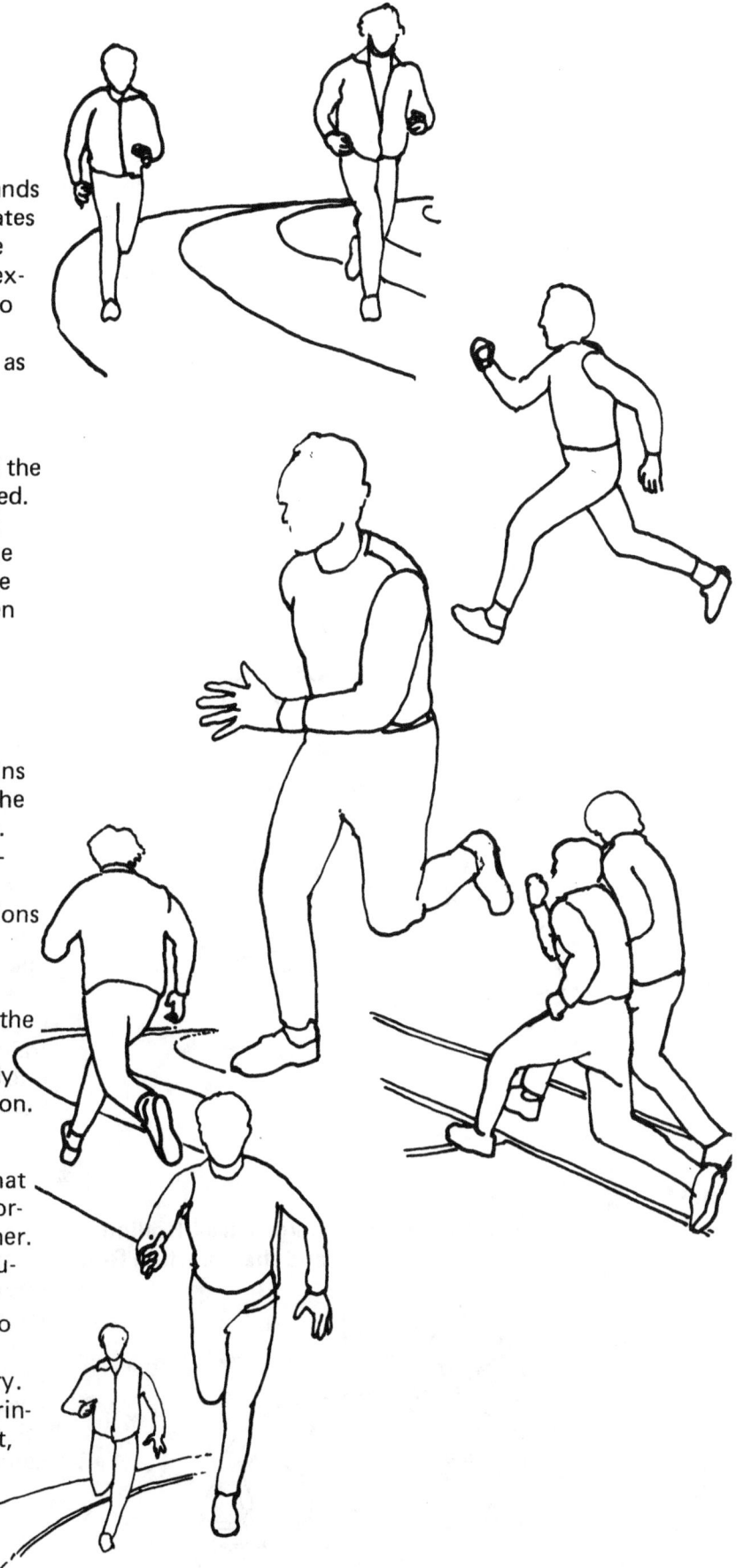

- As the leg-wheel opens from medium to full size, the periphery of the circle expands accordingly and a greater distance separates the space between the front heel and the back toe. Correspondingly, the C-curve extends its upward bend that much more to maintain the principle of the plumb-line center, with the lower spine functioning as the core leader of this activity.

- In the loping run, the arms are more extended, the hands more open-fisted, and the fingers more alertly reaching, as illustrated. Avoid clenching the fists or closing tight the spaces between your fingers. With the loping run, you should be able to feel the air "breezing" through finger spaces, even if those spaces are imperceptible to the eye.

- Make sure to steady your shoulders so they don't sway from side to side or jut back and forth. The same principle obtains to the head. You'll quickly notice how the arms and hands move in orb-like fashion. It is these arm circles, plus the spine connection to the under-thigh muscles, that trigger and actually generate the revolutions of the leg-wheel.

- Be careful not to bounce down on your heel. Bouncing on the heel is a shock to the heel-bone **and** to the entire body. It prevents smooth rolling and throws the body into a heavy, helpless, pre-falling condition.

- Be certain, throughout your loping run, that the body feels balanced and easy; that it does not intentionally **lean or thrust** forward or backward, to one side or the other. From the waist, the spine-curve just naturally "crescents" upward and forward. What you are seeking is least resistance to the **body in movement**, in order to optimize efficiency, effectiveness, and artistry. If you remain aware primarily of the intrinsic rhythm of your running style and gait, and tune in to the rhythm-feel of that

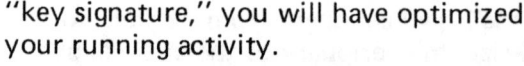
Energy and Relaxation in Movement

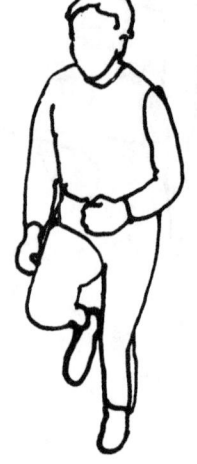

"key signature," you will have optimized your running activity.

- Practice the lope-run for the rhythm feel, and then vary it by alternately introducing buoyancy, radiancy, and potency energy.

- Apply the breathing process described earlier in this chapter. Start with a smaller norm if the one you used with small-wheel jogging was in any way strenuous. Recall the procedure: If you begin with a norm of twenty-five strides, repeat it once or twice; next, reduce the norm by complements of five until you reach five strides per breath; then repeat the last five and end with breath-sighs in and out until you feel relaxed. The entire procedure is done while running. Of course, in the beginning, if you need several breaths in between stride-count changes, do take them. Recall that the three-fold object is to build your endurance — to develop speed and agility — and to **experience the esthetics of running.**

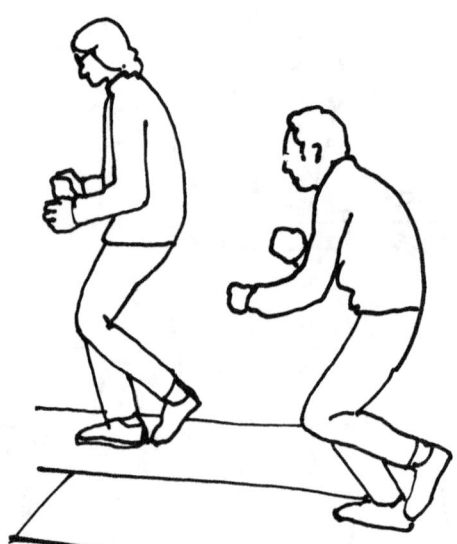

The instructions for distance running and sprinting are fundamental, but they are intended here for general application. Specific preparation and coaching for track meets and particular events encompass a broader, structural regime of creative training, diet, rest, etc., as well as a more intensive discipline in the applications of Body Wisdom.

Experiment Nine: **Large Wheel Rolling and the Sprinting Run**

In speed running, radiancy energy dominates inasmuch as lambent lightness is the basic body feel. To harness speed running to this radiancy energy state, keep reminding yourself of the role played by the spine and back in generating the lifting and smooth revolving of the large leg-wheels. Keep in mind that one runs with the energy-relaxer centers of the back and spine; that the rest

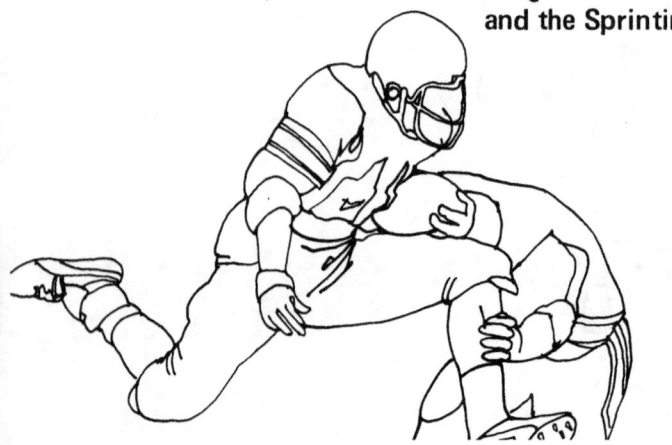

Perception of the Upright

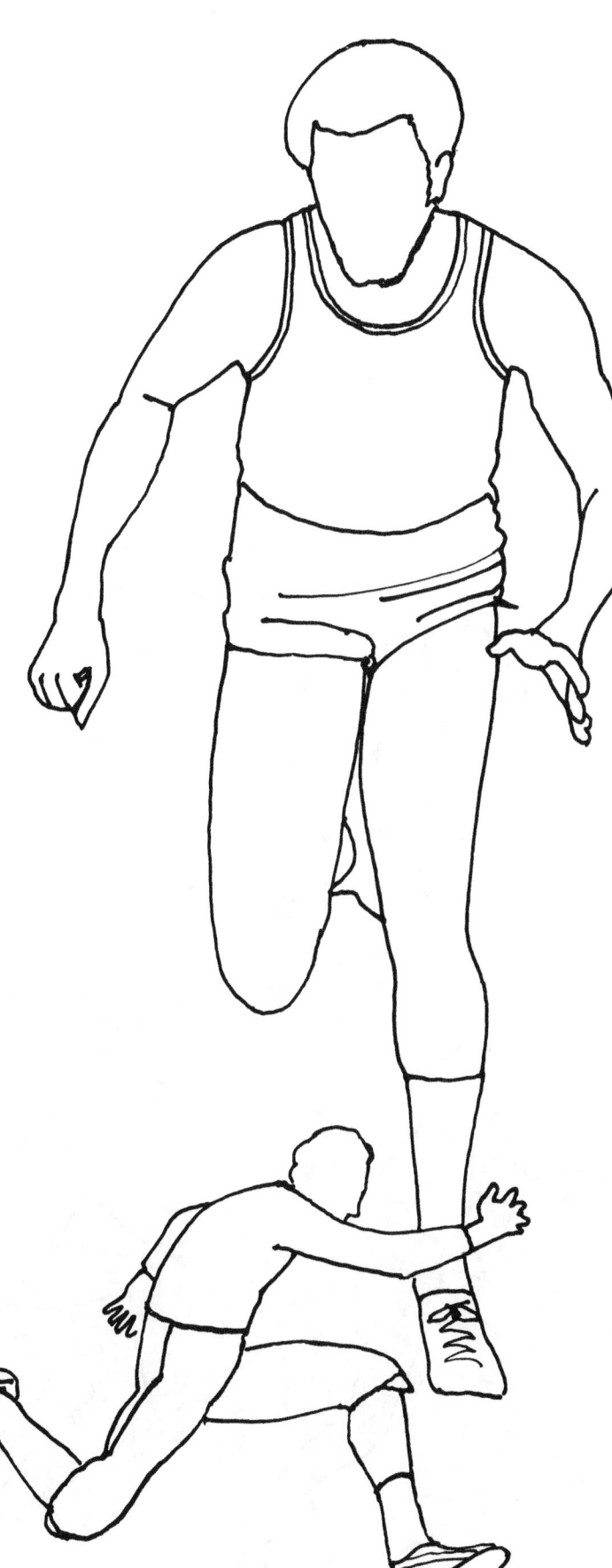

of the body simply enjoys maximum freedom, liberating the body in movement for full-fledged running. Your first key is the spine, then the arms, **and then**, your free-wheeling legs.

- For the sprinting run, envision your C-curve as an extended electrified coil-spring, with the two ends sending arcing sparks of vitality toward each other in an energy circle that may be imaged as a "traveling personal space sphere."

- Now, instead of your hands and arms moving in circles or orbs, they become rocker-rims, moving from one end of the rather long rocker-rim to the other. The hands are more open (never clenched), and lead with palms facing downward three quarters as illustrated. Your arms will rock naturally in front of the body. They should **not** be thrust all the way back and then, strenuously pumped forward. This only creates undue tension and tightness.

- In sprinting, you should actually feel an eased-up rhythm. It feels as though the larger leg-wheel takes a bit longer to complete its revolution even though the distance is covered more rapidly.

- Concentrate only on the rhythm. The intrinsic rhythm of the body in movement. serves as a signal system for the leg and arm muscles. The arms provide a sense of balance while the legs follow the rhythm cues. If you approach your running artistically, the feel of that rhythm esthetic will free and loosen every muscle, joint, and ligament in your body.

NOTE: Do not, in your sprinting, concentrate on the progressive, stride-changing breathing process we used for jogging, loping, cross-country and distance running. For short sprints no special effort need be exerted to breathe in particular key signatures. The beneficial accrual of your previous training and explorations will suffice. As long as you

Energy and Relaxation in Movement

breathe naturally and instinctively during the sprint, your body should not require practiced or specially planned inhalations to sustain the gait and rhythm with ease.

Breathe naturally with the "small of the back" (lower spine center) and let the front of the body take care of itself. For racing, this will keep the body light and free as you radiantly dart from the starting line and dash to the finish.

Experiment Ten: Hill Running

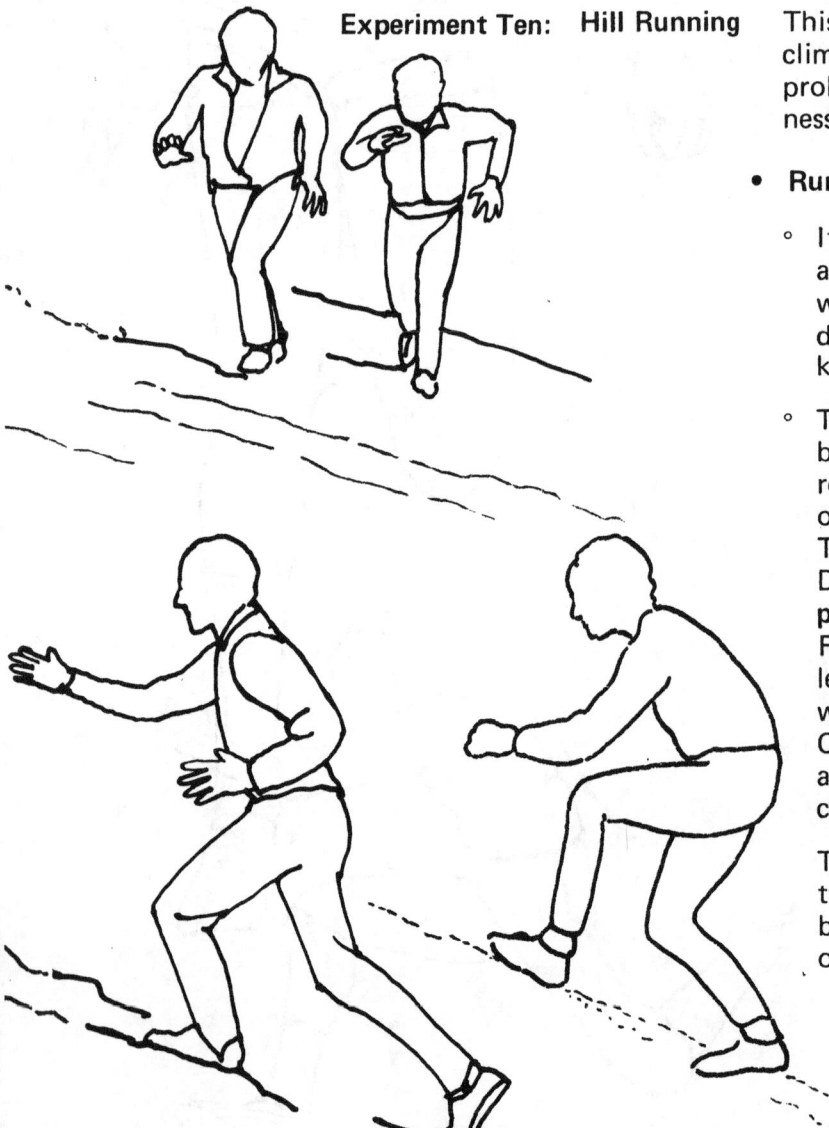

This is a common experience. We've all climbed hills and run down them, but probably with less efficiency or effectiveness than is available to us.

- **Running Up or Climbing a Hill**

  ◦ It may sound contradictory, but with the assistance of potency energy and our leg-wheels we can actually "**roll** uphill." To do this requires a sense of stretching and kinesthetic body-yawn.

  ◦ The key to running uphill is the "leveled" body position produced by balanced rocker-rim leg-wheels, following each other as quickly and, easily as possible. Translated into an organic instruction: Do not **push** with one leg in order to **pull** your body up with the other. Rather, stay in lambent balance on one leg-wheel while the other revolves upward, attended by a well-rounded, deep C-curve. As graphically indicated, as soon as that rocker-rimmed foot has made contact, the other wheel begins to revolve.

The feeling, here, is that of **rolling up** on two revolving wheels while the rest of the body remains in leveled balance. Instead of the usual pushing and pulling, huffing

Perception
of the
Upright

and puffing uphill, you'll experience a
series of pleasurable balancing acts.

° The steeper the hill, the more compact
the body sphere: As your C-curve bends
to accommodate the incline, always
maintain your plumb-line center.

° If you rock on your rocker-rimmed feet,
you will feel yourself rolling up. As you
roll uphill, breathe rapidly and regularly
through your lower spinal (relaxer-
energizer) center.

• **Downhill Running:**

° Running downhill is primarily a loosening
up and shaking exercise with **less than
medium-sized leg-wheels**, for optimal speed
and spontaneous functioning. Leg-wheels
that are either too small or too large will,
in this case, cause loss of balance and
control.

° As always, use your foot rocker-rims from
head to toe. The steeper the decline, the
more you should rely on rocker-rims to
balance your leg-wheels.

° Above all, avoid bouncing and landing
hard on your feet. In other words, do
not destroy the rhythm and balance of
downhill leg-wheel running by introducing shock stress or extra body
weight to the bones and joints.

° If you feel the rhythm, rather than the
running, of shaking down with properly
sized leg-wheels, you will control both
the rhythm **and** the running.

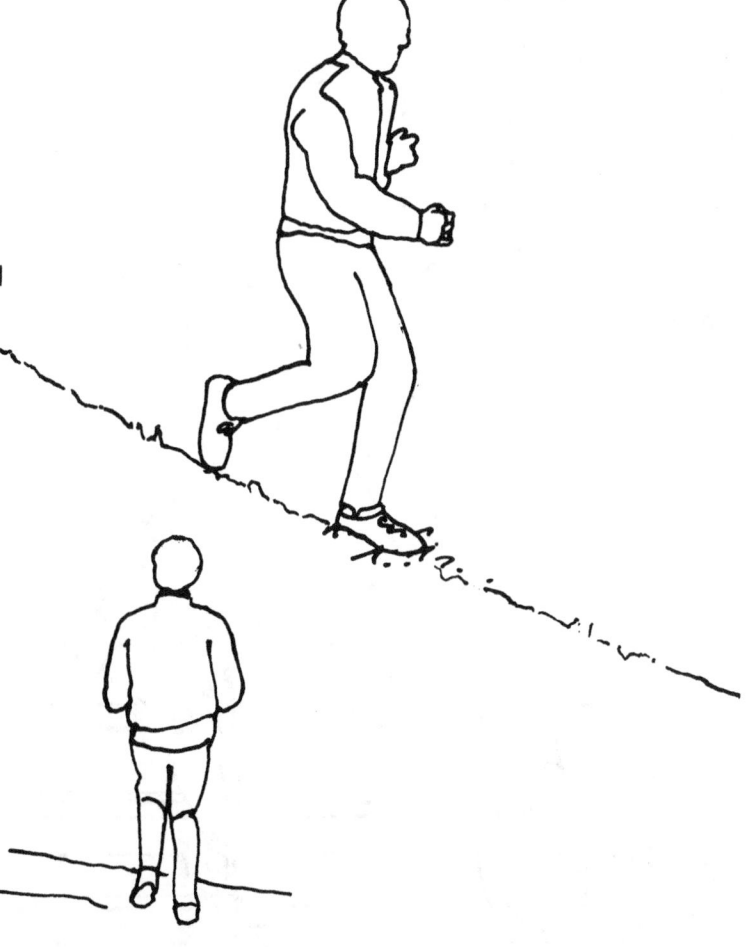

Elevators and escalators are our society's
technological admission that climbing
stairs, up and down, is a hardship no
"civilized modern" should have to suffer.
Climbing (or rolling) **up** the stairs is a unique
experience in body balance; dancing **down**
the stairs is a unique experience in body
agility and body radiance.

Experiment Eleven: Climbing Stairs

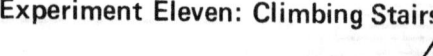

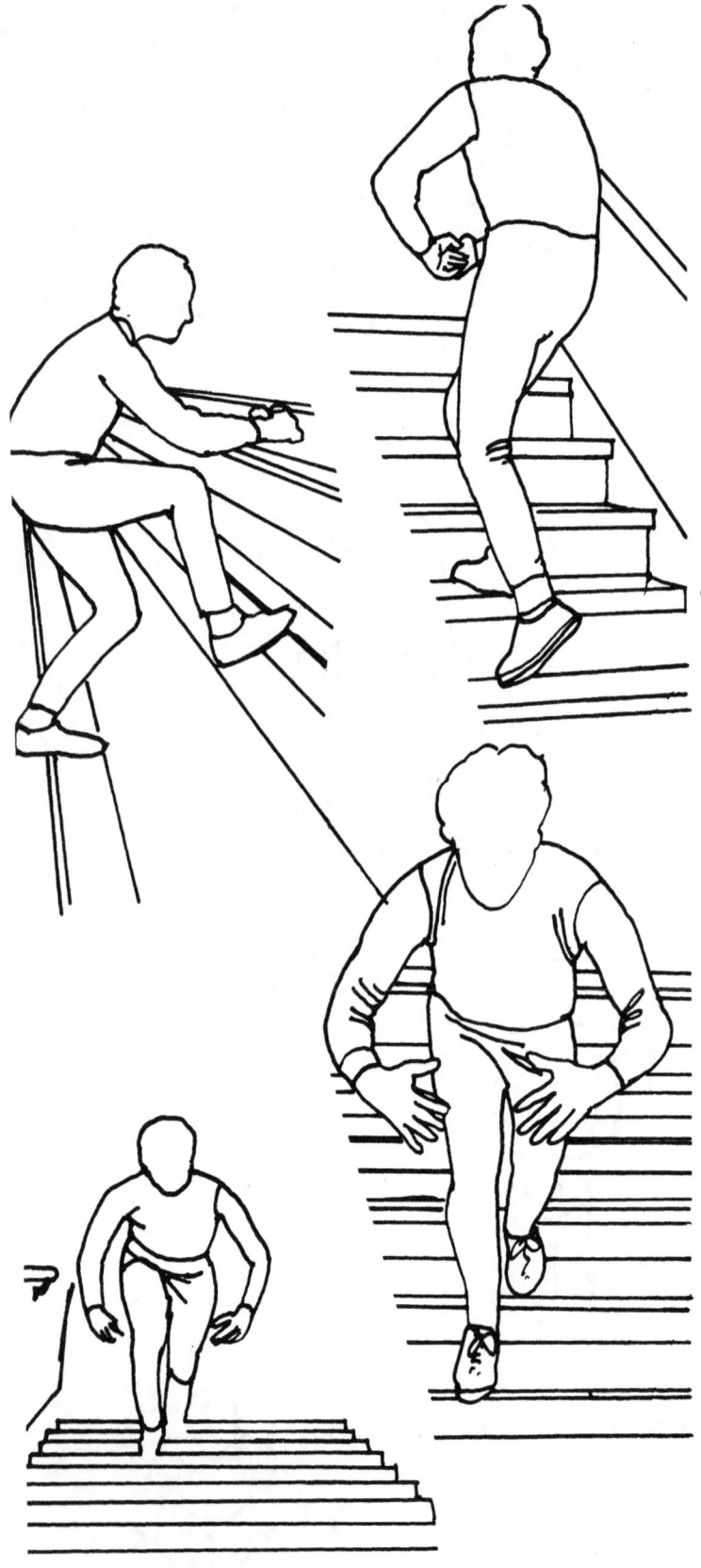

With us, climbing stairs is a psycho-physical exploration in energetic relaxation and relaxed energy at the same time.

If you recall the "in-place" (marking) exercises with the upright bow and leg-wheel set forth earlier in this chapter, you will find your way to applying that action to "rolling up stairs." **Indeed, climbing stairs with "bow and wheel" is nothing more than a balancing act!**

- **Climbing Up the Stairs:**

The kinesthetic strategy for stair-climbing is not to feel the weight of the body at any time. Follow the graphics and begin your practice on a stool or on a single platform. It will then be a simple matter of transferring the action to the flight of stairs, basically a series of ascending stools or platforms.

○ Start at the point where your lower foot completes the "foot rock" while the upper wheel begins its rocking action. Taste the feel of that preliminary rock and roll before stimulating the leg-wheels to "roll up" through a series of balancing acts.

○ The free wheel will simply roll itself up in moving balance while the contact leg sustains the body in delicate pedestal balance.

○ The body should not feel itself going up or down. It only feels **level**, as in rising buoyancy or gliding, upward levitation. The combination of breathing energy with buoyancy and radiancy energy states constantly "buoys" you up.

- **Climbing Down Stairs:**

This is a body shaking and loosening experience that has you toe-tipping agilely down

Perception of the Upright

the stairs with "vanishing contact feel." The radiant vibrations become especially important for smooth functioning of the ankle joints, knees, thighs, shoulders, elbows, wrists, and cervical joints of the neck.

○ As you dance down lightly and trippingly on the toes, feel your arms and body jiggle and shake like a dish of jello. You'll barely touch the surface of each stair as you nimbly "tap-dance" yourself down them.

○ Make sure to get the rhythm feel of every step. The lighter you feel them, the easier it will be to glide your way down.

○ Resist the temptation to skip steps as you do your downstairs shaking and vibrating. This is neither safe nor physically graceful.

• **Climbing (Rolling) Up Stairs Two Steps at a Time:**

Whereas you should avoid climbing **down** stairs two or more at a time, you can certainly learn how to roll **up** a series of stairs safely and smoothly on your leg-wheels. The strategy here is to employ a more deeply-flexed C-curve, resulting in a much shorter plumb line between eyebone and kneecap.

You'll be using mostly a body-yawn stretch energy, in comfortable combination with our other energy states. Your C-curved body will feel like a "slinky" coil-spring, anxious to uncoil itself. With two and three steps rolling-up, arm rocking action comes to the forefront.

As you are by now aware, we cannot in this text edition cover individual track and field or other related events and sports. These await separate treatment in subsequent, more specialized works. However, those of

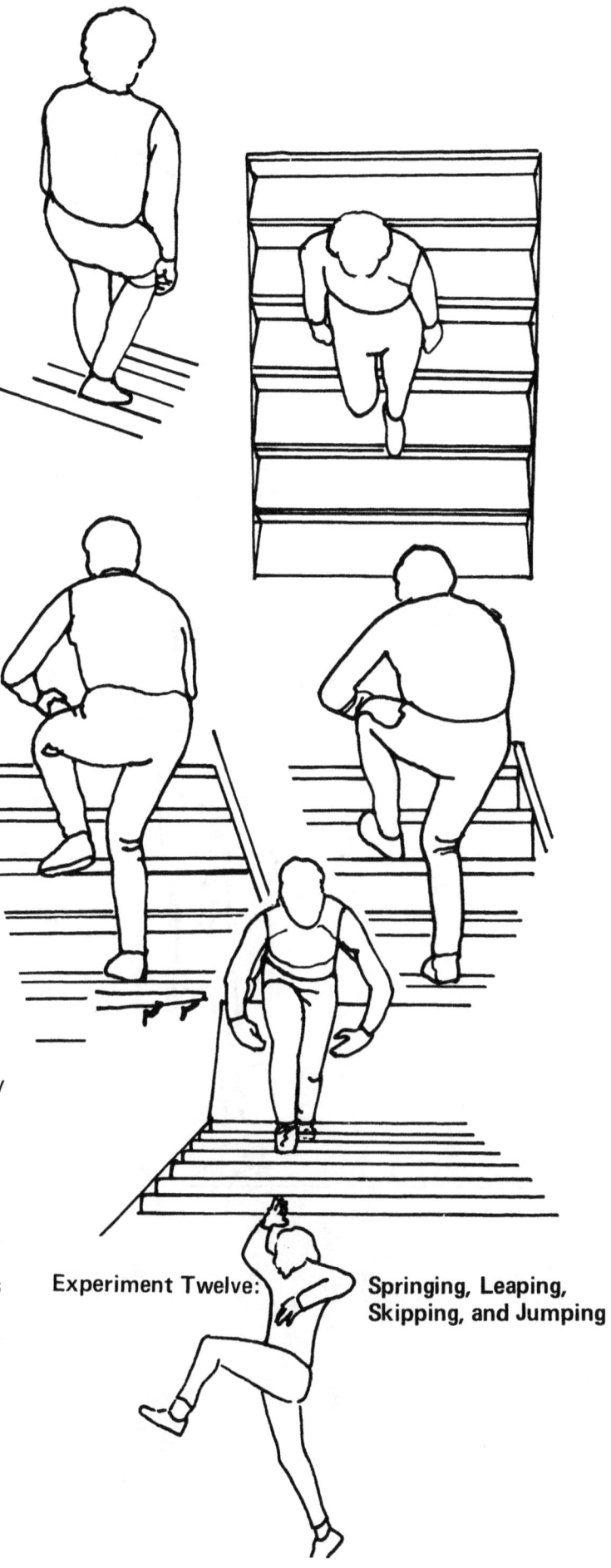

Experiment Twelve: Springing, Leaping, Skipping, and Jumping

Energy and
Relaxation
in Movement

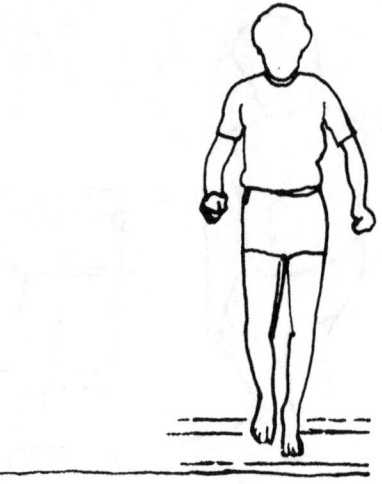

you involved in such activities can productively apply what we learn here to any and all of them, particularly in regard to the "feeling process;" the perception of energy states; relaxer-energizers; body esthetics; and general body intelligence. We will, however, devote considerable space and time to the general area of body springing, leaping, hopping and rope-skipping.

- **Pogo-Stick Spring and Jump**

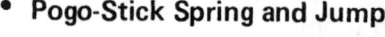

For springing activities, contact vanishing point, body weightlessness, and coil-spring agility are each, and together, the dominant chords. Let's begin with "pogo-stick" springing and jumping — essentially, gentle body-recoiling with radiancy energy.

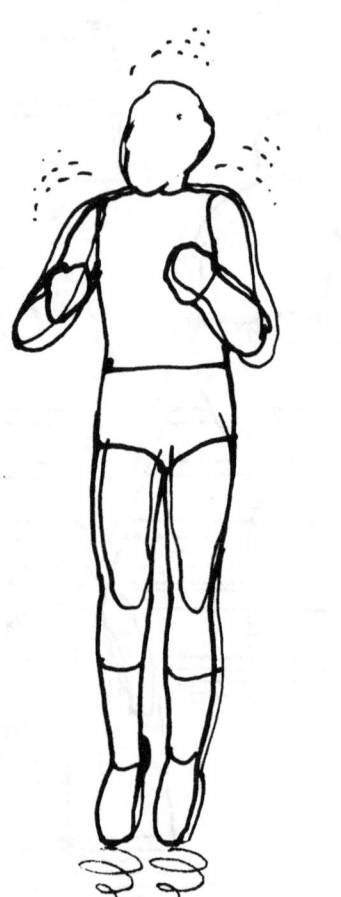

- Start with a rhythmic, coil-spring toe-stretch. Continue the up and down, dance-like toe-stretch until you feel your toes letting go of the ground surface. Take special note of this gentle, off-the-ground recoil as it will also constitute your first rope-skip action.

- Always using the ground as a "touch-off pad," let the gentle spring-offs take you higher and higher into the air. Focus on energetically "resting-up" and enjoying the upper space for that brief instant.

- The lighter you touch the ground, the more the "up-spring" will uncoil.

- Return for relaxation to the preliminary, pogo-stick recoil, and once more, gradually take off into the air, always aware of the rhythm of each jump.

- **Skipping:**

You have done this continually and spontaneously as a child. Now come back to this lovely body action with perception of its rhythm and movement, and enjoy it once again as "play experience." Wherever

Perception of the Upright

possible we have supplied graphics; check them out and relate to them.

° Begin by skipping lightly, then lambently with radiancy energy. Do this as long as it feels comfortable.

° When you need to rest, simply return to the gentle, pogo-stick launch pad and dance your way through the elastic, toe-stretch recoil.

° As the toe-stretch constitutes the first rope-skip action, so this skipping step forms the basis for the second, rope-springing activity.

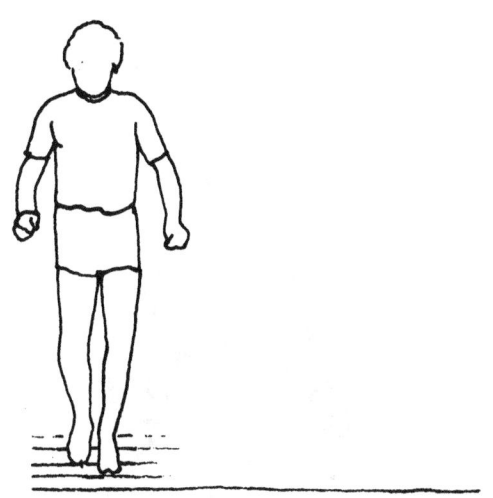

Experiment Thirteen: Rope Skipping or Rope Dancing

• I refer to this activity also as "rope dancing" in order to stress its body esthetics and artistic eurhythmics. Rope skipping is a powerful body-builder involving the total use of the body in natural exercise (see p. 173).
° It is a prime developer of the cardio-vascular region.

° It offers one of the finest ways to increase body endurance.

° **It provides a complete workout in fifteen minutes that equals a running workout of approximately three times the duration** —a superior workout in that the muscles remain looser and freer than in strong running.

° It approaches that dance-like resting and relaxing activity we recommend to relieve fatigue during running or in any other body building activity.

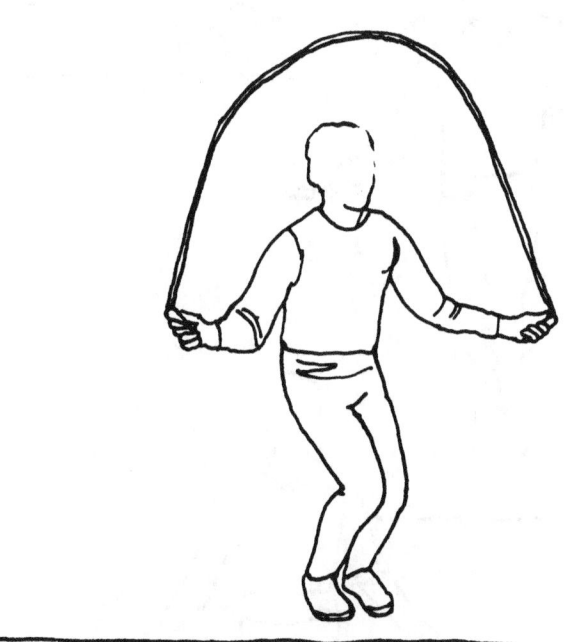

Rope skipping relates most directly to the C-curved back and spine; to the plumb-line center of balance; to rhythm and breathing; to the forceful awareness of the feel of body electricity and body buoyancy. It coordinates independent arm, wrist, and shoulder

Energy and Relaxation in Movement

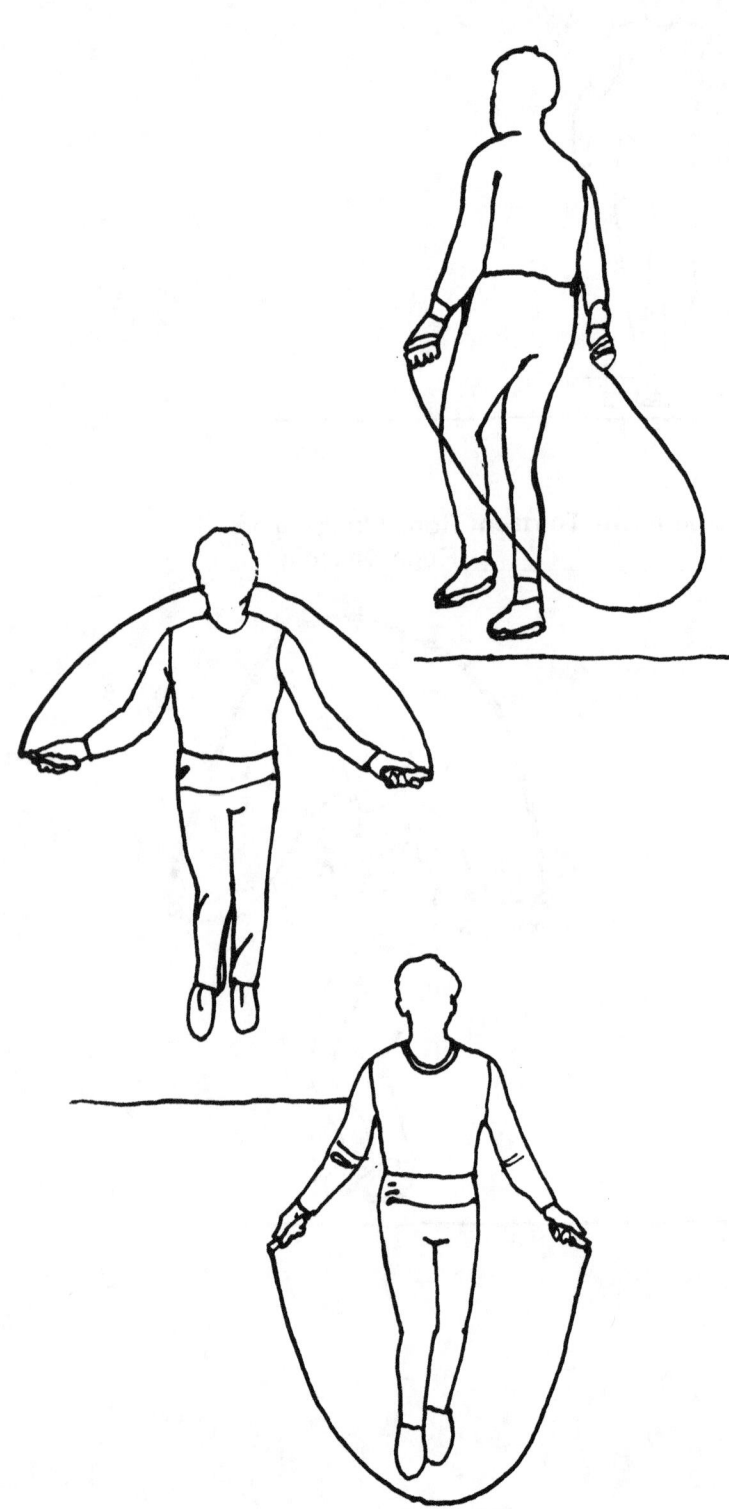

movement with jumping. And through rope skipping, the body can teach itself how to become more "spirited" by combining the radiancy and buoyancy energy states.

Before initiating the exercises below, a word about the skip-rope itself. Your rope should have "body" to it — not too light — and, like your own body, feel "live" and responsive. Too many of the skip-ropes currently on the market carry their own dead weight. So select your rope carefully.

It ought to be heavier than a clothes line. If, when you hold the handles waist high, as illustrated, the rope feels like a natural physical extension of your arms and body, and its size measures a comfortable sweep to the floor, then you've got a very good "live skip-rope." The importance of a rope with the right weight and size — the right fit for your body — to the following exercises, cannot be overemphasized.

- **Preliminary Coil-Spring Warm-Up:**
  (without the skip-rope)

  Do the light and agile pogo-stick coil-spring hop, on your toes, two feet at a time. Note that your C-curve may be a bit more pronounced in rope skipping than it was in pogo-stick springing.

- **Second-Stage Skipping Warm-Up:**
  (without actual rope-swinging)

  Do your gentle skipping, alternating one foot at a time. Do not spring too high — just enough to feel the rhythm of the jump, the hands, the imaged rope-swing, the rhythm of the whole body. Remember: you are dancing, not jumping. (Now use the rope.)

Perception of the Upright

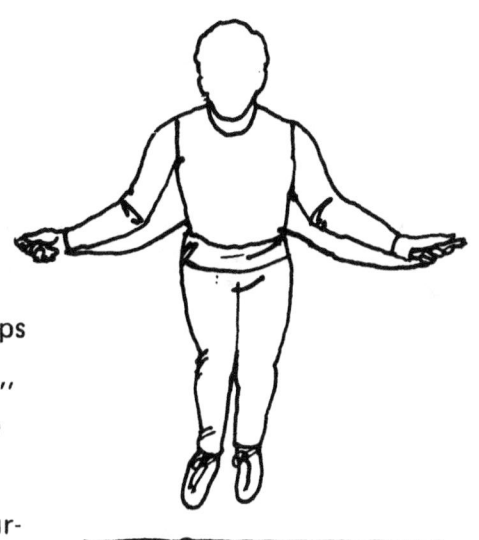

- **Combining the Coil-Spring Hop with Gentle Skipping:**

  Use the skip-rope and do the steps you've often seen youngsters do; alternate the skips first on one foot then the other. Skip with the same light feel of the "coil-spring hop." Guided by the feeling of rhythm, combine them into a rope-skip action for as long as you can. Don't be discouraged if at first your coordination is poor. Familiarize yourself with the style, quality, and rhythm by dancing the step swinging the rope in one hand; then resuming the rope-skipping with the identical rhythm feel. Once you have the basic swing, you can train for speed and endurance.

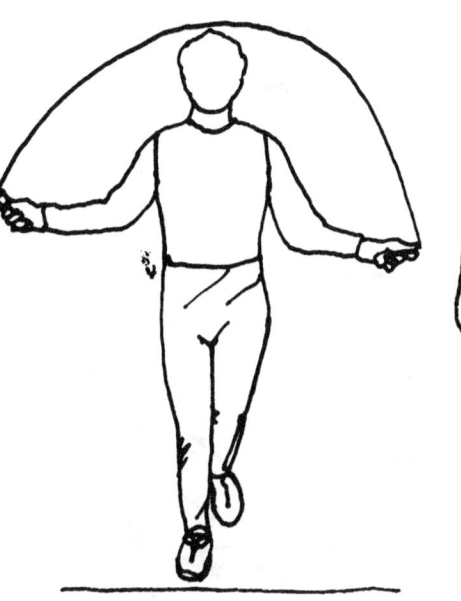 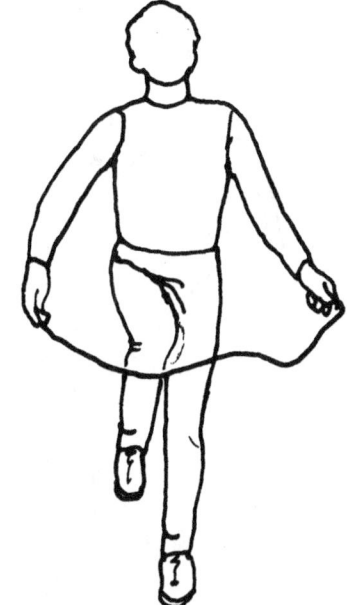

- **Rope-Swinging While Running and Jogging:**

  Small-wheel, medium-wheel, or large-wheel running, using the skip-rope, is an excellent exercise if you have the space. It requires a bit of timing and coordination, and works beautifully if you are sufficiently **carefree** to enjoy the esthetics.

- **Criss-Cross Rope Swinging:**

  ○ Spring with both feet at the same time, as illustrated. This is basically the pogo-stick jump, except that now the arms criss-cross the rope.

  ○ Criss-cross once every three or four jumps, at the outset. Then increase the regularity until you use it for every spring.

  ○ Criss-cross the left arm over the right; then change to right arm over left. Then alternate until you can make the shift on every spring.

  ○ Do not concentrate on foot actions. Let your arms feel the rhythm and the legs will follow.

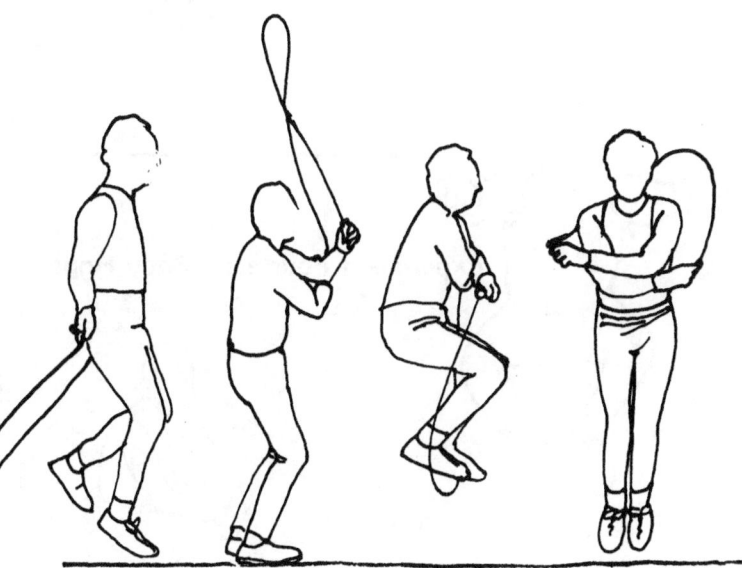

Energy and
Relaxation
in Movement

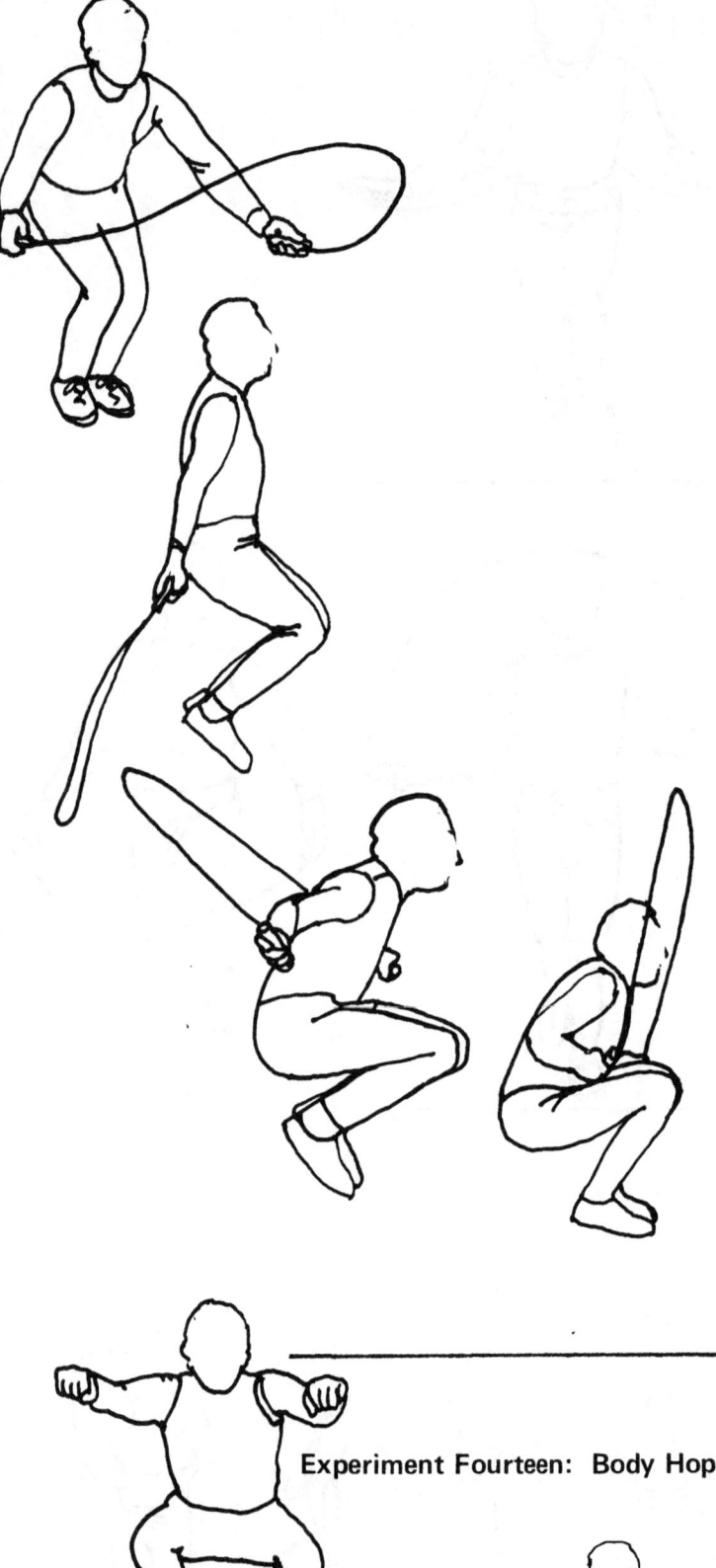

- **Double Rope-Swing on Single Spring-Jumps:**

  These are not easy, but great fun. You simply swing the rope twice on a single skip while maintaining balance and rhythm. Three swings on a single jump is also fun but very difficult — it is a challenge but certainly not a requirement.

  NOTE: If you have a heart condition, perform this movement sparingly as a dance experience, and only after a medical check-up.

  ° Keeping your muscles loose, jump weightlessly with your leg-spring, somewhat higher than before, and let your arms effortlessly swing the rope.

  ° Remain carefree. If you work too hard at this, it becomes an exhausting action. Double rope-swinging involves balance of a number of movements and an integration of several different body rhythms.

  ° At first, double-swing once every five or six jumps. Then gradually increase the frequency until you can do it rhythmically on several successive jumps. As with all of the exercises in this chapter, avoid hard landing on the feet or any heaviness in the jump.

- When you have completed all of the fundamentals, and feel entirely comfortable with each, create your own variations of artistic rope springing and rope dancing.

Experiment Fourteen: Body Hops

Body hop-leaps, integrating the squat postures you already know, are natural continuations of double-swing rope springing. These are primarily spine curving and thigh strengthening exercises that **protect the knee-joints by giving them breathing**

202

Perception of the Upright

space and "living room." Because our body hops emphasize the squat postures, we will begin with the squat-run.

- **The Squat Jog or Squat Dance:**

  Similar to the sit-walk, this movement incorporates free-wheeling, sophisticated foot-rocking, body rolling, and sliding at the same time.

  ° Imagine yourself "waddling" like a duck or goose and transfer that image to the feel of your own feet rolling on its rocker-rims. As you move, the body feels as if it is on thousands of tiny ball-bearings with your arms acting almost like tiny sails.

  ° Introduce inter-involvement energy to the squat run in everyday training. As you glide along, acknowledge the outside world: greet passersby; engage in window-shopping; tie your shoe laces; help a disabled person cross the street, etc.

- **The Sparrow Spring-Away:**

  Like the squat jog, this hopping variation induces the feel of inter-involvement energy. It should make you feel like a little sparrow or sandpiper — lovely to see, lovely to feel, graceful, beautiful, and **light as a feather.** Work with the graphics wherever available to develop the physical characteristics of the sparrow spring-away.

- **The Chicken Spring and Wing-Flap:**
  This is a relatively short-distance leap-spring, not very high off the ground but more than the sparrow spring-away.

  ° The accent is on quick, dartlike, hopping sensations.
  ° Coordinate your "chicken spring" with arm-flapping which helps keep the movement vibrated and light.
  ° Once again, introduce inter-involvement energy by practicing the "chicken

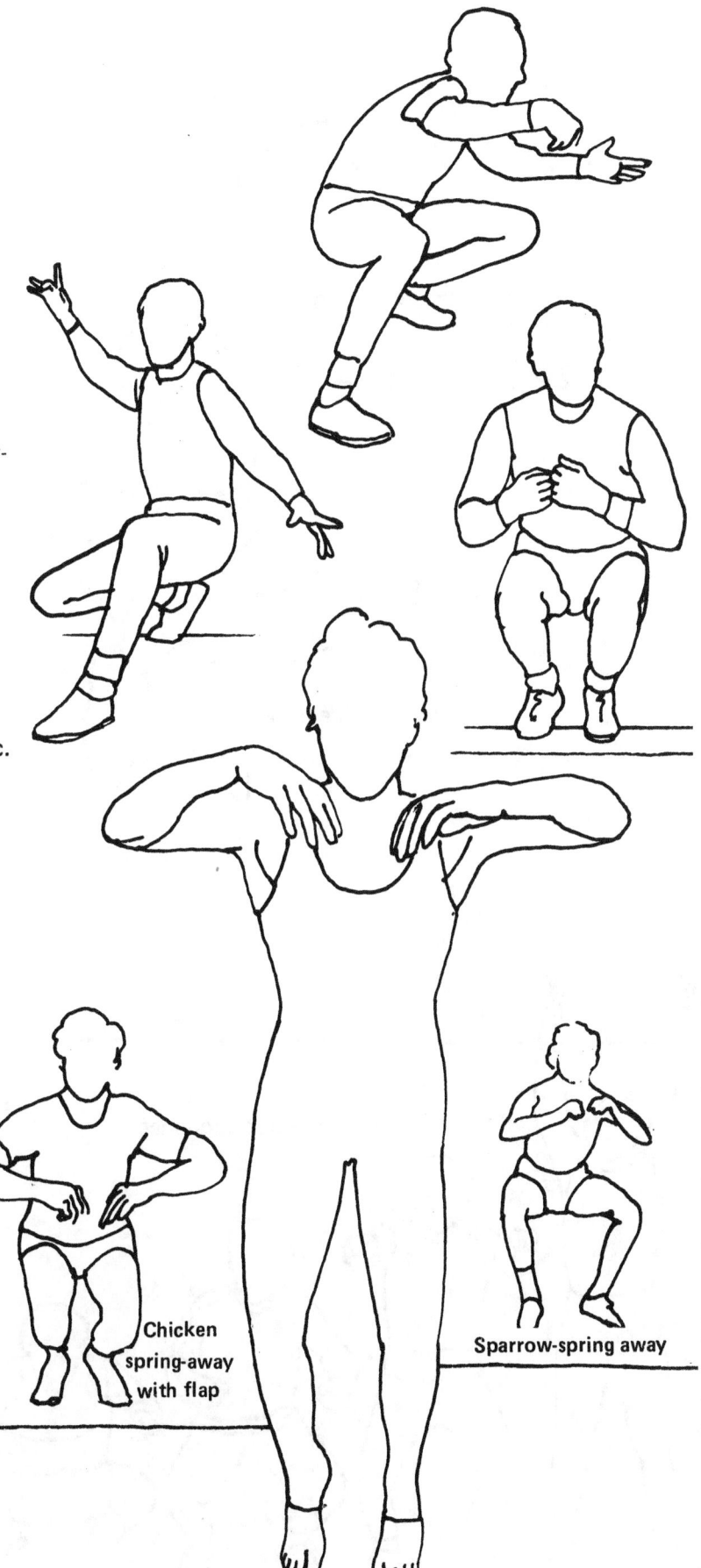

Chicken spring-away with flap

Sparrow-spring away

Energy and
Relaxation
in Movement

spring and wing-flap" in daily relations with the external environment. Check with available graphics and relate.

- **The Jockey-Ride Hop:**

We now approach a series of more vigorous hop-leaps. Don't be surprised if your front thigh muscles experience certain uncommon sensations the next day, and tell you so. They're simply responding to unfamiliar movement and requesting, in direct body language, more relaxer-energizer activity.

It is curious how even those of us who keep very active and eschew the usual conveyances in favor of climbing stairs, walking, bending, etc. for natural exercise, still underestimate the needs and potential of the thigh muscle. That is, until we do these vigorous hop-leaps.

So be judicious in the amount of time you initially allot to these next exercises. If you've worked well and easily through the upright experiments until now, with the right combination of relaxed energy and energetic relaxation, you should be ready for jockey hops, kangaroo hops, and one-foot hop-springs. But use your own good judgment.

NOTE: Again, I want to alert and urge you before attempting these more strenuous activities to be sure you've had a thorough medical check-up, to confirm that you are as strong of heart as you are of spirit.

- **Jockey-ride Hop:**

  ○ Start with a body-yawn stretch to the ceiling, as if trying to uncork your body from the waist up. Feel the elongated C-curve from the hollows of the knees to the tips of your fingers.

  ○ Continue the C-curve stretch into a water-skiing or horseback riding position, and

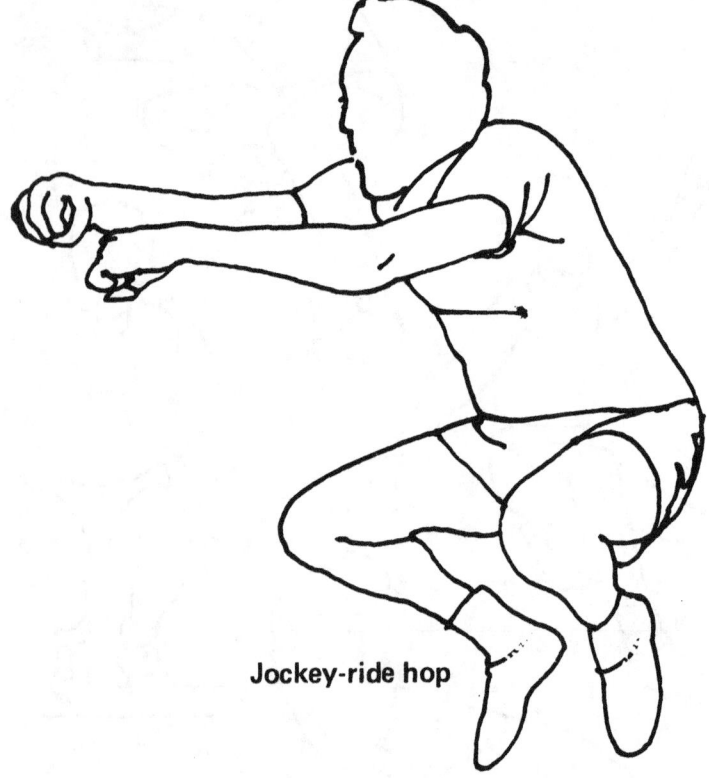
Jockey-ride hop

Start of Jockey-ride hop sequence

follow-through by holding onto the imagined reins or rope-lines.

○ Now, maintaining the riding posture — with feet high in the stirrups and body not really seated in the saddle, almost in squat position — feel yourself moving up and down with the horse's rhythm. As you get into a full jockey-seat squat, you'll begin to move. Through the use of your thighs, legs, feet, and arms, the "jockey hop" moves the body upward (and forward) in medium-sized spring-leaps.

○ Still "riding the horse," begin to take fairly long and higher leaps. Measure these by what feels secure for maintaining a light-weight body in perfect balance over a reasonable distance. Through a **series** of jockey leaps, you ought to cover a distance anywhere from 30 to 50 yards. Do not try to increase the distance of each successive hop, as this exercise is better served by more hops that are better controlled.

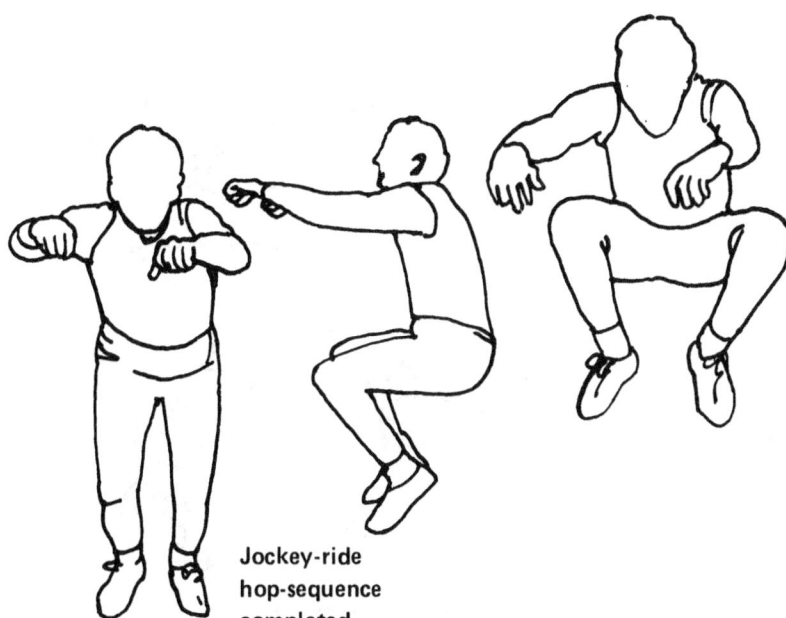

Jockey-ride hop-sequence completed

After three or four weeks of practice, you should find that the lighter your body, the higher you'll spring. And the higher you spring, the easier it will be to retain a fetal-like position with legs folded up at the height of the jockey hop.

- **Kangaroo Leaps:**

  Similar to the jockey hop, the kangaroo leap produces a somewhat higher spring. The feet and legs fold into squat position in the air and require fewer jumps to cover the same distance. Instead of relying on the jockey-riding image, your body is, itself the Kangaroo in action.

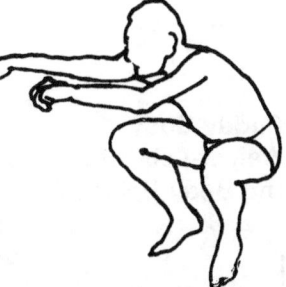

Kangaroo-leap

- **One-Foot Hop-Springs:**

  This is the springing away of the bird or the cat, or the dancer who leaps high into

Energy and
Relaxation
in Movement

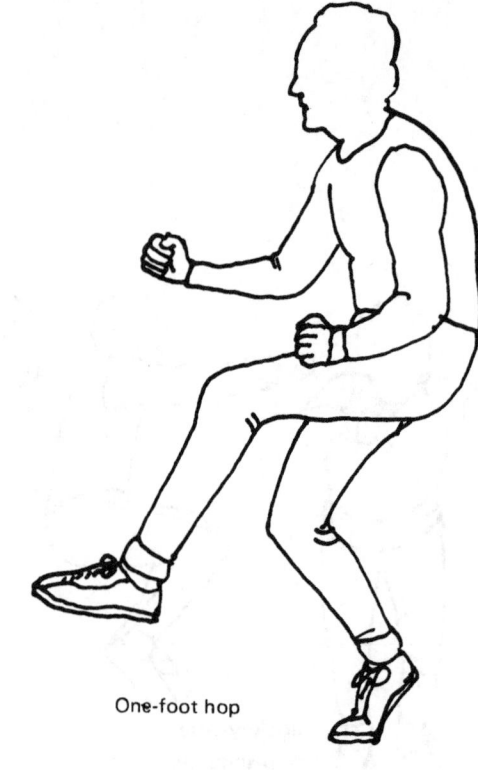
One-foot hop

the air with every intention of pausing for a second or two in vital stillness before coming down.

Not an easy exploit — the one-foot hop-spring requires gradual strengthening of the legs over several weeks. So approach it with preparation and good conditioning and don't, at first, stay too close to the ground.

○ Start in upright C-curve position with the knee flexed for comfort and looseness. Hop on one leg, not too forcibly, concentrating on lightness.

○ While hopping, gradually move lower (as close as comfortably possible) to sitting position; then, if you feel up to it, gradually return to a flexible, upright C-curve.

○ Borrow the image of staying in the air after weightless take-off. Avoid any distracting focus on either the landing or the height.

The work in the hop and spring section takes on the semblance of Russian-style folk dancing, especially with the squat springs and leg thrusts. In fact, when the work is comfortable, the carry-over to the dance activity becomes your creative exploring activity. All leaps or hops have the characteristic "feel" of springing away, not landing.

Experiment Fifteen: Buddy Body Weight-Leg-Lifts and Body Balance

The following exercises reinforce coil-spring stretching, resilient body lifting, buddy-balance, springing away, and catapulting skills through buddy work in variously combined positions.

- **Coil-Spring Action:**

  ○ Sit on your partner's feet, as illustrated, and begin a comfortable coil-spring,

Leg-lift coil spring action

206

Perception of the Upright

gently stretching up and down with easeful balance.

○ You should feel as weightless as possible as you ride your buddy's foot elevator in energetic relaxation, while your partner experiences restful energy in resilient, elastic leg and thigh movement from the lowest point of the ground to the highest.

○ Continue the coordinated coil-spring for as long as it feels mutually pleasant and enjoyable. To invigorate the activity as it progresses, the "rider" buddy will introduce a bit more off-the-floor body balance to the ride.

- **Lift-Up**

    After completing numerous coil-springs and before lift-off, your partner is ready to raise the foot elevator to its highest lift-up level with maximum equilibrium.

    ○ While your buddy prepares for "lift-off," both of you must cooperate with a skill-ful combination of moving, pedestal, and pin-point balance.

    ○ You may keep your feet adrift or rest them on your partner's thighs or seat. His/her hands may either hold on or remain free.

- **From Coil-Spring to Spring–Away:**

    Follow the graphics for this three-step procedure. With proper teamwork, you will eventually be catapulted by your buddy relatively high and far, landing lightly on your feet in squat position or C-curve up-right posture. This activity is a full event and makes complete sequential use of all the steps above. The accent is on resilience, grace, lightness, rhythm, and balance.

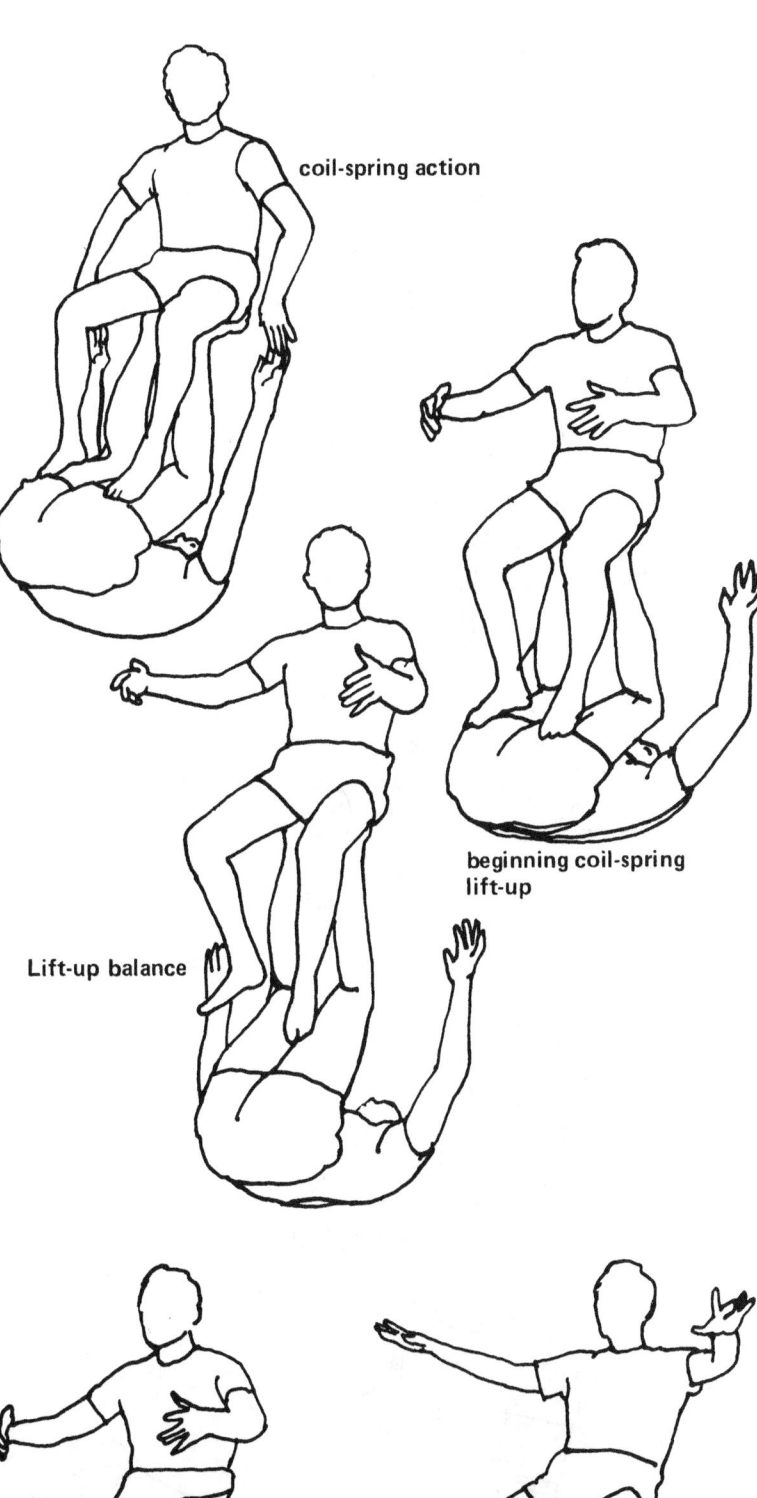

coil-spring action

beginning coil-spring lift-up

Lift-up balance

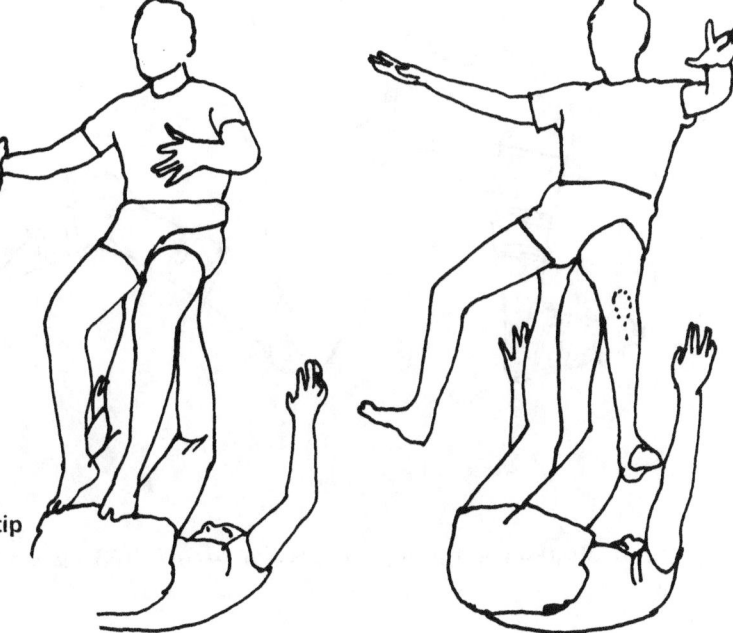

coil-spring toe-tip balance

Spring-away balance

Energy and
Relaxation
in Movement

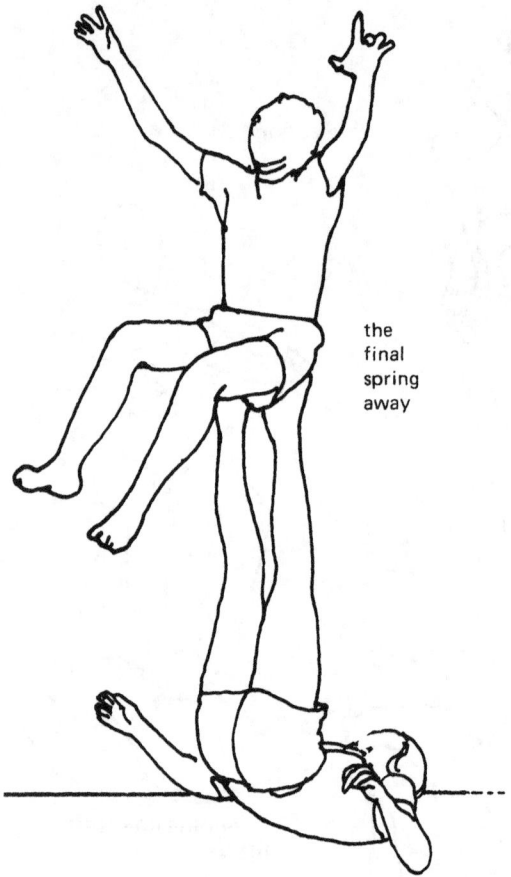

the final spring away

Some helping hints:

° Any time either of you feels the burden of weight or an impending loss of balance, counteract by applying the appropriate body energy states.

° Do not proceed to lift-up until you have both experienced the coil-spring action as a delightful, comfortable game; and certainly do not even attempt the spring-away until you have achieved the same degree of control with the lift-up.

° Before approaching the spring-away and catapult, make sure you can negotiate the lift-up of a partner at least fifty pounds heavier than yourself.

Summary Notes and Special Comments

1. **Breathing While Running:**

Different running styles, weather conditions, and body circumstances mandate different breathing cycles, rhythms, and techniques. What we need at **all** times is the quietest, easiest, most efficient, and most expansive, comfortable intake of air. This requires us to determine, at any given moment, which is easier: breathing through the nose or through the mouth?

The concern is not merely whether you can continue to breathe easily and freely, but also whether you are able, at any necessary moment, to alter the character, quality, or quantity of the breathing cycle, its rhythm and technique. If you find yourself in the untenable situation of panting and gasping for air that you cannot convert into salutary vigorous sighing, then you have clearly gone beyond your safety cushion and you should pause to walk or dance a bit for relaxation and then start over again.

If your safety cushion sends warning signals (such as a sensation of oncoming exhaustion) while you

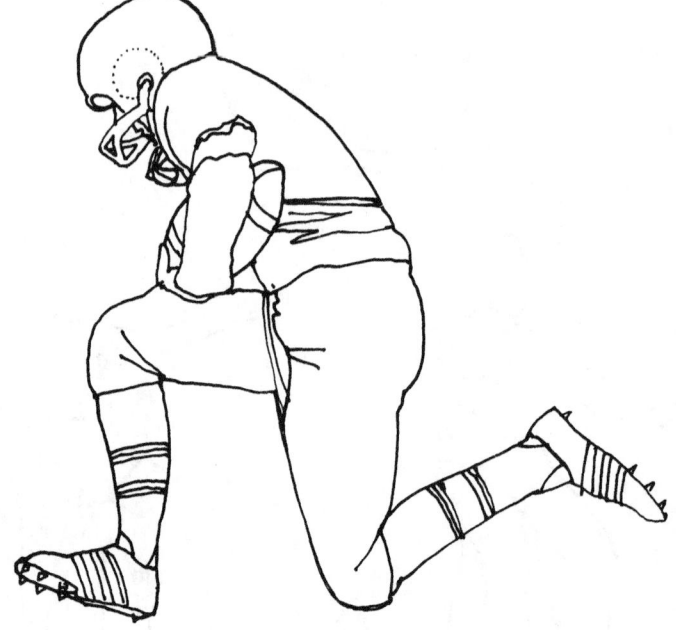

Perception of the Upright

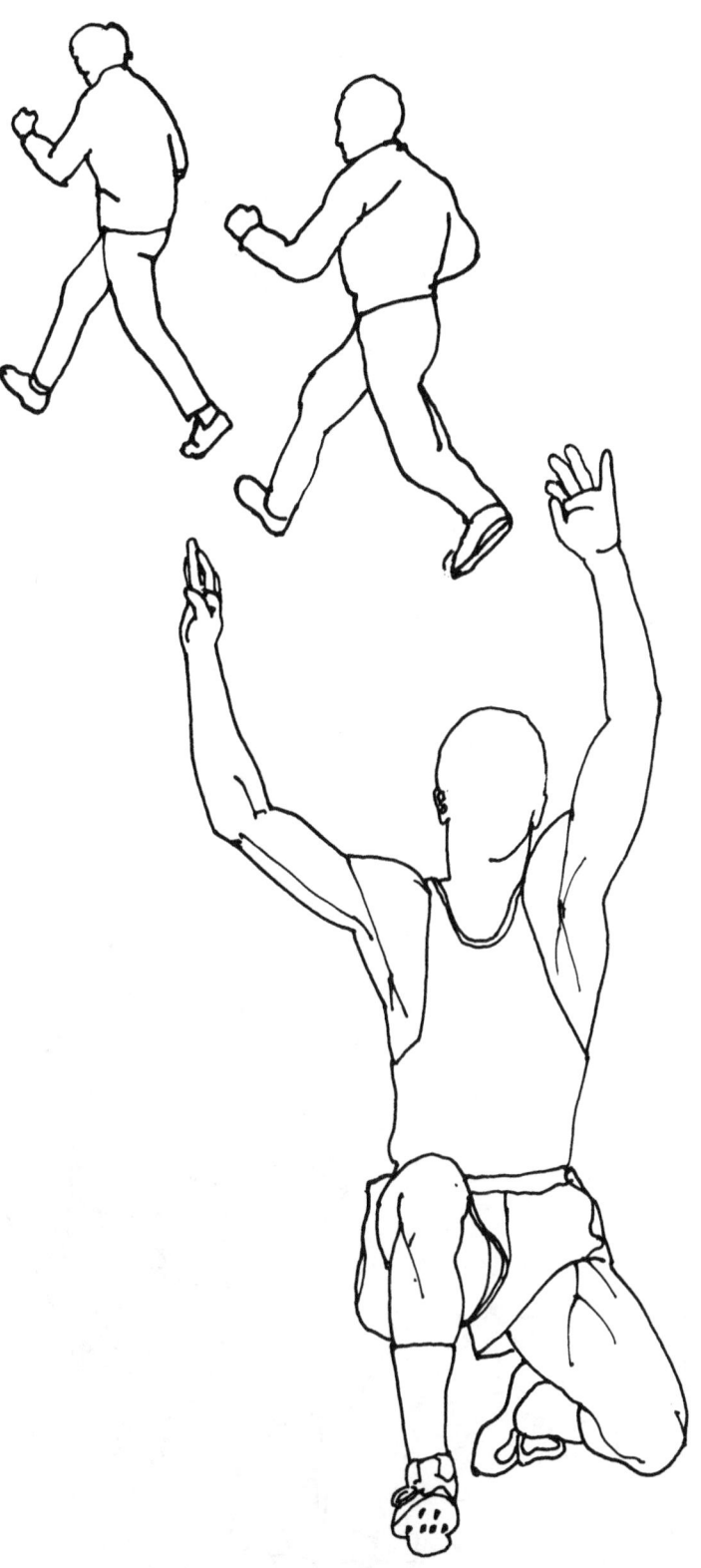

are running, jumping, or leaping, you should be free to change the breathing rhythm accordingly. You should feel free to move into breath-sighing or inhaling with legato buoyancy; to electric, short breathing or gently, prolonged breathing through the nose; to inhaling quickly through the mouth, etc. Adopt the rhythm that best meets the physical task at hand, at that very moment. And keep in mind that while nose-breathing is preferable, you should not breathe **only** through the nose any more than you should breathe consistently through the mouth.

Recall the breathing regime of our running and jogging experiments, and use it as a model for establishing a strong and potent cardio-vascular condition and a sensible, realistic breathing strategy. There, you ran at normal speed and counted the maximum number of strides in order to construct a base breathing norm for those particular activities. With practice, at least three times each day, you can progressively increase that starting norm by three to five strides every three weeks. But start with the smaller norm to build comfortably and pleasurably week by week.

2. Energy States in Running and Springing:

Except for particular exercises and special effects, our body energy states — buoyancy, radiancy, potency, and inter-involvement — seldom operate independently from one another. Generally, they "buddy-up" so that a more synergized and better integrated personality is functioning. This is especially true in everyday behavior and in sports.

In terms of the use and training of the human body in the upright: sprinting **must** incorporate both radiancy and potency energetics; distance running **must** combine potency with buoyancy experience; jogging and walking **must** utilize both buoyancy

Energy and Relaxation in Movement

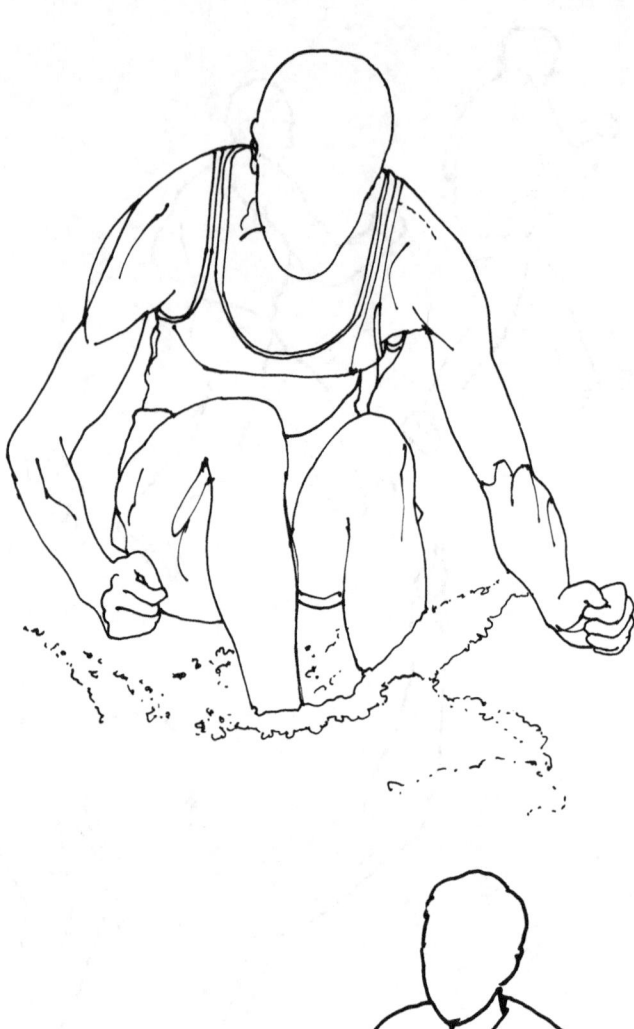

and inter-involvement energy; leaping and hopping **must** unify radiancy, buoyancy, and potency energetics, etc.

Moreover, the artistic sensing of one's own humor, one's sense of rhythm and balance, one's sense of perception, and one's ability to respond awarefully to the body in movement — all have direct relationship with the four non-derived, primitive energy states. When, for example, radiancy leads the sensing of humor, our rhythm, balance, and perception are not quite the same as when buoyancy or potency or inter-involvement is the dominating energy state. This inter-dependence and difference in shading between the body's various energetics cannot be overstated.

3. Arm Training While Running:

When you discover that the shoulders, arms, and hands can actually sail and steer the body, then you begin to sense the importance of arm training for running and as well, for total body development. In running or jumping, it is as important for the arms to feel light and loose as it is for the legs; perhaps more so. Once into their intrinsic, kinesthetic rhythm and balance, you are free to forget about the legs. It is as though the arms do the conscious work of the sails and rudder, so that the motorized leg-wheels can enjoy free-wheeling rhythm and balance in fuel-free over-drive.

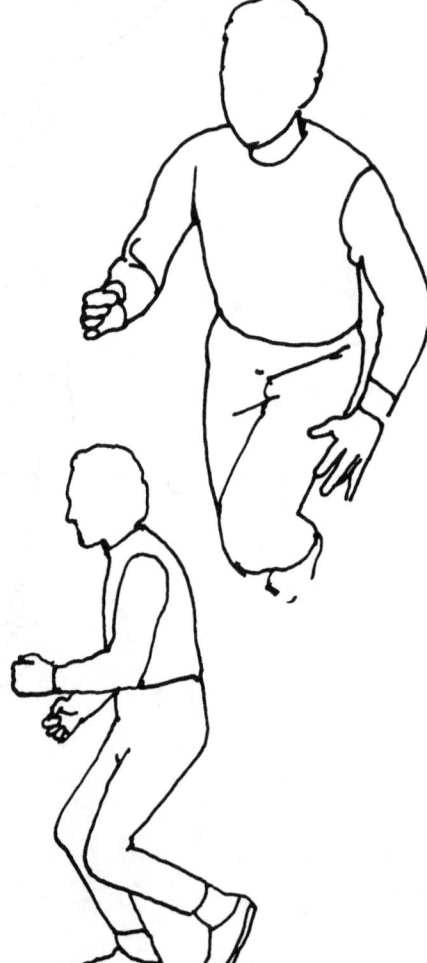

Primary awareness of arm and hand dynamics takes the mind off the work of the legs, thereby diffusing anxiety and freeing the leg muscles to "play" in smooth, coordinated movement. The shapes and forms and dimensions and rhythms made by the interplay between the arm and hand movements can positively or negatively affect the running. For instance, if in sprinting you make circular or piston-

Perception
of the
Upright

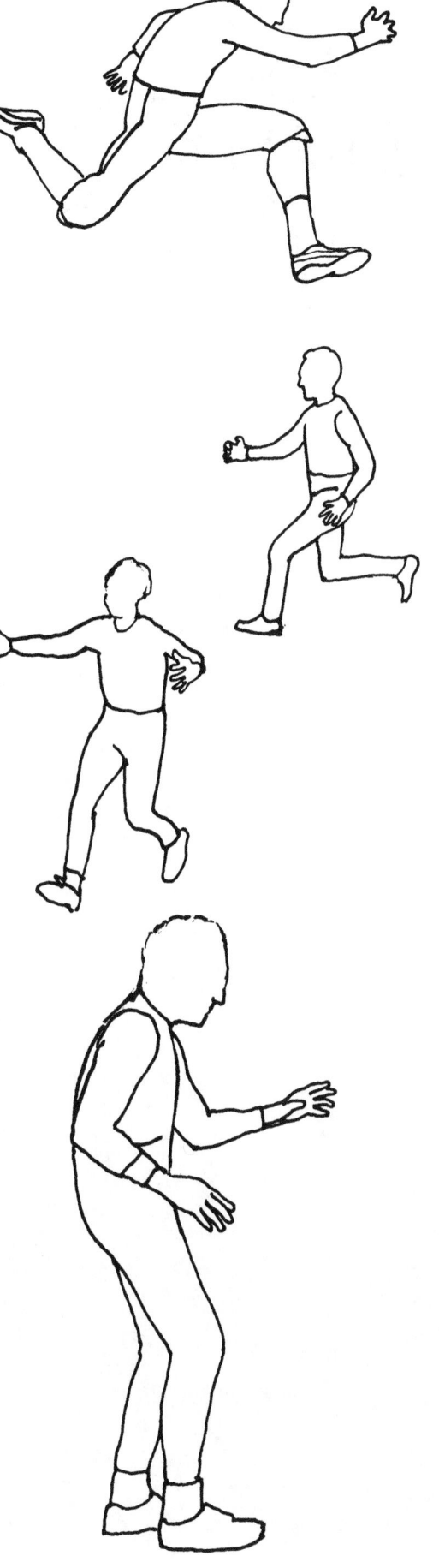

pumping movement with the arms, you will fare less well than if you use long, rocker-rim arm movements. If, in leaping, you neglect the shoulders and elbows, you lose optimal effectiveness. If, in hill running, your arms make looping motions instead of sweeping arc, you sacrifice some of your potential.

To further illustrate: if, in running, you clench your fists disallowing the air to breeze through open-cupped palms as you speed along, your running will tire you out prematurely. To put gliding grace into your running, hold out your hands, elbows, and arms, almost as though they were sails embracing the air and wind — never push-pull them behind your body.

There is, in fact, a different style and character of arm movement to dovetail with each body energy state. Through your explorations, you are now in a position to discover for yourself all the subtleties and coordinated assists that your arms and hands can provide to your running and leaping.

Begin to develop variations on all of our exercise themes. Add your own push-ups; your own cylinder roll movements; your own rope-skipping steps; your own stretch extensions. Discover your own personal, indigenous dance styles, mime techniques, and Tai Chi — by applying your own expressive interpretations to the universal concepts presented here.

4. **Recognizing Rhythms and Tuning Into Them While Running:**

For a helpful image, think of the modern jazz drummer whose body — whose whole being — truly **feels** the rhythms of his music. As he tunes in and gets a tap on his organic sensations and perceptions, he uses his sticks, more and more, as an extension of

Energy and
Relaxation
in Movement

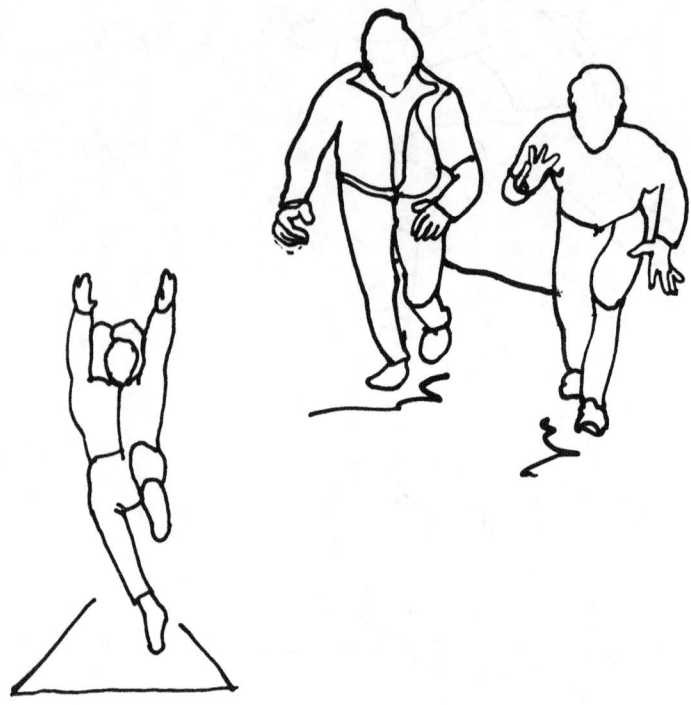

self. He uses them more easily and freely, with more spring-away, creative improvisation, and artistic control.

In like manner, but more directly, use your legs and arms and eyes as "dancing drumsticks" for running, springing, and climbing. Respond to the sensations, perceptions, and feels of those inner rhythms and balances that manifest themselves in the dancing, springing-away qualities of your natural extensions. And do this **without worrying about your muscles.** Your muscles will take care of themselves if you know how to make ecological and psychosomatic use of your body energy states, and of your natural body extensions.

5. **Running on Walls:**

My daughter has a cat — a slick, shiny-skinned, beautiful animal named Charlie who simply fascinates me. I would swear that as Charlie scampers over a wall on his way to the ceiling, he stops for a split second to wink at me. I wink back, but by now he is already on the ceiling, and I dream of having an automatic camera that could capture that instant when Charlie stopped his wall scampering to "wink" my attention.

And this puts me in mind of pictures I've seen of a fox running on walls and I try to explain to myself how they do it. After all, these creatures are not flies or birds! Why should an animal have the privilege of defying gravity, and a human being, that consummate animal, be denied even the thought that he can do it, too?

Well, as you can see from our illustration, we have thought about this. I know that some of our explorations seem far removed from familiar events in your own daily experience; some do appear quite difficult while others probably strike you as easy and elementary. Certainly, except in fantasy or day-dreaming, running on walls is not a familiar event! But if you are in the habit of turning fantasy into reality — if your bio-psychic intelligence permits you to experience that fantasy through your "harmonic overtone sensory system" and the organic feeling process — then you may just be able, through pre-programming your experiencing systems, to take a crack at it.

Needless to say, unless you have an authoritative, instinctive tap on your body energy states, your relaxer-energizers, your body esthetics, dialects, and intelligence or the sensing of your own humor — **don't try it!** Just keep enjoying it as an eventually realistic possibility in your mind's eye. But if you are determined to run on walls, I at least owe you some advice, if not my blanket consent.

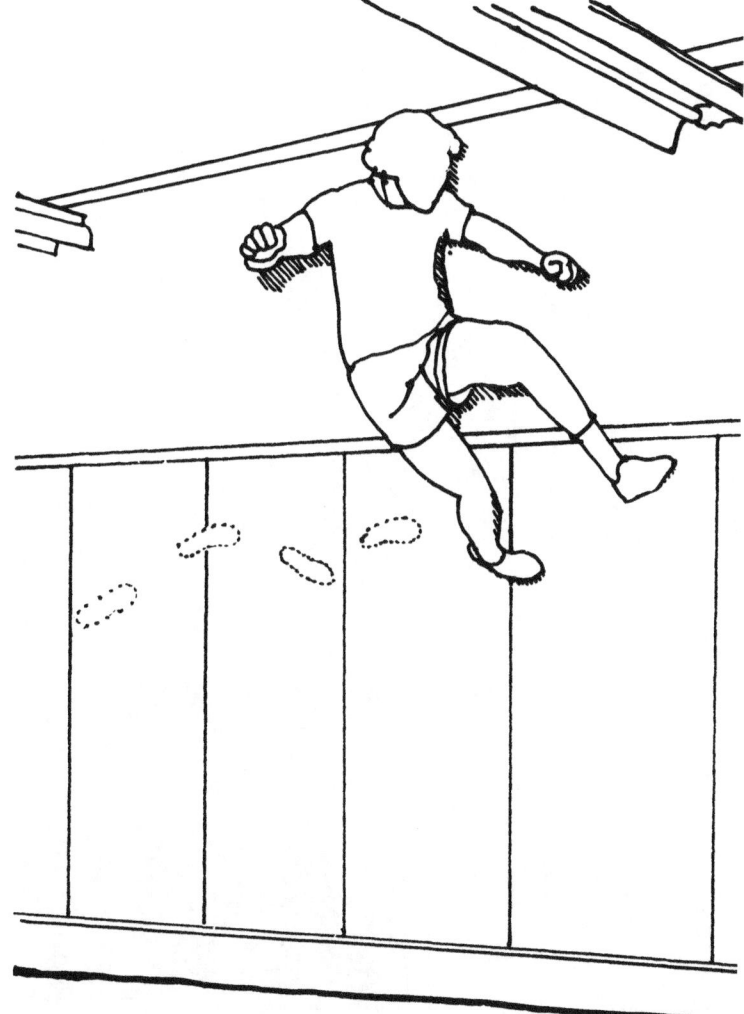

- First, the walls should be padded before you even begin your experimenting.

- Second, the floor should also be padded.

- Third, the walls should be minimally forty feet long and fifteen feet high.

- Fourth, mobilize your sensory intelligence to make your body so light and weightless as to feel yourself functioning in a gravity-free climate, ready to defy the existing gravity-pull.

- Fifth, ask yourself simply and seriously: "Can I fly?" "How high can I move on that wall?" "How high and long an arc can I make on the wall?" "How many steps along that arc can I make?"

If you can take three steps, you are running on walls! Of course it's difficult, but once you've done it the possibilities are unlimited.

Energy and
Relaxation
in Movement

If you really manage to run four or five steps on the wall, you'll be convinced that it is not "just a trick," but rather a lifetime experience telescoped into one fleeting second.

Perhaps not so exotically, but just as excitingly, we are now ready to explore and discover our "Personal Space Spheres" — those natural extensions of our body structure, vocal, visual, and auditory life — of which we spoke at the outset of Part Three. But first — a brief postscript on our exercise classifications that will serve both as final review and preparation for your independent study and practice.

POSTSCRIPT

TO CHAPTERS 7 THROUGH 12

By way of modulating the material of our work chapters toward a resolving cadence, I take this opportunity to summarize some of the objectives and exercise classifications of: **Body Building — Body Fitness — Body Power — Body Swiftness — Body Balance and Rhythm**; and **Diametric Exercising**, particularly as it relates to a) a "third force" approach to body training; b) sinistrality and bi-lateral body development; and c) the reserve cushion image.

BODY BUILDING

- **The general objectives of Body Building are:**

1. To look good, feel good, function well, and serve the internal needs of the small personal environment in its overall behavior.

2. To construct an attractive body form whose every muscle and dimension is proportionately developed to fit the size and shape of the whole; i.e. a balanced musculature and weight distribution, rather than exaggerated "muscle mass" and muscle groups.

3. To build a healthy body core with perfect body alignment, posture, and balance through an optimal breathing process that is integrated with proper spine extension and form.

4. To develop exercises that avoid muscle-punishment in order to assure free and easy muscle movement. These exercises exploit primarily: the potency of body-yawn stretch for building muscle power and strengthening the body, and the concept of working with live weight versus dead weight. Hence, weight-lifting exercises are performed with one's own body and/or with a partner rather than with dead weight barbells.

Of course, these objectives are generalized throughout our work. However, they are listed here as specific Body Building objectives because of their special relationship to building body musculature and perfecting optimal alignment, posture, weight distribution, and breathing regimes.

...one does not stutter and stammer with speech alone; one can, and does, stutter and stammer with voice with eyes with fingers with feet with the thought process with memory with the whole body!

Exercise Classifications for Body Building:

a. Primary use of the potent body-yawn stretch for body strengthening and body building in activities involving stretching, lifting, pushing, pulling, and carrying of heavy objects.

b. In the repetition of these exercises, we work not for speed but consciously and deliberately for tempo, rhythm, balance, and control. Furthermore, we consider the "return trip" from the initial action (push-up, chin-up, sit-up, etc.) as much a primary event as any other part of the exercise.

c. The use of moving, "live weight" ropes, pulleys, springs, pedals, and oars as props or images to support the re-training of the body to instinctive behavior; organized around progressive exercise plans structured to reasonable limits and individual limitations. Exercises that employ these moving props or images incorporate self-teaching mechanisms for progressive pressure build-up.

d. As regards weight-lifting, we discourage the use of outside dead weights at least in the beginning, until our energy states and training regime have taken hold. In kinesensics, weight-lifting means **body weight-lifting** and refers principally to lifting one's own live body weight and/or that of one's partner. Thus, we try to exploit the weight through a counter-energy or through the coordinated body esthetics of our assisting partner.

BODY FITNESS

- **The general objectives of Body Fitness are:**

1. To be "in condition," not "to be conditioned."

2. To provide the body with fuel power for optimal physical performance. This relates not so much to food and diet as to "breath power," to direct and indirect breathing strategies.

3. To train for stamina, durability, and strength of physical constitution.

4. To supplement training for the musculature with exercises that increase and improve the fitness, function, and free "living space" of our internal organs, systems, terrain, and climate.

5. To provide self-protection against strain, (dis)stress, fatigue, undue force, and resulting overload of body wear and tear.

6. To keep the body in good working order, resistant to negative influences and breakdowns, so that it can progressively mature rather than deteriorate through premature obsolescence.

Exercise Classifications for Body Fitness:

a. General breathing exercises designed to build body potential, control, endurance, and internal hygiene.

b. Specific breathing exercises for body weight distribution and postural alignment, as well as in connection with running, dancing, skipping, climbing, and walking.

c. Springing-leaping-hopping exercises embracing: squat jumps and hops; skip-dancing; rope-skipping, rope-running, and rope-dancing; uphill and downhill running; stair climbing and nimbly skipping down stairs; walking, jogging, and running.

BODY FLEXIBILITY

- **The general objectives of Body Flexibility are:**

1. To improve and sustain muscle elasticity and spontaneity.

2. To understand and apply all the energy "feels" of body extension, body bending, and body expansion.

3. To achieve optimal, flexible use of body joints and hinges, aiding "flex-ability."

4. To move the body into the **use** of space, rather than merely existing within it.

Exercise Classifications for Body Flexibility:

a. The body-yawn stretch, augmented by buoyancy and radiancy energy, to expand the "stretch-ability", and the "swing-ability", and therefore the "flex-ability" of the body.

b. Rocking, rolling, and slow-motion balance; cat, fox, and other animal exercises including walking, leaping, landing, and stalking; also pole climbing, ring swinging, horizontal bar and ladder swinging; trampoline activities; throwing, heaving, and catapulting.

c. Plastique body movement ranging from T'ai-Chi-like exercise-dance, space sculpting, and mime training to fantasy expressiveness, dream dancing, and organic imaging.

BODY SWIFTNESS

- **The general objectives of Body Swiftness are:**

1. To develop optimal speed, alertness, and agility through the "kinesensic" feel of body humor, body esthetics, body energy states, and body relaxer-energizers.

2. To achieve good and alert coordination among **all** body systems through the integrated use of total body intelligence.

3. To develop the sensory skills for penetrating a seemingly gravity-free space field, and effortlessly cruising through it as your own center of gravity.

4. To register the kinesthetic feeling of internal rhythm and balance, and tap into this feeling for increased nimbleness, agility, speed, and momentum of the body in movement.

Exercise Classifications for Body Swiftness:

a. Applied buoyancy and radiancy energy to running, rope-dancing, gymnastics, skating, etc.

b. Applied use of the spinal C-curve, leg wheels, and the concept of resting up and resting down simultaneously — to develop a power-producing looseness in your stretch.

c. Techniques for defending against attack that like Japanese Aikido, use a science-art of ducking, weaving, dancing, rhythmic responses, and advancing without touch-contact — but now allied to a completely new system of organic/sensory learning. The reacquisition of instinctive body skills for self-defense against attack, without relying upon physical contact, communicates a psychology of security, artistry, and relaxed confidence in any physical confrontation.

BODY BALANCE AND BODY RHYTHM

- **The general objectives of Body Balance and Body Rhythm are:**

1. To become aware of outside space as a "feelable substance," and to perceive **the body moving through it and fitting into it.** The truly balanced body, feeling the stimulation of its rhythm dynamic, has a sense of cruising in "over-drive" with the efficiency of minimum fuel and minimum work — producing maximum speed and maximum relaxation.

2. To use body energetics and body esthetics to develop optimal coordination for greater psycho-physical security, fear diffusion, and imaginative, pleasurable reinforcement of our movements in space.

3. To promote the fullest understanding of the body as a sphere and its follow-through into body curves and wheels.

4. To internalize the feeling process of sensation-perception-awareness-response, supported by appropriate images, and to utilize this process as a means to organic body control. Such organic control provides the individual with a new appreciation of the body's performing grace and natural beauty, while reinforcing the sense of satisfaction, enjoyment, and maturation that accompanies this positive, personal self-image.

5. To develop through body balance and rhythm, the awareness that equates: **power** with grace and form; **speed** with lightness and alertness; **strength** with balanced muscle tonicity; **potent force** with the body-yawn stretch; and **momentum** with exhilaration.

6. To discover the art and science of harmonious and expressive body movements (eurhythmics) and body forms, accomplished by kinesensically combining balance/rhythm/symmetry with tempo/strength/flexibility.

7. Finally, to instill an emotional and evaluative appreciation of harmonically experiencing the physical "feels" of almost limitless energies, balances, and rhythms — as these inter-mix and interchange by kind and degree.

Exercise Classifications for Body Balance and Body Rhythm:

a. Perceptual imaging, and reserve cushion exercises.

b. Easy and vigorous breathing to overcome fatigue.

c. Live weight versus dead weight as related to body pressure.

d. Graceful and slow-motion rolling for tension-relief.

e. Exercises promoting body alertness and agility to cope with exhaustion.

f. Relaxer-energizer activities involving rolling, reaching, springing, landing, dancing, standing, and sitting.

g. Use of salutary and pleasing physical action, encompassing a new and healthy **esthetic perception** of "image trips" as part of the exercise strategy to defeat the feelings of ennui, tiredness, and body collapse that often result from imposed exercise conditioning.

DIAMETRIC EXERCISING

Throughout our body training, you have been learning how to balance and unify seemingly opposite dynamics and different energy esthetics. Elsewhere in your studies, or personal explorations, you have no doubt come across such terms as: **aerobics** (breathing and body exercises where fresh air and plentiful oxygen are taken for granted); **anaerobics** (body activities in which you are capable of functioning for a time without air, by drawing oxygen from oxygen compounds for body metabolism); **isometrics** (exercises involving movement against, or resistance from, an immovable object, or pitting muscle groups against each other within your own body); and, **isotonics** (exercises involving free body movement).

Kinesensic training leads, in an interesting way, to a graduated concept of creative exercising that I call **diametrics**. While the term is newly suggested here, we have in fact been working with diametric exercises throughout our experiments in Part Two and especially, Part Three.

Diametrics refers to body activity and exercise that work in equilibrium with at least two dynamics at the same time, much like balancing a see-saw. Our work does just that, as it equilibrates the opposites of **resting up** with **resting down; force-power** with **grace-power; muscle-strength** with **muscle-looseness; action** with **resting**, etc. As such, it combines the advantages of isotonics and isometrics, the benefits of both aerobics and anaerobics into a single "third-force" strategy.

* **For a Single "Third-Force" Strategy:**

Related to our concept of the "generalization of energies," the "third-force approach" reduces over-specialization in body training and the time wasted in separate investigations of opposites that more often than not lead to confusion and internal conflict. Our "third force" concepts, which are bi-polar in character, result from the **organic need** to integrate and reconcile various forces operating within the body into a unified direction, a new path that guides the body toward optimal functioning.

In vocal training through kinesensics, one such third-force dynamic is the feel of consonants as orchestral instruments. Those familiar with **The Use and Training of the Human Voice** will recall the "consonant orchestra" and how it helped to: a) clarify all consonant activity as an esthetic experience; b) save all that time and practice of separate, repetitive consonant drills; and c) introduce a new music, rhythm, and balance into various speech situations. It did so by working with both ends of the music/diction spectrum simultaneously or by combining two complementary energies at the same time.

Similarly, our experiments with running, jogging, sitting, walking, springing, leaping, etc., adopted the third-force strategy in unifying body esthetics with relaxer-energizers and synthesizing the dualities of equilibrium and energy into a new balance. Hence, diametric exercising produces from two opposites a kind of "binary coordinate" that operates within the body as a multi-dimensional **gestalt**.

But **diametrics** does much more. In our system:

° It makes exercising a qualitative experience rather than a regime of quantitative drills.

° It clarifies, for any particular exercise, both the advance **into** the action and the return **from** it.

° It offers the possibility of performing an exercise in reverse as well as in forward direction; e.g. in walking, running, skating, pedaling, swimming, riding, steering, etc.

Diametric Exercising (Sinistrality)

○ It brings into new perspective the advantages of bi-lateral body development as opposed to segmented, isolated, or dominance-exercise training.

○ On the one hand, it demonstrates and exposes the vicious cycle of "sinistrality" or one-sidedness within the body, and on the other it emphasizes and moves forward, the benefits to be derived from important, new split-brain research.

To illustrate with several examples that are by now familiar from our training experiments:

1. Feeling some looseness in your muscles while chinning (up or down) is a **diametric** combination.

2. The feeling of resting while doing push-ups is **diametric** exercising.

3. Feeling buoyancy while running is a **diametric** experience.

4. Feeling radiancy in your leap is another.

5. Sensing movement in your balance is another.

6. Experiencing speed through inner body rhythm is a **diametric** perception.

7. Tasting internally both the sharpness and softness in producing the "S" consonant as an orchestral "sound effect," is a **diametric** feel in speech training.

8. Feeling the darkness of tonal color as "something-ness" and the lightness of the body of tone as "nothing-ness" at the same time, is **diametric** experience in voice training.

9. Feeling legato-buoyant reaching as an integral component and follow-thru of the potent body-yawn stretch, is another.

10. Sensing a constant space cushion between the upper and lower teeth as good, preventive medicine — sensing the whole lower jaw as an unconditioned reflex — or sensing the rich **color, resonance,** and **shape** of vocal tone all at the same time — these are powerful **diametric** activities.

And these are just a few. The combinations, permutations, synergies, and synesthetic conversions are virtually limitless.

- **Sinistrality and Bi-Lateral Body Development:**

When the body is divided into two halves — one dexterous, the other "sinistral" — we have a body in vicious conflict with itself. The most

...inner
"harmonic overtones"
are offspring
of the outer
"fundamental five senses"
and create
their own esthetic qualities,
dynamics,
essences,
intelligence....
...these harmonic offspring
do their own intrinsic seeing,
hearing, smelling, touching, tasting;
and in various subtle nuances,
produce indigenous resonances,
wave reflections,
vibrations,
impulses,
currents,
rhythms,
images!

Remember!
"Harmonic sensing" is a
bio-psychic system of:
intelligence gathering...
memory retrieval...
internal reserve cushion...
and
built-in contol valve system
serving the body's
vocal equipment,
emotional equipment,
physical equipment!

Postscript
(Chapters 7-12)
Diametric
Exercising
(Sinistrality)

obvious, and in a sense, superficial example of "sinistrality" is handedness. Left-handedness is no longer considered a sign of congenital retardation or insanity — a shameful blight to be hidden from public view by locking the victim in a dark closet or casting him adrift on a "ship of fools" as was once the custom. But even today in our "enlightened age," left-handers are still restricted and imposed upon by the dominance and technology of a right-handed world.

"Sinistrality" or dominant sidedness occurs not only in the hands, but as well in the feet, the hips, the thighs, fingers, lips, eyes, ears, **and** the brain! The left side is no more the "wrong side" then the right side is the correct side of the body. Right and wrong, as concepts for body functioning or body training, have no place in organic, sensory development; especially for the young child **whose individual rhythm, so essential to creative exploration, is destroyed by the intrusion of these non-organic values.**

The same holds true for the adult interested in recapturing some of the child's instinctive body behavior and natural talents and skills. Quite literally, your left hand must **know** what your right hand is doing, in order that it may do it too — in its own way. And your right hand has much to learn from your left in terms of artistry and special skills.

Especially in body training, it is a disservice to the organism to let any physical activity promote the dominance of sidedness or sinistrality. Anything that tends to overdevelop one part of the body leaving another part underdeveloped or less developed, is creating relative deformity and contributing to a misshapen, misaligned, imbalanced body! What's more: it effects "closure" of part of the brain's functioning potential, relegating closed parts to a perpetual state of relative dormancy.

Diametric exercising — bi-lateral development — multi-dexterity. These should be the constant watchwords for body training, especially where the body is perceived as a psycho-physical totality. Creativity and dexterity are as natural to the left side of the body (the right-brain) as to the right side of the body (the left-brain). It is only by tradition and conditioning that the sinistral side appears to function less efficiently and less effectively. It is not an organic given.

Hence, we must learn to exploit both sides bi-laterally as a way to experience another example of **natural diametrics**. In all probability, it is our harmonic overtone sensory system that responds to advanced activities in the internal environment, and it is probable that it is the

Diametric
Exercising
(Sinistrality
Reserve Cushion)

"inner sensory-perception system" that awakens the body to the use of the brain as a whole sphere, instead of as opposing hemispheres. It might just be the means by which we can eliminate sinistral functioning in our general behavior, which is more culturally conditioned than biologically pre-determined. After all, it is our particular culture that has determined which side is "normal and natural."

By the same principle, I am convinced that sinistrality applies not only to "handedness" and "footedness," but also to the body's thinking, hearing, seeing, feeling, and emotional experiencing systems. It is sidedness that is dangerous, not its particular locale. Perhaps the **inability to perceive** something that **does** exist and is available to our powers of perception and response, is just another form of one-sidedness and ought to be included in our broader definition of sinistrality.

In sports such as paddleball, an interesting exercise for increasing bi-lateral perception is to use two paddles instead of one, and to let the right hand challenge the left and vice versa. You will be pleasantly surprised at the galvanized gathering of fresh ideas and the physical excitement generated, as your individual "self-image" perceives and responds to the competitive challenge of skills and strength between the left and right "body images." This bi-lateral perception should lead to a more sensitive awareness of the brain's role in directing actions. And you will recognize this as a familiar awareness, identical to the experiments of Part Three where the brain and muscles worked in harmony to neutralize dominance — permitting you to run backwards as well as forward; climb downhill as well as uphill; roll up stairs and down them; and begin to entertain the possibility of running on walls.

To be ambidextrous is not necessarily the answer, if this means sanctioning the development of two, identical **ordered** sides, functioning like siamese twins within a single organism. That condition would produce a double dose of sinistrality. Clearly, we do not need two right sides or two left sides, any more than we want one "good," dependable side and one "inferior," retarded side. We need **both** dominances as two inter-dominant branches of body wisdom, organically cross-feeding, with each influencing the other, through cultural, scientific, artistic, and perceptual exchange.

- **The Reserve Cushion Image:**

Every body energy state, relaxer-energizer, and body esthetic discussed and taught in this work serves a triple purpose, contributing to: 1) salutary and vital energizing; 2) psychosomatic health; and 3) a reserve cushion for extended activity.

To what degree these safety reserve cushions are psychological, to what degree physiological — is a question still open to discussion. Whatever the relative degree determined by future research, it is clear that the reserve cushion can be represented at least symbolically (typologically) as a psycho-physical phenomenon, with definite psychosomatic cause-effect relationships.

Let us continue our discussion of the reserve cushion, begun in the **Midword Break**; the following observations should be more meaningful to you now that you've completed several additional experiments in the upright.

In athletics and other forms of strenuous physical activity, we require a built-in control valve. We need the reassuring knowledge that we can call on the feel of our stretch, balance, rhythm, alertness, and anticipation energy — all fundamentals of our physical training — to perform with maximum efficiency without heroics or "do-or-die" marathons. The breaking of long-standing records, over and over again **once the record has been broken a first time,** does not represent supreme, emergency effort. Rather, it should be understood as a creative, esthetic achievement that uses the "cushion image" as insurance and reinforcement of both safety and performance. In this instance, the mind **must** cooperate with, and follow the lead of the body, instead of vice versa.

You have noticed that nowhere do we use the terms "make a greater effort" — "push yourself to the limit" — "run as fast as you can," as organic instructions. This is not because we consider ourselves limitless, but because the **awareness** of unknown limits is in itself, limiting. It entails a negative instruction to the body, and is self-defeating and contradictory to the cushion image.

The fact is: You go as far as you like with impunity, as long as you feel the harmonics of the experience and perceive its body esthetics. That is the cushion! Far from "mind over matter" or anything nearly so mystical, **your body illumines your mind** by educating it to the full possibility of body potential despite the brain's outer-conditioned message that the limit may already have been reached. Until one recognizes that there is more potential for relaxed energy and energetic relaxation, regardless of the mind's contradictory opinion, one can never even dream of the full creativity that lies latent and largely untapped within the organism.

Diametric Exercising (Reserve Cushion)

- Getting a conscious tap on inner balance and rhythm when the body approaches fatigue, will provide you with revitalized energy. **This is part of your safety reserve cushion.**

- When running fast and feeling increasingly exhausted, you fall back on smaller leg-wheels that bring your C-curve closer to the ground, producing renewed comfort to your lower spine energy-center and adding a "rest-quotient" to your body, **without breaking stride. This is creative use of your reserve cushion image.**

- When you accomplish this without disrupting body rhythms, you can smoothly return to the larger wheel and faster sprinting for the home-stretch. **This is part of the inner control valve of your safety reserve cushion.**

- If, when any physical activity such as stair-climbing or carrying heavy bundles induces strain or heaviness, you are able to tune into a light-weight, balanced buoyancy feel, you will quickly realize that you're breathing more freely — that you've found your "second breath." **This is another of your reserve cushion images.**

What are the alternatives? These, I think you already know. Losing the umbrella of the reserve cushion image or never having it in the first place means: tightened joints; tense body; heavy body weight; poor breathing; pained, strained facial posture; and impingements on nerve and bone structures that starve and use up the body, rather than sustain and nourish it.

13
THE BODY'S PERSONAL SPACE SPHERES

The body requires "living space", both within and without. So far, we have explored in detail the living space of the inner environment; evolved its basic curvo-linear structure; and demonstrated its indigenous, instinctive behavior and integrity, quite apart from the strictures and conditioning imposed by the outer environment. But we have also seen, in delineating the feeling process and evolving the body curve, how instinctive behavior establishes ecological balance with the outer environment; how the body's experiencing systems, when restored to health, can rebuild an organic-perceptual bridge for relating to the different creatures, climate, terrain, phenomena, and institutionalized conditions of the outside world. In a phrase, that organic-perceptual bridge aids us in reaching a stage of rapprochement with the outer environment.

Because we now know how to keep the body relatively safe from imitative behavior and other extrinsic hazards, we need not ever feel like registered aliens existing within the outer environment. Not only can we safely co-exist with the outside world, we can now, constructively, though critically, fit into it and move through it with psycho-physical control and untethered creativity. Because we know how to use the body for optimal functioning and protect it from premature obsolescence, we can better ascertain our own realistic living space — our own expressive "personal space spheres" — based on **output to the external world from the vital inner body environment.**

By "personal space spheres," I do not mean some mystical other space or the simple space-disbursement taken up by actual bulk-size of the body structure. Rather, I refer here specifically to the body's "follow-through energies" and its configurated physicality; to dimensionally controlled body spheres,

Chapter 13

The Body's Personal Space Spheres

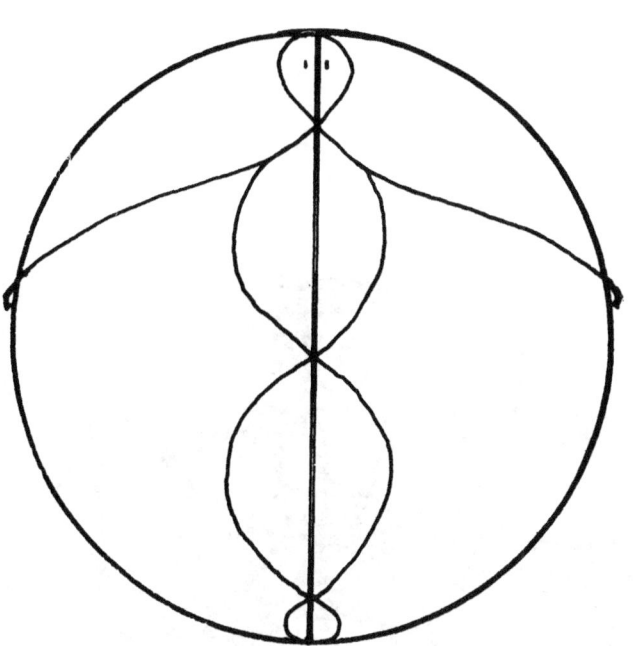

The Body's
Personal
Space
Spheres

arcs, wheels, and curves naturally extending into outside, physical living space.

Our "personal space spheres" derive naturally from the body in movement and movement in the body. Resulting synergistically from renewed exchange between the harmonic overtone sensory system and the five fundamental senses, they become logical extensions of the body as a small ball, an expanded sphere, a crescent lying down and standing upright.

"Personal space spheres" are always defined by the boundaries extending from our ACTUAL PHYSICAL STRUCTURE, our VISION, HEARING, VOCAL LIFE, and CAPACITY FOR INTER-INVOLVEMENT. Through our communicating and experiencing systems, they vary in nuance and dimension according to the relationship we establish with the objects, creatures, and natural phenomena of the outside environment. And ultimately, as we shall see in the final chapter, "personal space spheres" extend into the formation of new, healthier "self-images" shaped and nuanced by the individual curvo-linear body in movement.

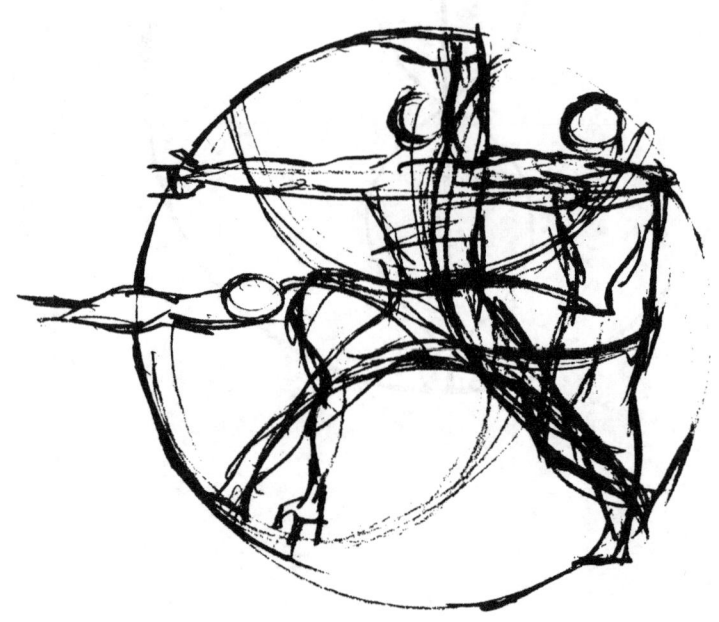

Each of us has the capacity to reach out with five organically-related, "personal space spheres."

° **Your Structural Space Sphere** is the follow-through of the body's actual physical dimensions. In the structural space sphere, you are primarily alone and relate mostly self-to-self.

° **Your Auditory Space Sphere** is the follow-through of your hearing faculties.

° **Your Tonal** or **Vocal Space Sphere** is the range and circuity of your vocal life.

Structural
Space
Sphere

○ **Your Visual Space Sphere** is the curvolinear compass of your seeing and observing capacities.

○ **Your Traveling Space Sphere** is the follow-through of the body in **planned movement**. In the traveling space sphere, your body's curves and wheels constantly adapt and readapt to the space sphere in movement — becoming a sphere within a sphere, a space within a space.

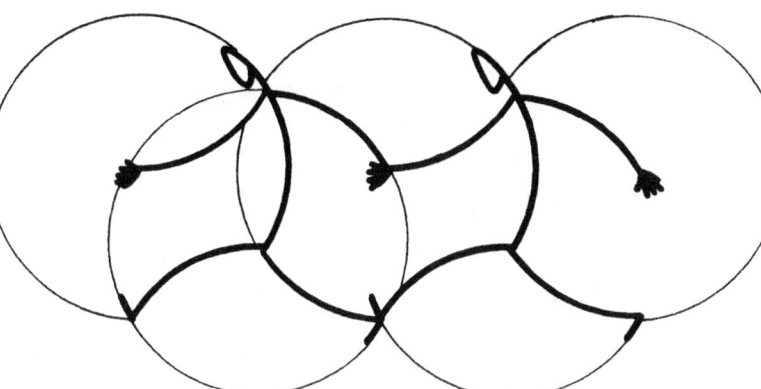

- The structural space sphere grows out of our live body, our vital bearing, our moving posture. To initiate awareness of your structural space sphere, recall the body's five major energy **circuits**: the neck and head — the torso (back, stomach, chest) — the legs as wheels — the feet as rocker-rims or loops — the shoulders, arms, and hands as circles. Check graphics on p.176. Note once again, how the neck/head and arm circles tap into the upper spine energy-center; how the torso, leg-wheels, and foot loops tap into the lower spine energy-center.

A. **The Structural Personal Space Sphere**

The actual size of your structural space sphere will depend upon your posture and body alignment, and upon your response to the kind and measure of energy — real or imagined — that flows through your body's organism.

To identify your structural space sphere:

○ Try to image the rolling and moving of the structural sphere through the five, coordinated energy circuits as one interrelated configuration;

○ Explore the image of "alternating current flows" of the double figure-eight forming a single "forward direction."

○ Through the movements of these currents and the extension of these energies,

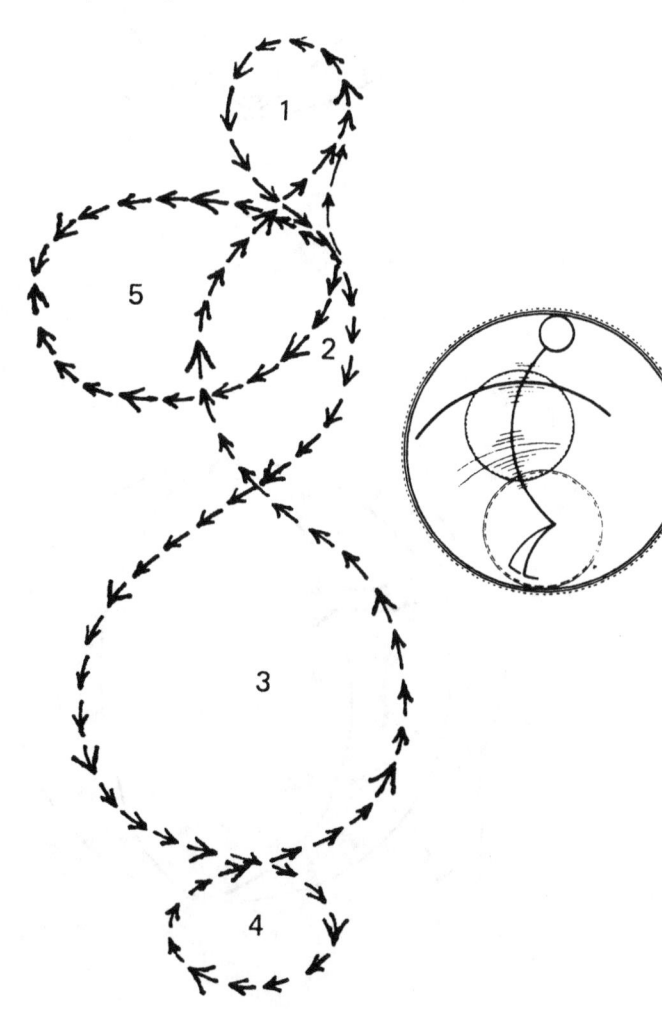

The Body's
Personal
Space
Spheres

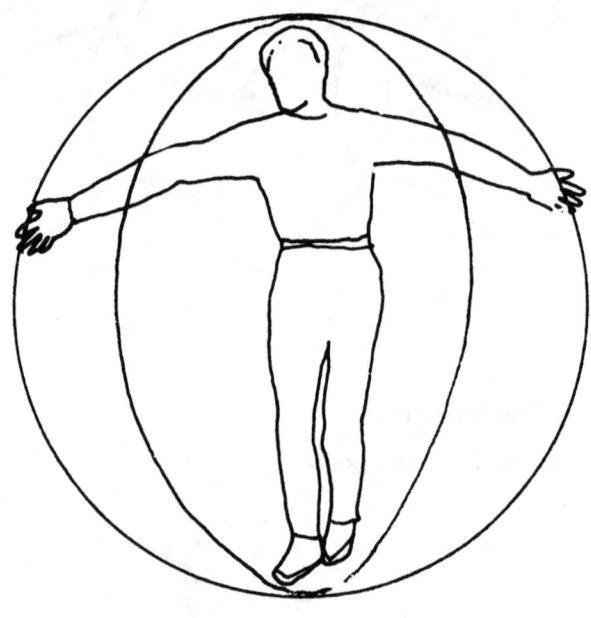

From the outside looking in

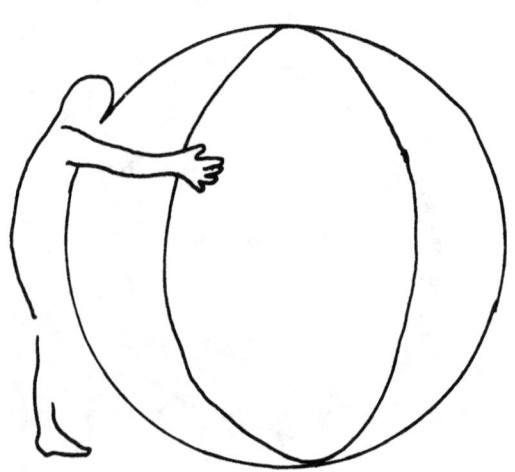

suggest to yourself the completion of the horizontal arm circle and the follow-through continuation of the spinal curve into a vertical perfect circle that extends from head to toe and from toe to head.

From the outside looking in, your structural space sphere is a clear, see-through air space. From the inside looking out, it seems to form, in front of you, a kind of transparent bubble fashioned by a resilient membrane or flexible, elastic skin.

Test this concept first by exploring the outer membrane of your structural space sphere. Your face, front of neck, chest, stomach, abdomen, front of thighs, knees, legs, insteps, and toes all form contiguous parts of your structural sphere. You feel as though you are rolling this graceful bubble of which you, yourself, are a part.

° You roll it forward, obviously with no push, as though travelling on ballbearings. You motivate the movement of the sphere from the outer surface; your back alone touching external space as your front participates as a contiguous part of the inner rim of the structural sphere.

° As you explore, and as you become fully extended, loose, and buoyant, you will be a little taller than you normally are. Your structural space sphere will also be larger. The dimensions of the sphere ought to be two to four feet taller than your normal height, at the highest point in the upper arc of your space sphere. Thus, a person five feet tall would have a structural sphere measuring roughly seven feet in diameter; a six-footer would own a sphere about nine feet in diameter, and so on.

229

Structural
Space
Sphere

- Of course, if you are so loose and extended as to feel weightless, like a bird about to "take off" or a runner waiting for the **GO!**, then you can feel ten feet tall in your body dimensions, and perhaps fifteen feet tall in your space sphere.

- If, however, you hold your body in a careless or depressed posture, your space sphere will be proportionately starved and sparse. It will seem small and antiquated, like an early model that has become obsolete by neglect. So the choice is yours.

• Now, image yourself **inside** the structural space sphere, and use the roll, glide, and walk to test the feel. The structural extension remains the same except, as illustrated, the membrane now forms around the **back** part of you and continues the back extension through the rear of the head — down into the upper and lower back — the pelvis, the inside of the thighs — all the way to the calves, ankles, heels. Now, it is these body parts which become contiguous partners of your structural space sphere.

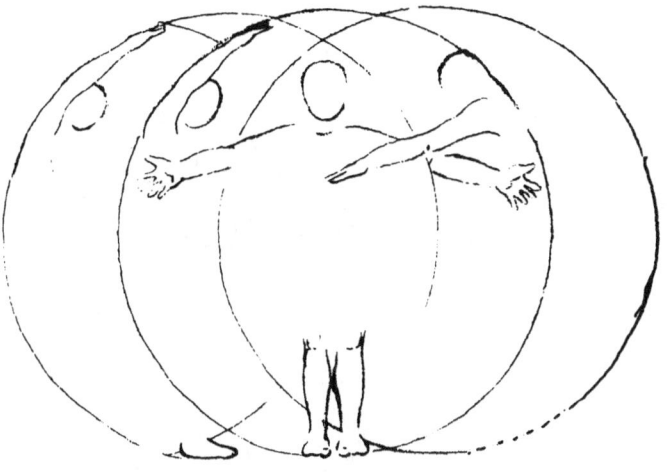

Inside your structural space sphere

As you roll, glide, and walk, the experience feels quite different from the first experiment. This time, you feel as though you're gently drawing the sphere — leading it from behind while simultaneously maintaining a frontal perspective of its movement. It's like carrying your child piggy-back rather than holding the babe in front, cradled in your arms. It is also perceiving, in a more private sense, the "inside" accommodation and dimensions of your structural space sphere.

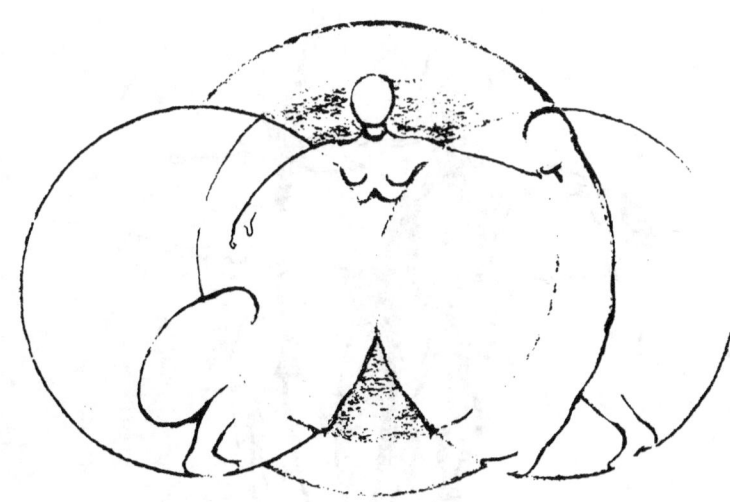

- What was previously a bubble is now an individual special space for you to live in, swim in, reach through. As you move through it, tune into one or more of our body energy states, beginning

The Body's
Personal
Space
Spheres

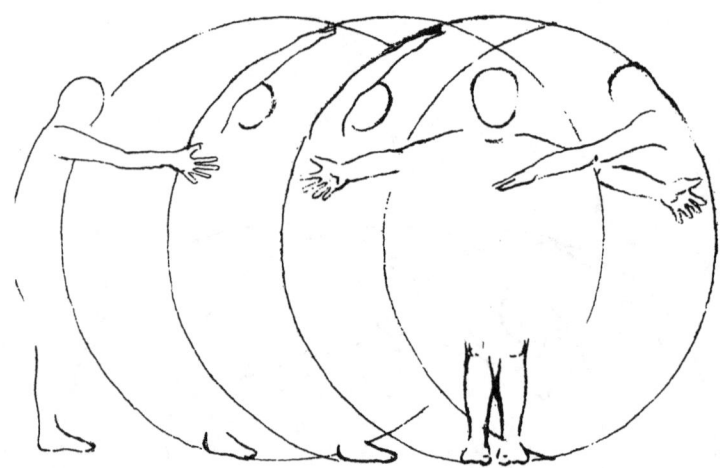

with the buoyancy feel. It becomes emphatically apparent that your space sphere, both within and without, is the kinesthetic extension of your individual body structure embracing all the characteristics of your respiratory, nervous, and "calculating" systems. As you work with your "extended self," note how the structural space sphere strengthens and validates our experiments with correct alignment, crescent and C-curve postures, natural breathing, balance and rhythm, etc.

○ Make sure that wherever you are, there is enough room for you **and** your structural space sphere to move. It won't do to pretend that your sphere can disregard wall boundaries and simply dissolve through the walls. Be realistic. A nine-foot structural sphere cannot be comfortable in a room that is nine feet square — it has no place to go!

○ If a room is smaller, then adapt to fit by making your body structure, and therefore also your personal space sphere, proportionately smaller. **If a room is too small for your structural sphere, then it is probably too small for you to work in. It will certainly be too small for your moving and expanding "self-image."**

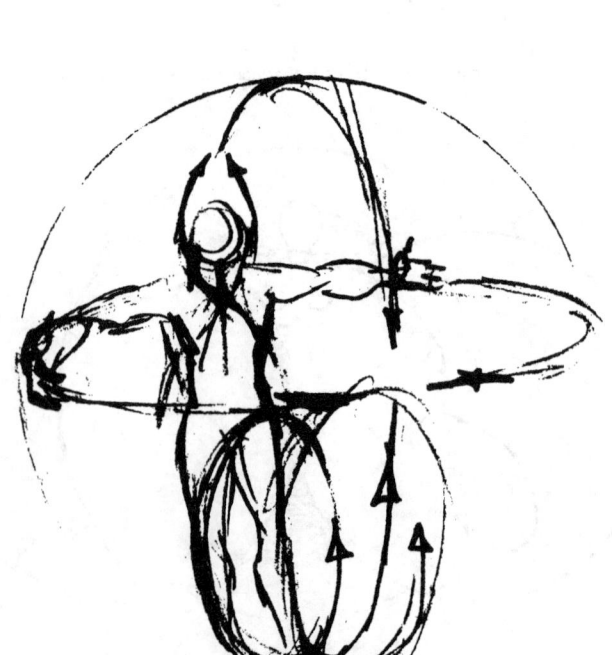

• Outdoors, as well as in spacious indoor areas, you should have little problem of accommodation, unless, of course, the social distance prescribed by cultural custom inhibits the natural size and movement of your structural space sphere. This raises an interesting question concerning the relevance of our personal space sphere concept to cross-cultural learning. Too seldom do we respect "the body culture", the "silent languages" or other adaptive

Structural Space Sphere

processes of the visitor, the immigrant, the refugee; and too often is the information misunderstood even when perceived. I believe that exploring and mastering the multi-faceted concepts of the body's personal space spheres presented here can serve to sensitively reach out, and "bridge" into the less familiar personal space spheres from different parts of the world.

- As you work with the structural space sphere, you begin to realize that others need not physically touch you in order for you to reach out or be reached. Nor do you need to touch another's musculature or body surface. "Communication and response" is not just between bodies, but much more intimately, in a psycho-physical sense, between individual structural space spheres.

- Hence, your structural sphere becomes an orientation space; a transition space; a benign protective device wherever you are. It is a conducting medium through which attitudes, perceptions, and energies can reach you with new, reinforcing rhythms. Received first by the structural sphere and transmitted through its space, they reach you already warmed by apprehension and awareness so that you can handle them with curiosity, with interest, and with a sensing of humor.

- Your structural space sphere offers you the options of privacy with yourself or intimacy with others. You may keep the door closed or open. You can extend welcome to guests and friends, or you can reserve and protect your personal solitude. The structural sphere's empty space now truly belongs to you. The vital force that you inject into its atmosphere is part of you. It's akin to finding yourself, for the first time, as a fish in your own pond where you can instinctively experience visceral enjoyment — float, shimmer, curve — and in your own way, listen, observe, and feel.

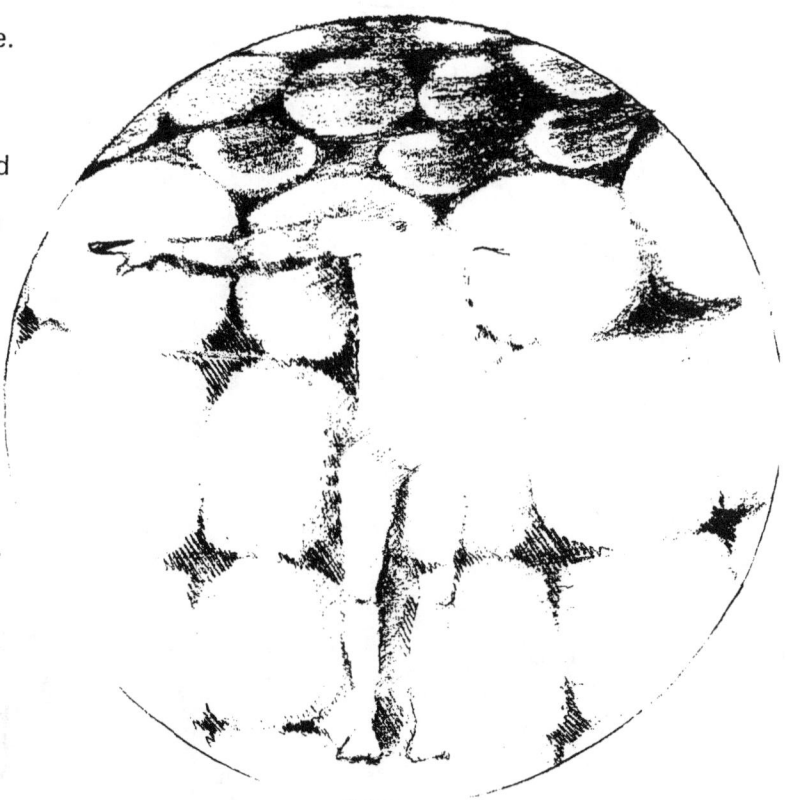

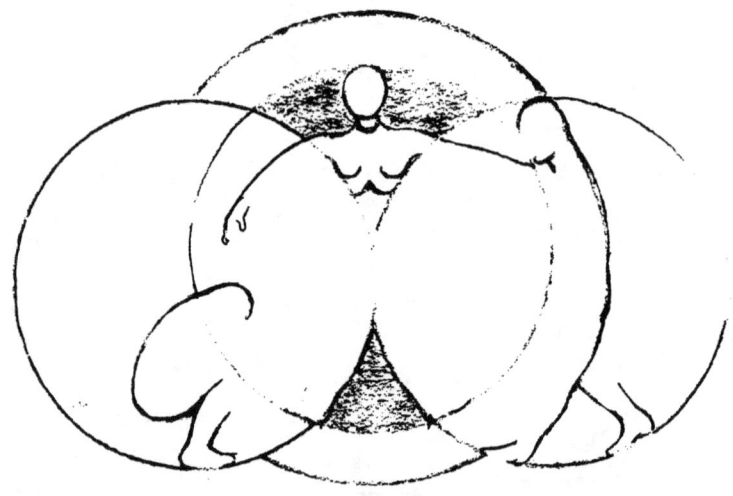

- Finally, the structural sphere is your private space where innocence, ingenuousness, fantasy, naive exploration and inventiveness, uninhibited plastique movement, day-dreaming, and self-expression of all kinds, free from comment or criticism, can be accommodated.

• Let us look, then, to our **body expressiveness in movement.** Let us explore our instincts and discover our responses:

- How do I accept or reject another's structural sphere coming close to mine — becoming acquainted or familiar or friendly or inquisitive?

- How does my emotional experiencing system respond and react if someone seeks entry into my structural space sphere? Is it an intrusion or an event?

- How does it feel seeing someone enter while I am functioning on the **outer** circumference of my sphere? Would I feel differently if I were **inside** my sphere or if I were separated from the wall and moving within the sphere — if some animal entered it — or a bird flew into it?

- Would I feel differently upon entering **someone else's** structural sphere?

- What are my emotional reactions to social intercourse within my private and close-quartered structural sphere as compared with the same social intercourse if it occurred in my auditory or visual or vocal space sphere?

• Explore these perceptual questions as a way of becoming positively familiar with your personal structural space sphere — its size, its form, its extension of your structure, your experiencing systems and values. Explore these primarily in self-to-self involvement:

Structural
Space
Sphere

1. Experiment until you succeed in feeling broad and tall in your structural sphere; then very small in that same structural space. Decide whether you have a choice in making these changes. Introduce varying emotional currents and attitudes that may influence the outcome.

2. Within your personal structural space sphere, experiment with different responses to your use of space, and to that same space **using** you. Does the use of your arms sculpt space, or does space shape the use of your arms — and when is there a voluntary choice? Can you sense space affecting the architecture and the way that the body parts tend to influence your response and relationship to space?

3. Infuse your structural space sphere with the feels of the different body energy states: first buoyancy, then radiancy, potency, and inter-involvement. Use these states to turn your space field into an energy field in which **you** are the center of gravity. What are the experiences of body rhythm and body balance within these spherical space/energy fields?

4. Work in your structural sphere with eyes closed. Then ask: Does the outer space disappear? Do you stop using the space and simply exist in it? What is light and what is dark? Use all your imaging faculties to answer these questions.

5. Now open your eyes. Do you light up the space outside of you, even in a dark room? Does the balance experience differ with eyes open, when the inner space no longer dominates or shapes the body's activity in the same way? Do you find yourself temporarily turning out the lights on the outer space and

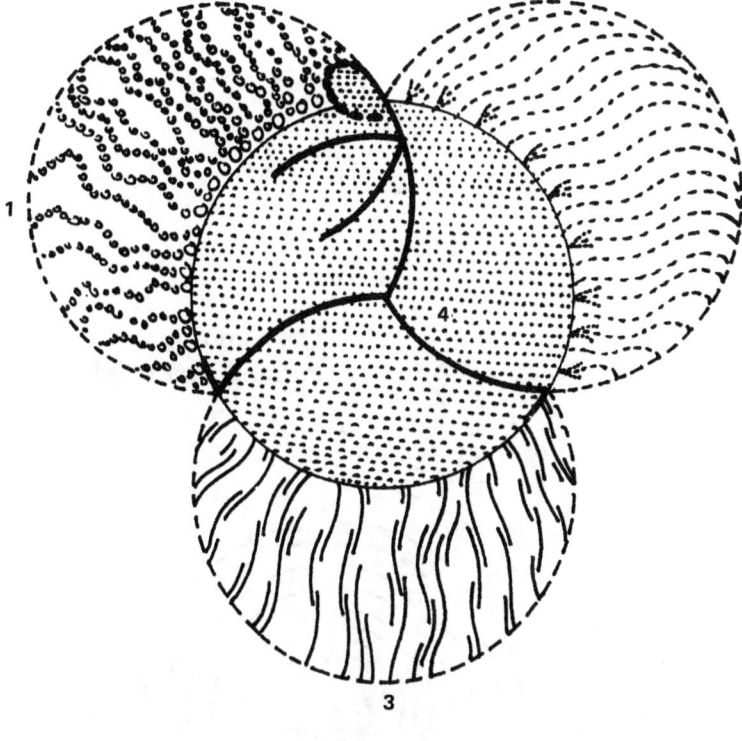

An image of the 4
Body Energy States:
1. buoyancy
2. radiancy
3. potency
4. inter-involvement

returning to illumine your inner space with its own dark glow, its own aura?

6. Like our progenitors the fish, begin to breathe, float, swim, shimmer-quiver-vibrate inside your structural space sphere. Listen **within**, as a blind person listens, or even as a deaf person listens. Catch the nuances in tone and different, perceptual shadings. Listen to the "smell of things" within, as an animal does; and relate the sense of smell within, to the sense of touch. Fill your structural space sphere with the dark of night — an atmosphere that makes listening easier and more exciting. Listen within and "taste the feel" of different vibrations and breathing experiences that lead to perception of inner rhythm, melody, and harmony.

7. Above all, become aware that it is the SPHERE of space, not space itself, that is significant. And it is body action, suffused by body energy, that declares the needs of your communicating structural space sphere and helps it to increase as it matures.

B. The Auditory Personal Space Sphere

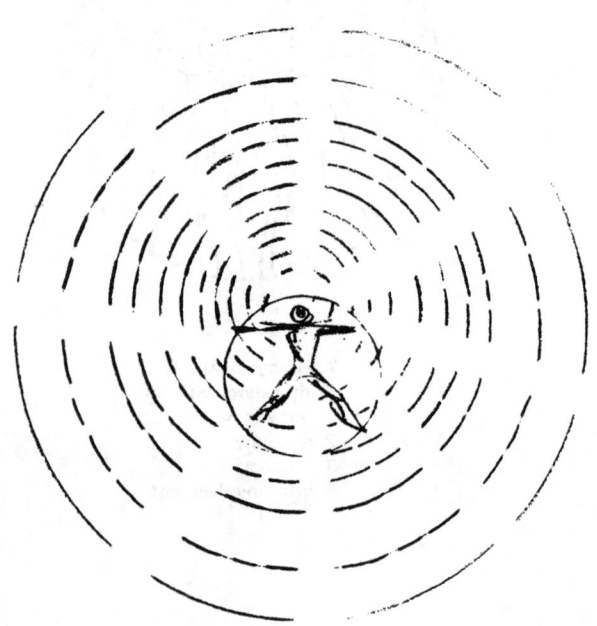

Once we can "feel what we hear" and "taste our listening," we can project the concept of an auditory space sphere. Listening within one's space sphere is a natural extension of our sense of kinesensic hearing, and expands the faculty to inwardly "see" the space behind us and surrounding us.

The auditory personal space sphere, while not so intimate as the structural sphere, is much more private than the visual space sphere. Indeed, the visual space sphere is the most externalized and in that sense, offers the least personalized perceptions. Unlike the visual sense, auditory sensing

Auditory Space Sphere

seems to originate from within; you not only hear something inside, you also **see** it there.

When it comes to listening within one's personal space sphere, we enjoy no superiority over the deaf. Rather, we can learn from them. As we feel what we hear and taste our listening, our auditory space sphere begins to teach us the feeling of extension, beyond structural space, through an expanded consciousness. We hear ambient noises never observed before and learn to listen to the design, dimensions, color, and qualities of these noises, and hear their rhythm and balance **in movement**. If these seem strange and inaccessible explorations, it's because we are literally unattuned to them, not because, as the deaf well know, they aren't there to discover.

As you now begin to experiment in the auditory personal space sphere, realize that your engagement to it comes from the extension of your "hearing energy," not from the extension of your body dimensions. Thus, from the outset, your auditory space is both behind you and in front of you.

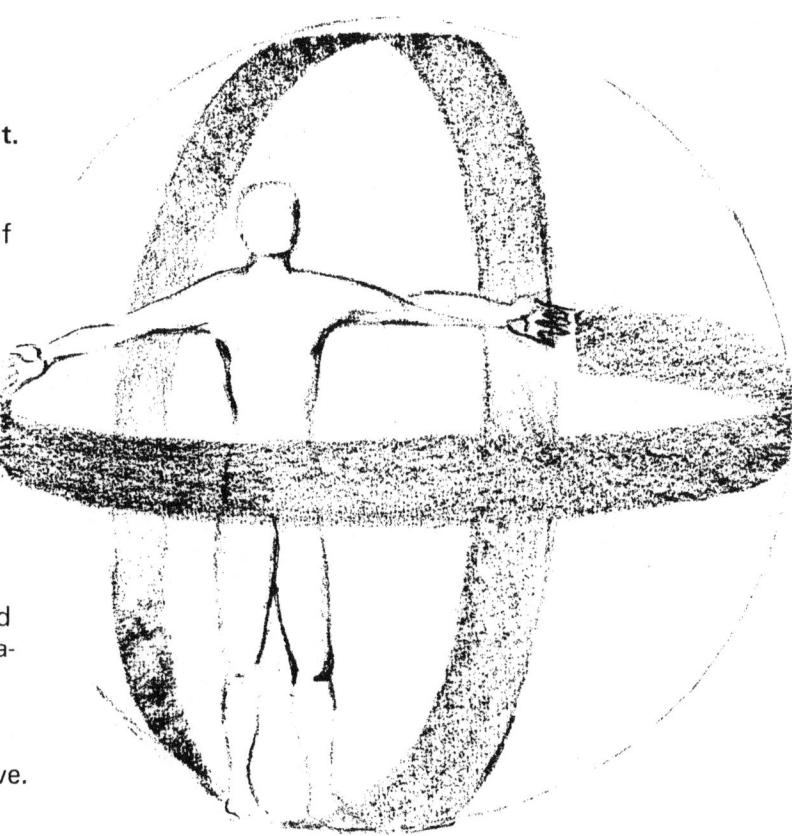

- Start by exploring auditory space all around you until you can register the exciting sensations of **hearing through eyes** in your back, your spine, and the lower crown of your head. You'll begin to auditorily visualize all those ambient noises we referred to above.

  ○ Test your responses and awareness to these perceptions. Relate to the scope and size of your auditory space sphere, first with eyes closed, then open. Study this same phenomenon when the outside space is very dark — during daylight hours — in artificially lit surroundings, and compare your responses. Check out the cues and signals you receive from the body in relating to what you hear.

The Body's
Personal
Space
Spheres

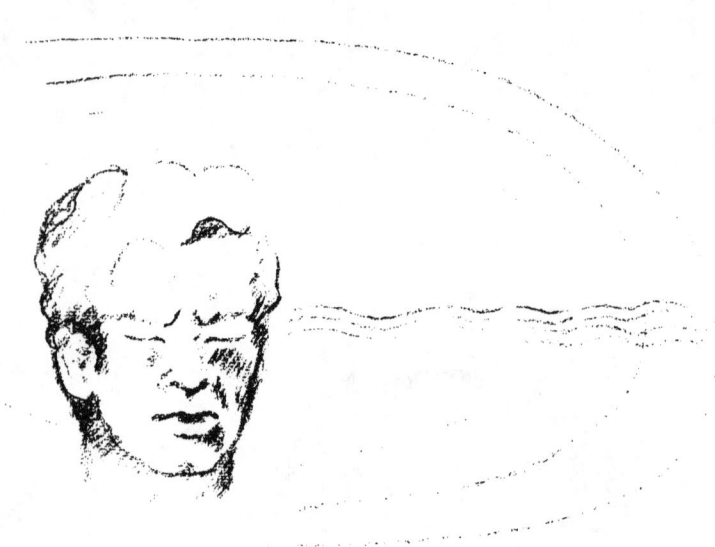

- Check also for strain, tension, or discomfort. With your eyes closed, does your auditory space sphere grow larger – smaller – does it remain the same? Are the changes in any way a challenge to your sense of equilibrium?

- Explore the sensations and perceptions resulting from the dynamics of your auditory space sphere:

  ○ Note how the perception of auditory space appears to flow **from** you rather than from the space itself. A sixth-sense energy reaches out to gather in whatever sounds are being transmitted to you. This out-reach is, itself, an extension of your inner energies, creating pathways and range-finders for your auditory experiencing system. This is not to say that your ears act as antennae or radar screens, but rather that **out** of your inner ears, energy flows in the direction of sound and brings it back to you and your harmonic, sensory receiving center. In fact, this sixth-sense energy appears to flick out not only from your ears, but as well from your head, skull, neck, face, and other parts of the body. The kinesthetic effect is rather extraordinary. You can tell yourself with authority, that through this kinesensic "feedback," it was your **finger** that heard the sound; that it was your **back** that attracted and brought back the sound to your body. By all means, continue to work on this level with this caliber of body intelligence and communication.

C. **The Visual Personal Space Sphere**

Being the most externalized, the visual space sphere is the largest and the least intimate. Visceral "looking and listening" will always take place in the "touch" or

Visual Space Sphere

"smell" of your structural space sphere and in the "blind" acuity of the auditory space sphere. The visual space sphere is where you not only 'look out in order to see,' but where you "feel what you see," and "taste what you look at."

Test this out:

- Explore the nature, character, and identity of what you see, and get a tap on its movement, rhythm, balance, color, and other visual esthetics.

- Discover the size and scope of your visual space sphere. Can you hear and read all the way to its periphery? If you cannot, is this due to your body's inadequate or deficient communicating system, or to the sheer expanse of your visual space sphere?

- As you relate to what you see in your sphere, respond to the cues and signals from your body. Is there a sense of strangeness, or any tensions — either psychological or physiological — that influences or affects your equilibrium while responding and reacting to the dimensions and boundaries of your visual space sphere?

- Note that this space sphere is an extension of your "looking energy," and vision is limited only by structural boundaries or by "as far as the eye can see." In the visual space sphere, you in fact see what you have always seen — but differently. **And you see what you had never seen before in the same place, though it was always there.**

The voice, in a one-to-one relationship with the emotional experiencing system, puts all the space spheres together, allowing us to reach, relate, and fully communicate with inter-involvement. It incorporates touch and

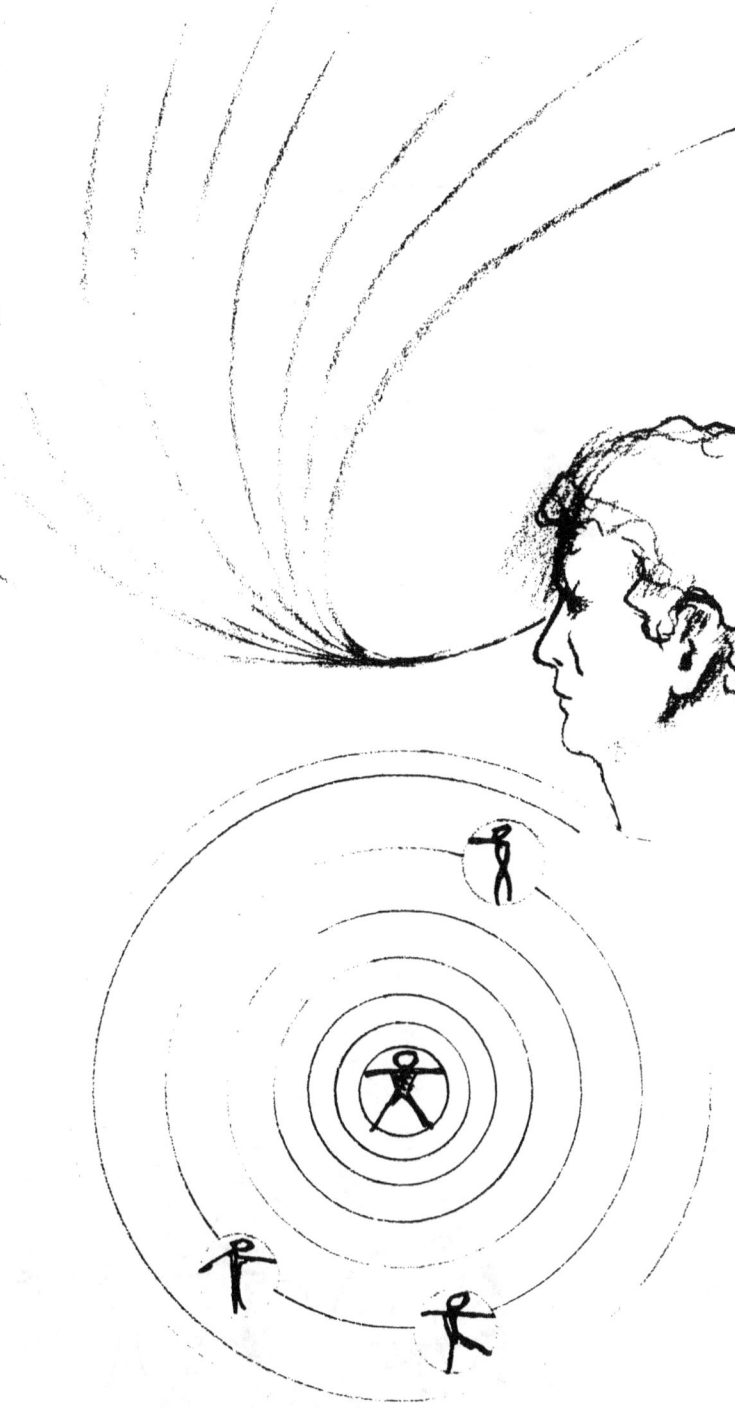

D. **The Vocal Personal Space Sphere**

The Body's Personal Space Spheres

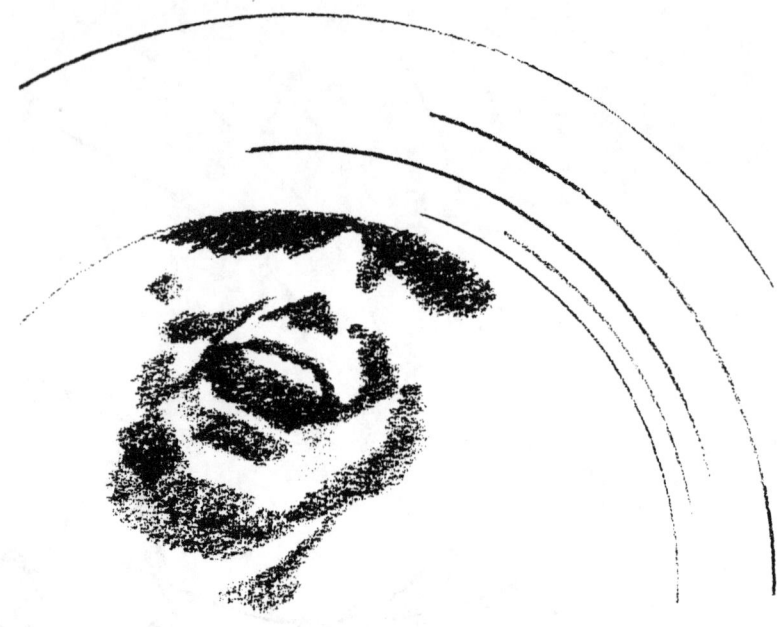

smell, hearing and listening, looking and seeing, feel and taste in balanced combination. Hence, it acts as a spatial and thermostatic, organic control valve for determining the optimal proportions of any of your personal space spheres where **self-to-other** communication takes place.

The voice is the final determinant in arranging a space sphere that is not too large to hear and listen; not too expansive to see "what" or whom you're addressing; not too small to crowd your vision. It is the voice that incarnates your speech, and reflects your body energy states and your emotional experiencing system.

When we speak, as we do at length in **The Use and Training of the Human Voice** and at various points in this work, of the vocal experiencing system or the "feeling process of the voice," we refer to the difference between hearing and listening to what one **thinks** is the feel of vocal registration — the feedback of the sound of one's voice — and to the feel of the **original** organic sensation of the voice — **before** outside feedback occurs. The former is negative vocal registration; the latter is positive vocal production. The first permits us to hear and listen only after the act; the second allows us to experience during the act. A personal space sphere, whatever its form or shape, is far better filled with what **is** rather than with what **was**.

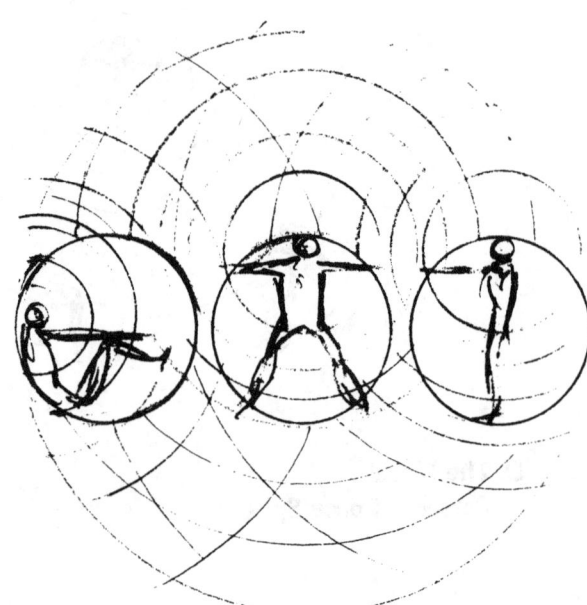

As you fill your vocal space sphere:

- Try to sense the distinction between "hearing" your voice and "feeling" your voice. Do you feel the body esthetics of bone-conducted tone; or do you feel the anesthetics of breathy, throaty, forced tone? Can you actually feel the difference between "forcefulness" and "force?"

Vocal
Space
Sphere

- Try to determine when your space sphere is too large for vocal life to flourish, and when it is too small for vocal tone to function efficiently. Does the space sphere adapt to your vocal life or does your vocal experiencing system adjust to the sphere? Is it perhaps part of a combined movement?

- Can you give your voice, eyes, and ears — distance and dimension guides — extensors through which to reach out, i.e. to **reach through**, rather than to or at, an object, creature, or other human being?

- Discover the distinctions in character, dynamics, and feel between the extension of your auditory and visual energies and those of your vocal energies. Compare those extensions of the body that reach out in order to receive, with those that reach out in order to give and send.

- Work on feeling the full extension of your organic-tonal arc in order to fill a larger space sphere. To fill a smaller sphere, you have only to sense the reduced tonal arc. Can you fill a large space sphere with sophisticated resonance/vibration and still be audible, intelligible, and believable? Can you excite a smaller space sphere with mature, dense resonance/vibration without getting noisy or losing intelligibility and esthetic quality?

- Check to see whether vocal strain or pressure influences negatively the auditory and visual aspects of your personal vocal space sphere? Do you recognize any necessity to modify or expand these qualities for better balance?

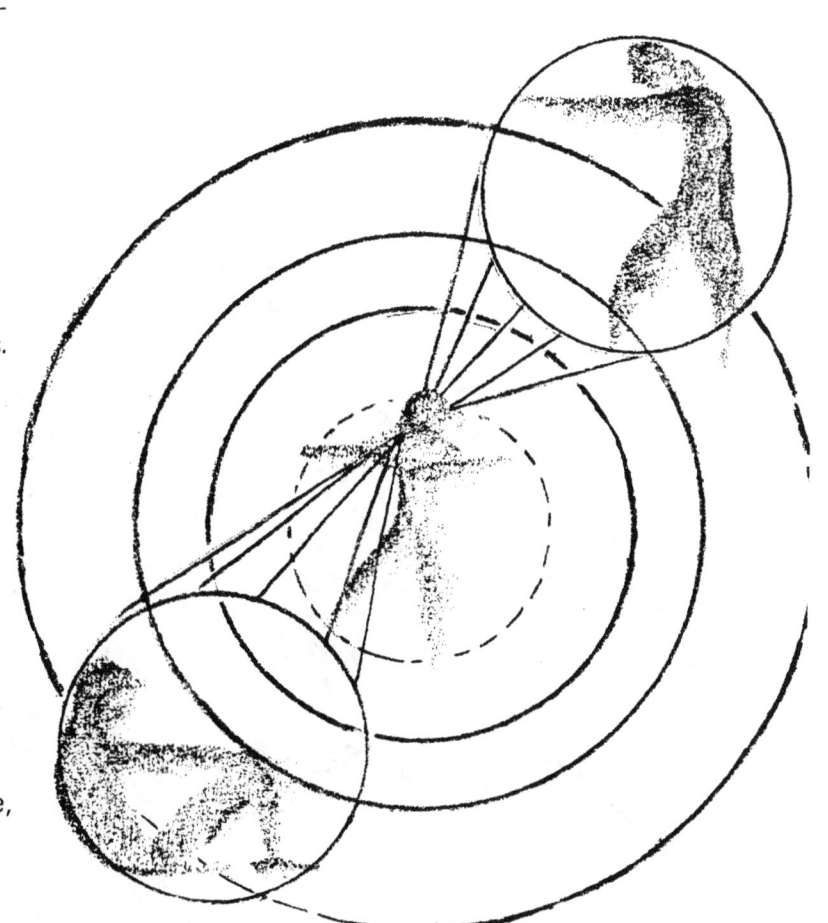

- Test whether your vocal life adds to the noise around you or reduces it — or perhaps simply **changes** the noise.

Can you see your voice? Can you weigh it, touch it, taste it? Does it touch you, taste you? Can you follow it, chase it, think with it? Do you need to hear yourself speak before you know what you're thinking?

How does your vocal space sphere function when you sing, chant, hum: at home — on-stage — in the shower — on the playing field — at work — in the crowded street — by your child's bedside?

E. The Traveling Personal Space Sphere

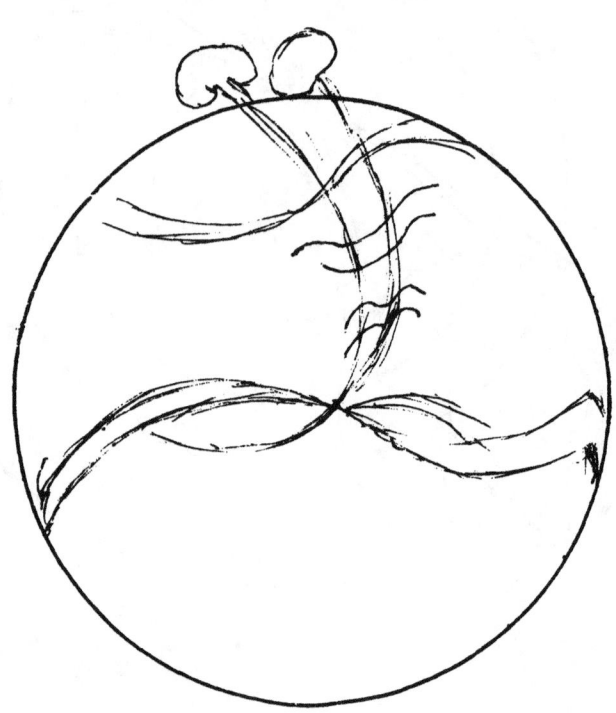

The concept of the mobile or traveling space sphere has special relevance for body movement in sports, dance, and personal pleasure-exercise activities. It applies to situations in which the individual moves through space over varying distances at varying speeds and pressures; as when you run, skate, ski, swim, swing yourself, sail, ride horseback, soar in a glider, or swing on ropes.

The question is: Do we divorce ourselves from our personal structural space spheres in such situations; or do our personal space spheres roll along with us during these activities? Does the more rigorous, physical activity preclude the use of any of our personal space spheres? Do they become obstacles or handicaps?

Definitely not! During any conscious behavior, one ought never lose contact with a personal space sphere, particularly the structural space sphere, any more than should one lose contact with perception or the sensation of awareness or one's self-image.

Bringing the structural space sphere along carries many advantages, especially when

Traveling Space Sphere

traveling fast. The moving quality of the structural sphere is a security device. It relieves tension and releases inhibitions and creative potential. Moreover, the structural sphere acts as a private, insulated space within which it is much easier to exercise the various body energy states — their rhythm follow-throughs and artistic carry-overs into optimal functioning.

This becomes crucially important for **sports, dance, creative exercise,** and **physical recreation.** The esthetics of balance, agility, rhythm, muscle tonicity, flexibility, strength, and body durability in these activities are much more closely allied to the structural space sphere than to any other. An athlete's awareness of grace, form, lightness, potency is nothing more than his awareness of the structural space sphere and its rhythm. The runner's structural sphere always runs with him. The mountain climber, distance walker, bicyclist, pole-vaulter all require the healthy co-assistance of the structural sphere.

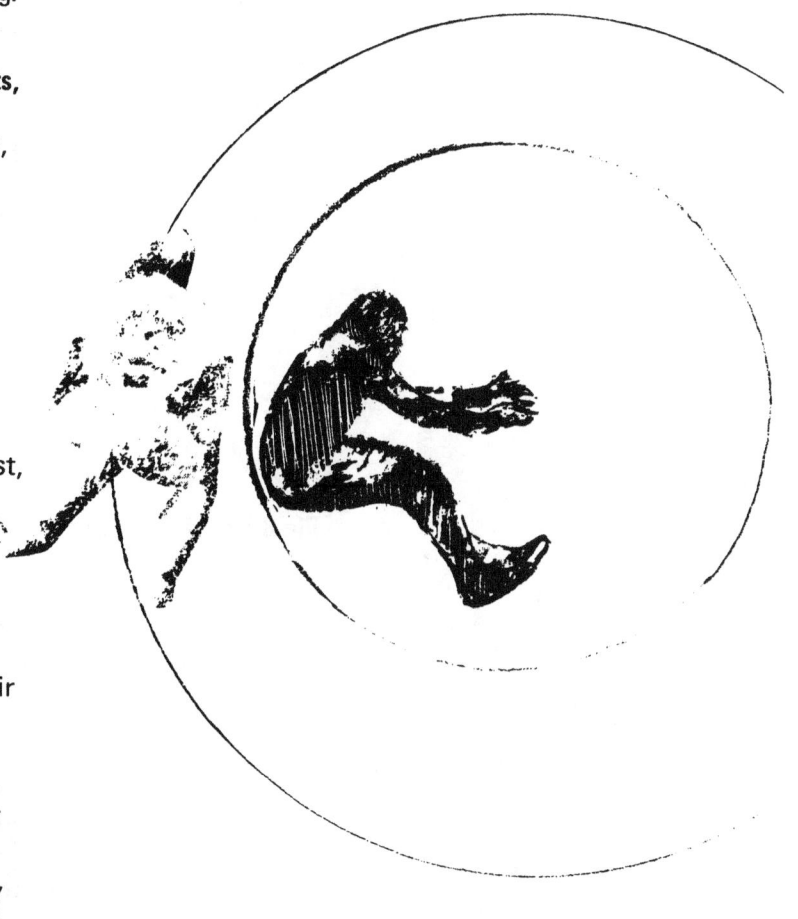

The instinctive understanding and awareness of buoyancy, lightness, and anti-gravitational sensation seem to thrive in their accommodating atmosphere. The runner, for example, can benefit from the psychological implications of structural space. It is truly easier to feel the rhythm of your leg-wheels — to sense them climbing uphill — to experience the floating, gliding, buoyant qualities that hold off fatigue and exhaustion, when you have succeeded in transforming the space around you into an accompanying personal space sphere. But the runner must feel that the sphere moves with him to experience its special benefits. Within the relative comfort of the structural sphere, there is a psychological diffusion of threat — be it from fear, competition, insecurity, or bodily injury.

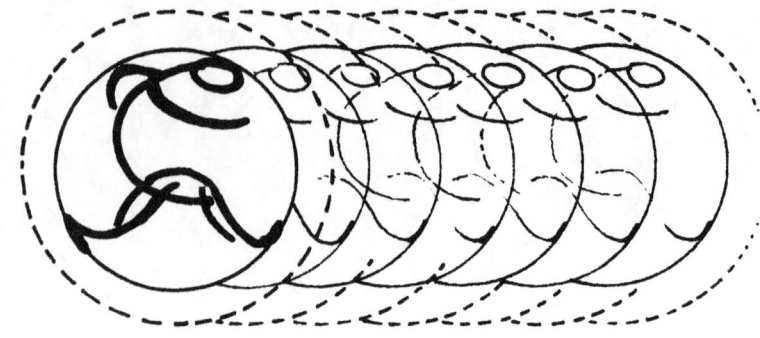

The traveling space sphere then, is the larger, encompassing sphere that directly surrounds structural space "on the wing." It is body movement in space — whether on its own, in a vehicle, on the back of an animal, on skis, or attached to an object traveling through space.

Because traveling carries with it the image of moving through space from point to point, the traveling space sphere extends our primary space spheres — structural, auditory, visual, vocal — into positive, finite relationship with the outside world. It provides, perhaps, our first experience where the outer and inner environments are not in competition or conflict: the outer environment is now in position to offer a "cushion" of psycho-physical security and equilibrium both to the body and its structural space sphere in transit.

Final Considerations

We have seen that personal space spheres come in various sizes, depending on the structure or faculties of the body and the nature of the activity.

- The structural space sphere could have a central axis measuring about nine feet when extended from your body's upright posture. That same sphere might be reduced to four feet in diameter when you're bent over or sitting; and perhaps to three feet when you're in squat or crouching posture. In all these structural space sizes, visual-auditory-vocal coordination is relatively simple. The only challenge might come from a forced or noisy vocal production that tends to overload the other energy circuits.

- The auditory space sphere, with eyes open or closed, is correspondingly larger than the structural sphere in

Personal
Space Spheres
Final
Considerations

relation to the sharpness and
range of your hearing extension.
The auditory sphere works like an
accordian, moving back and forth in
curving lines to explore the latitudes
within a limited distance.

- The visual space sphere, especially
without the use of your voice, can be
the largest of all. Visually, the sphere
might be reduced in order to meet the
needs and balancing capabilities of
vocal and auditory coordinates. But if
the eyes alone are involved, the sphere
could conceivably expand beyond the
size of the room, the auditorium, or
the stadium.

- The vocal space sphere is both limited
and controlled by tonal production and
vocal "reaching-thru" as it is released into
the conducting space. In the process of
using vocal life for relating and responding in self-to-other communication, your
tonal space sphere can span sizes from
touching distance to a huge arena.

- Each of these primary space spheres
represents a relatively stable set of
conditions, serving as a kind of transition
to connect the smaller, inner environment with the larger, outside world. That
connection is completed by your personal
traveling sphere as it dissolves the
competition between the two environments when one moves through space.

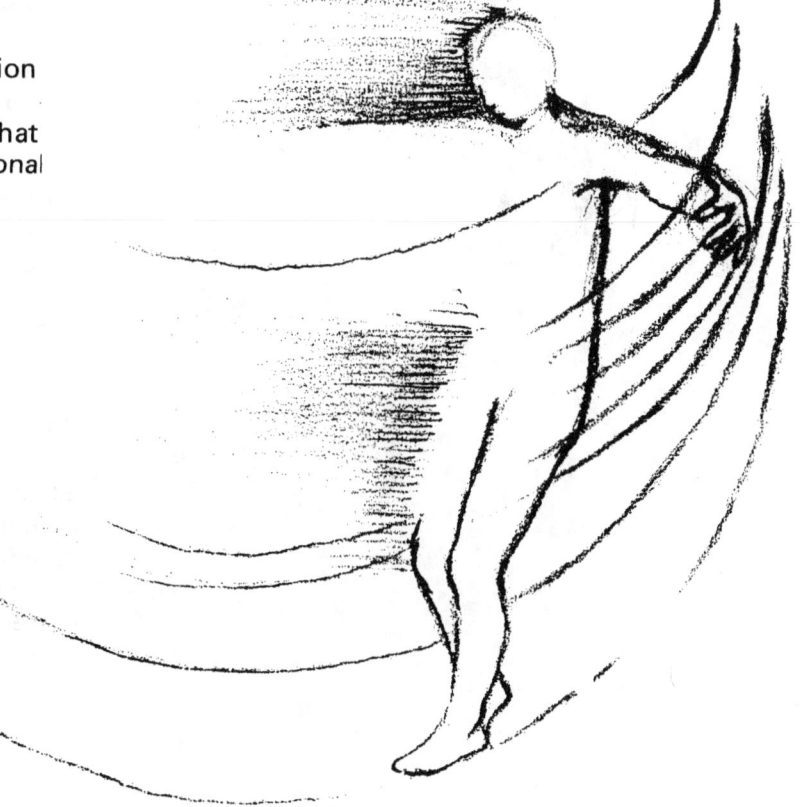

The Body's
Personal
Space
Spheres

In general, filling in and occupying any and all of our personal space spheres depends upon gradual discovery and awareness of the different aspects of outer and inner perception:

> How **much** can we see?
>
> How **well** can we hear?
>
> How **efficiently** can we speak?
>
> How **far** can we reach?
>
> Can we **see** inside what we see outside? Can we **behold** it?
>
> Can we **hear** within what we hear? Can we **perceive** the harmonics?
>
> Can we **say** what we think? Can we **sense** it?
>
> Can we **mean** what we say? Can we **believe** it?

Ultimately, can we inter-relate and communicate what we see, hear, think, and mean — with impunity and reinforcement — through a feeling process concerned with quality in social and inter-personal relations?

So far in the development of this process, we have found that the follow-through of self-to-self response is, indeed, self-to-other communication. Put another way, our perceptive experience with the inner-environment organic feeling process proves optimally efficient and effective in coping with outside influences and forces. All this keeps pointing to further search and discovery of the curvo-linear body in movement.

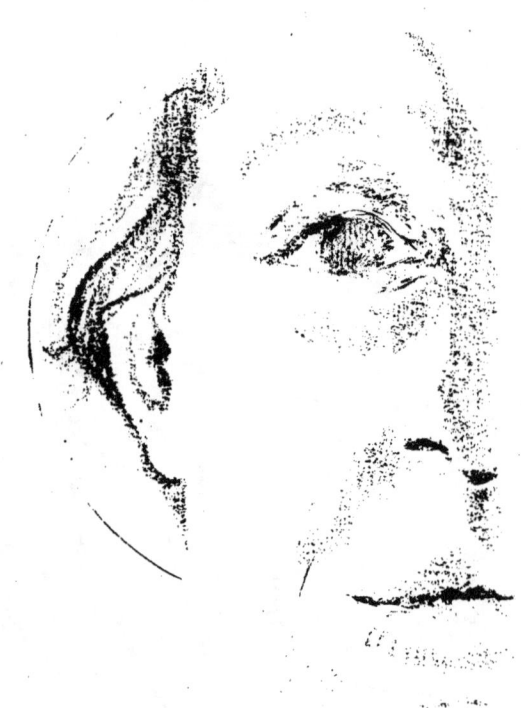

So, in conclusion: think of your personal space sphere as a globe and of yourself, as a live flame inside the globe that cannot be extinguished. Experience that live-flame of breath, of growth, of relating, of creating — and let it lead you, through its curvo-linear movement, in search of your self-image.

14
IN SEARCH OF A SELF IMAGE

Chapter 14

In Search of a Self Image

In terms of the "feeling process," and organic/sensory learning, what does it mean to be "in search of a self-image?" Clearly, something more than the phrase, a commonplace of "pop psychology," would suggest.

I use the word "search," here, to imply a process of **maturing** — a mode of **moving** naturally and progressively toward a self-image. It is not a hunt or a quest after something vaguely known or "anxiously" sought, but, in the classic sense of the term, an "inquiry" leading to (or back to) what we know is there and ultimately available. The mood of the "search," in our construct, is identical to that sense of **gentle turbulence** which characterizes the body — the self — in perpetual movement.

We also refer selectively to **a** self-image rather than to **the** self-image. To search for **the** ideal love, **the** perfect job, **the** self-image would be a "fool's errand." Kinesensic training is not a utopian panacea. It's a learning system posited on realistic possibility. Moreover, **the** self-image, as a concept, denies the principle and challenge of **evolving** creativity and invention that is central to our training method.

In reality, of course, there is no such thing as a singular self-image. Whenever we talk about an "integrated personality," even in common parlance, we assume the many sides of a person's character; the many facets of an individual's tastes, talents, professional capacities; and the multiplicity of roles played out daily by the average human being. It's only the clinical language of abnormal psychology, when overstated or borrowed without a card, that leads to confusion and underestimation; i.e. when we assume that "personality" is singular and observe plural manifestations as indicative of a "split personality" or schizophrenia.

A self-image in the singular is limiting, diminishing, unrealistic, whereas a pluralistic self-image is open-ended — always sending and receiving, giving and taking, with constant challenge and excitement. At best, a singular self-image is a finished product, and all that remains is to keep polishing it. A pluralistic self-image is never finished and never polished — it remains always vulnerable.

Thus, the notion of self-image as a collective noun is part of a conceptual grammar closely related to synergy and the "third-force" approach we've been discussing throughout BODY WISDOM. It is also a more fitting formulation for a system concerned not with psychosomatic disease, but with **psychosomatic health.**

Our work together has been leading, step by step, to this understanding of a self-image that lives, breathes, vibrates, and is con-

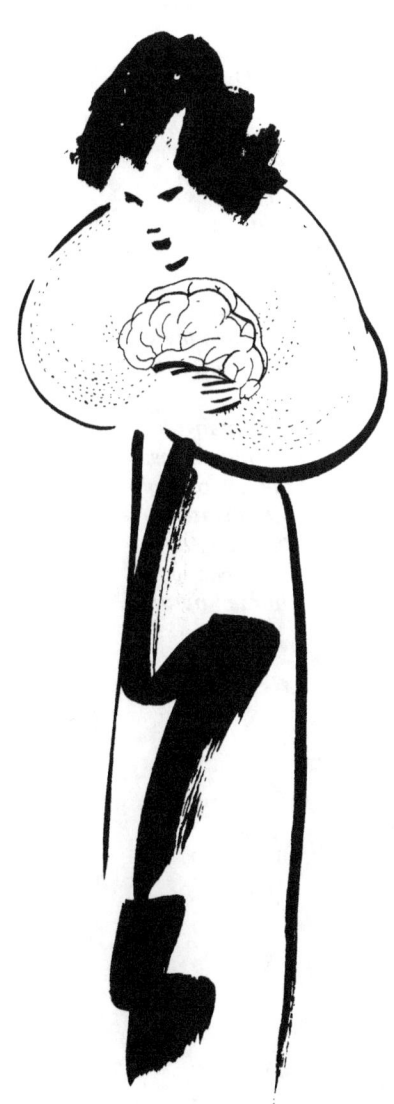

stantly re-energized **in movement.** All of our experiments have implied that at root, a person's "self-image" stems from his/her "body image", and is therefore **an image in action** — and an image in action does not get lost; it waits to be found.

Images only **appear** to fade. Breath just **seems** to evaporate. Rhythm can give the **impression** of having withdrawn. Vital energy may prove, at times, **elusive.** And a self-image may be **misplaced.** But they all exist. More than exist, they **live** as constants, as harmonic overtones fully accessible to our inner senses — provided our body environment is not deaf, blind, or dumb to them.

By "image", I do not refer to outer conditioned or habit-patterned imitations, likenesses, proto-types, or carbon copies. These are fixed images and lack the "movement" and experience of design, idea, color, and the gamut of shapeless migrations of nerve-fed substances.

... human laws and rules are human inventions; the law of logic that states "you can't change human nature" is a human invention!

It is therefore essential that the understanding of self and the respect for self be inextricably linked to **the psychological image of self as a moving picture, not a snapshot!** Your self-image is not something that can or should be translated onto a piece of paper. You can't read or judge what another person is feeling, or even who that person is, from stills or photographs of that person's face. You have to watch those expressions over time — in action! Why shouldn't the same be true of your own self-image? Why shouldn't the process of "feeling" awareness provide us with new ways of understanding "self-awareness".

Self-awareness, originating with the body-image and flowing rhythmically into the self-image, returns to the body-image in a state of energy. This rhythmic exchange between our body-image and our self-image, essentially a feeding back and forth of self-awareness, reinforces the knowledge and experience needed for us to cope more effectively with the outside environment.

The notion of follow-through is important here, particularly in relation to the **image of self as curvo-linear and moving.** It suggests a process which relates to your experimenting and exploring:

a) with movement that originates in, and flows out of structural and instinctive body curves; b) with movement that extends into our primary personal space spheres — (structural, auditory, visual and vocal); c) with movement that encompasses the five fundamental senses, the body's primitive energy states, and the follow-through functions, which combine to re-restablish healthy contact with the outside environment; and d) with movement from the extension of that over-all "follow-through" which nourishes our self-ego.

Hence, the self-image stems from the moving images derived from our curvo-linear body form, and is characterized by our functioning behavior within the personal space spheres. **In a very strong sense, the way we respond and relate, through the feeling process, in our personal space spheres becomes the frame of reference for our individual self-image.**

The follow-through principle representing movement **from** the body and **back to** the body is clearly opposed to anything static or imitative. If the body is constantly in motion and all body movement, in terms of functional behavior, must feel good, salutary, and fertile **during** movement, then everything connected to our self-image must be understood as part of the follow-through.

In the same way that we try to teach ourselves how each muscle unit **wants** to work (not how to work) and how different parts of the body **want** to behave instinctively, so can we teach ourselves how to relate the feel of movement with optimal functioning. That is, if the body in movement makes us **feel** very, very good, then in all probability, the individual components of the moving body **must** be doing everything right; must, in fact, all be functioning in optimal dynamic balance. This esthetic self-awareness feeds and becomes part of our creative self-image.

So let us not respond to the outside environment as a mirror source for self-image that we may cease living as mirror images of the external world. They are all, more or less, artificial reflections — they are all imitative. What we need are motivators that **maturate** behavior, not reflectors that mirror it.

Otherwise, the forebrain message, "You are what others think and believe you are," will come dangerously close to the mark! Is the bargain of self-fragmentation, as you try to sift and select from others' perceptions and opinions of you, really worth the price?

An outer-conditioned self-image is always in danger of petrifying. Like a hardened, uncracked shell, it can **encase** a gasping and choking inner sensory system. All glistening armor on the outside, all corroding rust on the inside, that shell has an astounding capability to keep out creative change and imaginative, courageous, daring exploration — if that's, indeed, what you want!

One thing more: the image you picture to yourself (e.g. your voice, your speech, your walk, your posture, the way you "carry yourself") is not necessarily — in fact, seldom is — the same as your self-image. Though it may appear to be realistically arrived at, it may still be only a reflection of your genuine self-image, which results from a delicate balance between your personal experience and your moving body-image. It is this last of balancing acts that allows each of us to manifest our personal uniqueness and originality. Thus, even while body-images may **possibly** resemble one another, self-images — **real** self-images — never do. Body-images are the "fundamentals"; multi-faceted self-images are the "harmonics and overtones" of our individual sensory systems. And it is your multi-dimensional self-image whose potential is unlimited!

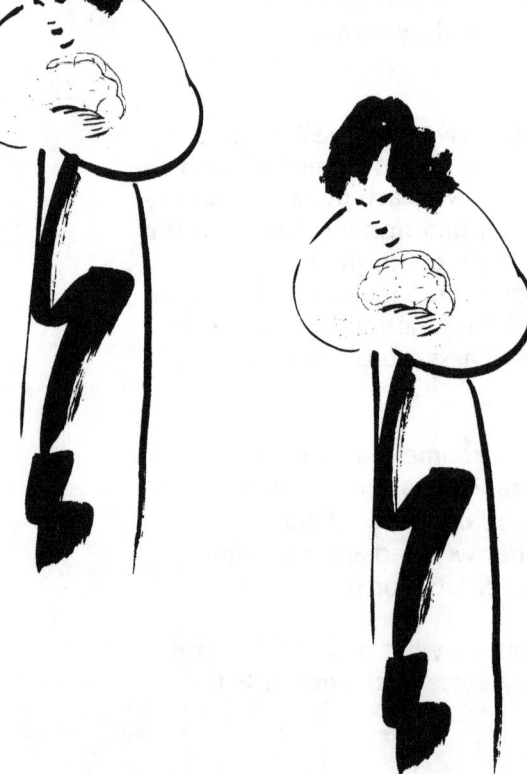

CODA
AN AFTERWORD

As you now begin to apply your self-teaching to everyday life, remember that our organic instructions to the body to dissolve fatigue are not so different from those used to dispel fear which, in turn, are not so different from those hired to fashion the products of imaginative creativity. The parting thought, here, is that we are speaking of an organic process of behavior that is transferable to multiple contexts; an over-all process of body functioning that is determined by, and has been developed from, the explorations and investigation of how your body **wants** to function.

CODA
... an afterword

With this in view, we conclude the present study with a brief afterword, designed to suggest several of the areas where you can begin to exploit those instinctive body skills and natural talents inherent to a many-sided self-image rooted in Body Wisdom. The picture essay and graphic illustrations that complement and complete the **Coda** offer a wide range of realistic possibilities where you can apply your experimenting and experience in the benefits of our body training: AT HOME — AT WORK — AT PLAY — IN SPORTS — IN THE ARTS.

We also take this opportunity to indicate several directions of our ongoing research that point toward innovation and major change in the ways we, as a society and a global community, can better meet the challenges of shared problems and concerns through applied Body Wisdom. The Coda is intended to be suggestive, not definitive; and, like the body curve itself, it forms part of a continuing, constantly evolving sphere of work where every end-point is, in fact, just another beginning.

If you have read carefully, experimented honestly, and internalized the accumulating perceptions as you've moved through Parts One, Two, and Three — then you have really begun to initiate your own self-teaching in the feeling process. You realize that Body Wisdom is not a grab bag, but rather an inherent potential and resource that exists within each of us whether we use it or not; that if we choose to waste that resource, over time it wastes away by itself and can be restored only by training.

Hence, the "democracy principle" intrinsic to Body Wisdom combines benefit with responsibility. It has nothing whatsoever to do with privilege, franchise, economics, personal endowment, or surface "beauty." All that matters is that the whole body environment remains **unravished, untortured, unabused.**

Moreover, Body Wisdom applies equally and completely with the same integrity and pleasure to the individual body environment whether at play, at work, at home, in the streets, on the platform,

CODA
The Body's
Constitutional
Democracy

stage, assembly-line, or sports field. Only the purpose and intensity of application differ by degree. The basic "esthetic tap" — once you have it — remains intact. It is this "esthetic tap" that puts things back into perspective and leads us to a sensing of humor and natural play, as well as to a retention of personal convictions and dreams. The "esthetic tap" lets us know, regardless of context or situation, when we are "out of humor or sustenance," i.e. when the body-whole is feeling and making disturbing statements.

How many practical situations, related to your interests, profession, job, daily activities, or recreational outlets, can you project where the "esthetic tap" would allow your body to function more efficiently and more easefully, with optimum balance between energy output and relaxation? Certainly the actor, dancer, and singer **must** have it, and athletes **should** have it! It is regrettable that so many professionals turn body esthetics into such a technical discipline that they tend to lose it again. The fact is, we all need it, in practically any situation, but certainly whenever a sense of psycho-physical equilibrium, endurance, strength, flexibility, and a way of dealing with our emotions and fears is required. To have an "esthetic tap" really means using Body Wisdom to tap all our **defects** as well as our skills, so that we can actively develop **all of them into talents.**

Furthermore, the same principles of Body Wisdom that apply to different situational contexts obtain whether used as preventive medicine, therapy, or as natural food and fuel for the body to grow, mature, and endure. But for Body Wisdom, just as for democracy, to flourish, it must first be practiced; to grow and develop, it must be nourished "care-free-ly" on a featured diet that categorically excludes man-made future shocks, conflicts, contradictions; and deals with addictions, crippling anxieties, and anesthetic conditioning as unhealthy body ingredients.

Those of you who have started to work on yourselves, practicing the exercises and experiments on a regular basis and beginning to apply them to various daily activities, should feel unthreatened by the alarming statistics offered in the Introduction, on common body ailments suffered needlessly by most Americans. You are already aware of how our concepts of posture, alignment, breathing, balance, energy states, balanced muscle tonicity, and relaxer-energizers can alleviate, if not eliminate, many conditions of low backaches, distorted spine and back conditions, serious bellyaches, digestive discomfort, headaches, high-back strain, neck tension, jaw tension, as well as the psycho-physical distresses of dry throat, nausea, itching, scratching, weariness, paling, helplessness, fear of falling, etc.

CODA
The Body's
Constitutional
Democracy

Now ask yourselves how you can use your self-teaching to:

... keep in closer touch with your emotions;

... control and communicate along with your emotions;

... experience unexplored feats of physical artistry;

... recapture some of the beauty, grace, control, and endurance of the cat, the fox, the child — i.e. recapture the ingenuous inventiveness that leads to ingenuity.

... cope more effectively with nervousness and competition, wherever they occur;

... confront large groups of people with stimulated curiosity and alerted body energy states;

... deal genuinely with small groups where the situation calls for negotiation, arbitration, or conflict resolution;

... replace exhaustion with exhilaration and, where exhilaration is improbable at least sit without tedium, or work without the effort that produces exhaustion;

... enjoy your body image in sports, in the arts — in running, sprinting, skiing, tennis-playing, golf, swimming, writing, painting, singing, dancing, etc.;

... better understand and sense cross-cultural differences, so you can better sense and appreciate individual differences among people;

... relate psycho-physically to differences in culture and react to them without losing your own individuality — therefore, without losing your sharpness of thinking and your sharpness of instinct

but at the same time, understanding and feeling whence derive the other culture's sharpness of thinking and sharpness of instinct;

... apply the C-curve, natural breathing, and body balance to overcome the routine dis-stress of carrying heavy bundles, lifting heavy objects, doing housework, standing for long periods of time, climbing steep flights of stairs, etc.

All of these potential applications deal with the self-image in movement and, as such, with the relationship between image and action. All assume primary Body Wisdom: the intelligences, communication networks, language energies, instincts. In short, all the wisdom that commands, instructs, and allows the body to function efficiently and effectively with full freedom and control **wherever the body happens to be.**

But, while we know very well how to apply the C-curve, natural breathing, and body balance to the areas listed above, as well as to the onset of fatigue or even the awkwardness of pregnancy, (which should be anything but awkward), we still need additional and more specific documentation in each case.

While we know how to adapt our physical environment to the needs and curvo-linear structure of the body, for better body functioning, we still require considerable research and development before making serious recommendations for the design of chairs and tables; beds and reading lamps; toilet facilities; shoes and clothes, that respect the body form and respond healthfully to the small, inner body environment. All are technologically feasible and long overdue.

It is actually a matter of integrity, and in that connection, it seems just about time to re-evaluate, unsanctimoniously, present day codes regarding hypocrisy, dishonesty, prejudice, double standards, and other such contaminants to the inner body environment. With some genuine re-defining we may, **with integrity**, teach the meaning of these "behaviors" to our children and at the same time **re-teach them to ourselves** to help avoid the "future shock" of becoming ethically insensitive; lacking organic esthetics; and functioning without kinesensic balance between body, intellect and spirit. **Conflict resolution with capitulation does not reflect human betterment.**

The experiments and pilot programs already conducted, using **applied kinesensics** in clinical and rehabilitative therapy, preventive medicine, executive management training, athletic coaching, and actor and ensemble theater training, need to be multiplied, further validated, and supplemented by new programs for pre-literate education, teacher inservice training, second language learning, and the whole field of cross-cultural or multicultural education.

It would be most interesting, for example, to explore the relevance of "personal space spheres" to problems of conflict resolution and acculturation. Why are people's structural space spheres so easily threatened and so different across cultures? Is it because the movements and the vocal qualities are objectively different, or is it purely a cultural overlay that we're missing or misreading? How do you decode another culture's personal and group space spheres towards: improvement of international relations; building "universal empathy" between peoples of different cultures (often in the same nation);

CODA
What's Ahead?

assisting the processes of acculturation and reception without destroying the integrity of the first culture; completing the concept of a language/culture universe with the recognition of personal space spheres as functional components and expressive dimensions of both language **and** culture?

Is it conceivable that those who have experienced and explored communication within their own structural space spheres will more instinctively adjust to those of different cultures; that they will more organically relate and perceptively respond to both universal rhythms and culture-specific frequencies? Is the follow-through of self-to-self response, through Body Wisdom, an out-reach to the harmonics of a more perceptive self-to-other responsiveness? Is it possible that, as we transform "stage-fright nervousness" into "creative excitement value," we can teach ourselves to so "feel" the sensations of hate or corruptness, that we may convert them into authentic anger and honest forcefulness in the interest of positive change?

These questions point not only toward specific levels of training for those concerned with the welfare of the international and intercultural community, but also toward a new kind of research and development institute that brings together the pioneer studies of many different disciplines (including bio-feedback and split-brain advances) around a set of common causes. It should be a vital function of that institute also to train a highly select corps of field advisors and instructors who, on an ongoing basis, can work with labor leaders, educators, urban planners, health care specialists, business executives, designers, architects, and artistic directors, on plans and strategies for incorporating applied Body Wisdom in their respective training and service programs.

Industrial, factory, and agrarian workers, teachers, professional and allied health personnel, managers, office staff, operators of heavy construction equipment, airline pilots and control center staff, sales personnel, actors, dancers, musicians, and athletes in every area of sports — all have the right and the need to know how to labor with less effort; enjoy greater equity; achieve optimal performance; **and at the same time,** develop so complete a repertoire of instinctive body skills and natural talents that they can at will, infuse any aspect of their work with endless variety, satisfaction, and pleasure.

Many of these suggested applications of Body Wisdom will strike a familiar chord within each of you. Several will receive special attention in subsequent studies and self-teaching guides. The graphic essay that follows is designed simply to suggest the range of realistic possibilities. In that sense, it constitutes both a finish and a prelude.

You and Your Body at Home

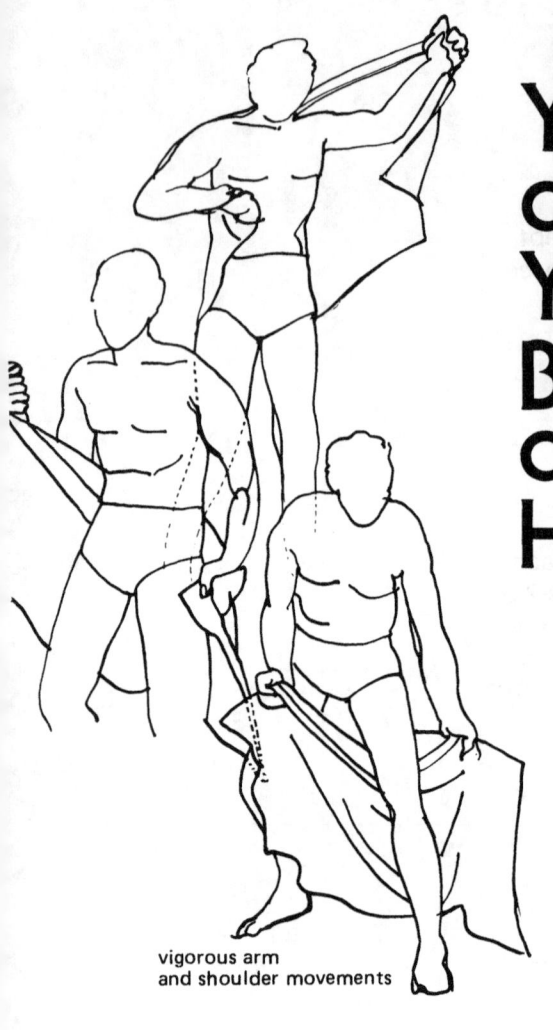

vigorous arm and shoulder movements

For excellent back, shoulders, arms, and finger exercise-workouts, take advantage of the shampoo, massage, rub-down, and drying activities:

...While shampooing apply extra strong and vigorous finger pressure and rubbing.

...Dry and massage your hair vigorously with strong finger-tip pressure.

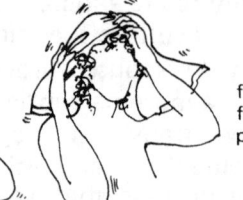

firm finger pressure

...While drying yourself after bath or shower with Turkish towel, use vigorous, rapid "rub-down" movements in all directions.

For excellent back, thigh, and leg workout:

...When picking up an object (light or heavy), use any variation of the squat posture — never bend as in illustration **b**.

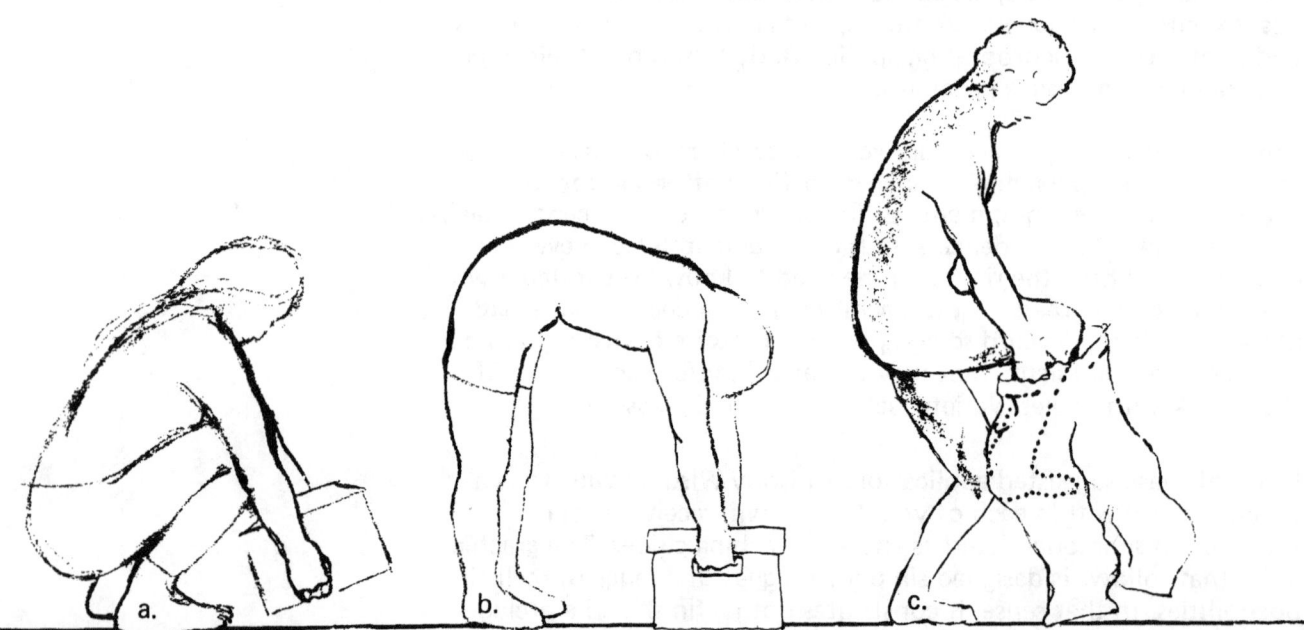

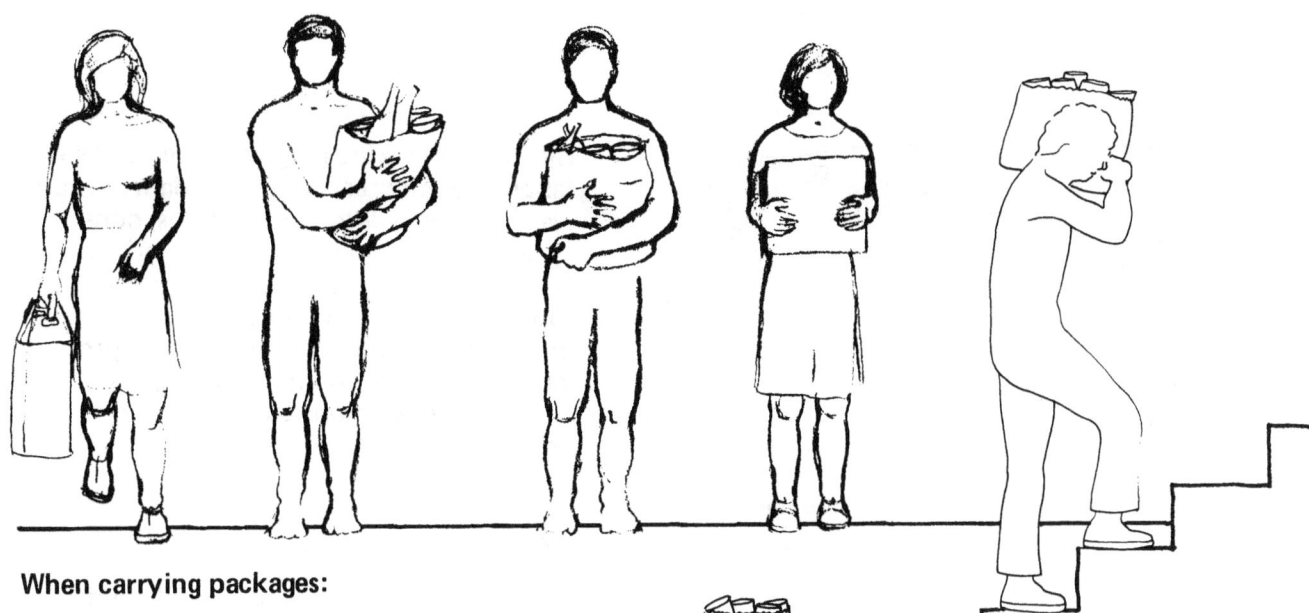

When carrying packages:

...Alternate hands, arms, shoulders, sides, hips, etc., whether packages are heavy or light.

...For back-pack use shoulder-girdle as a fulcrum center.

...Feel free to carry object on head but remember to alternate arms whenever using only one at a time.

...a "shower-head-vibrator" and/or a "whirlpool-massager" are excellent attachments to soften-loosen-lengthen-shake the body musculature, particularly at the upper and lower spine centers.

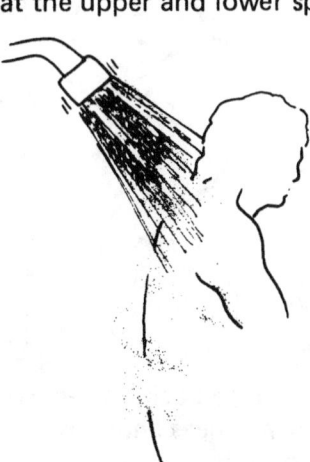
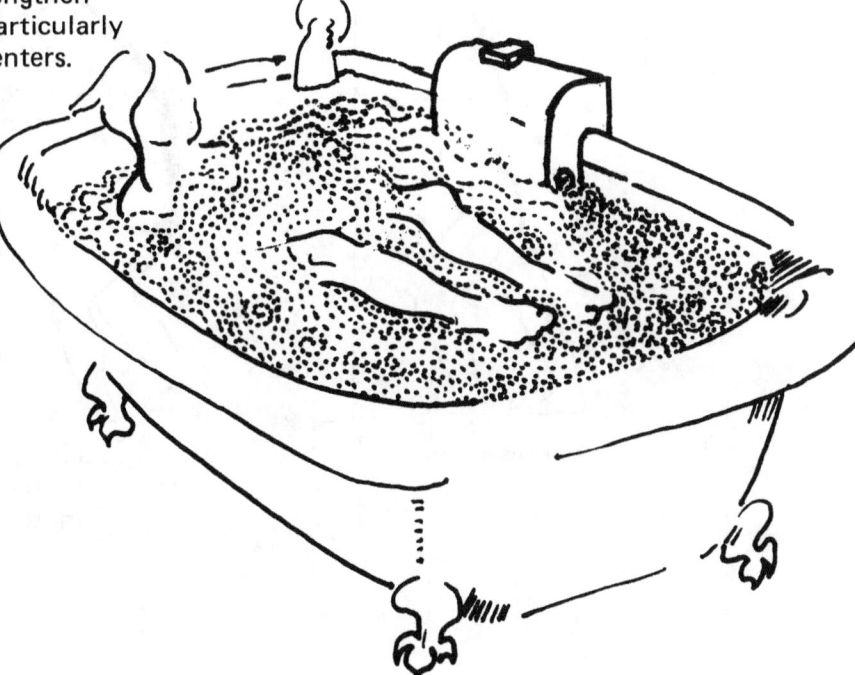

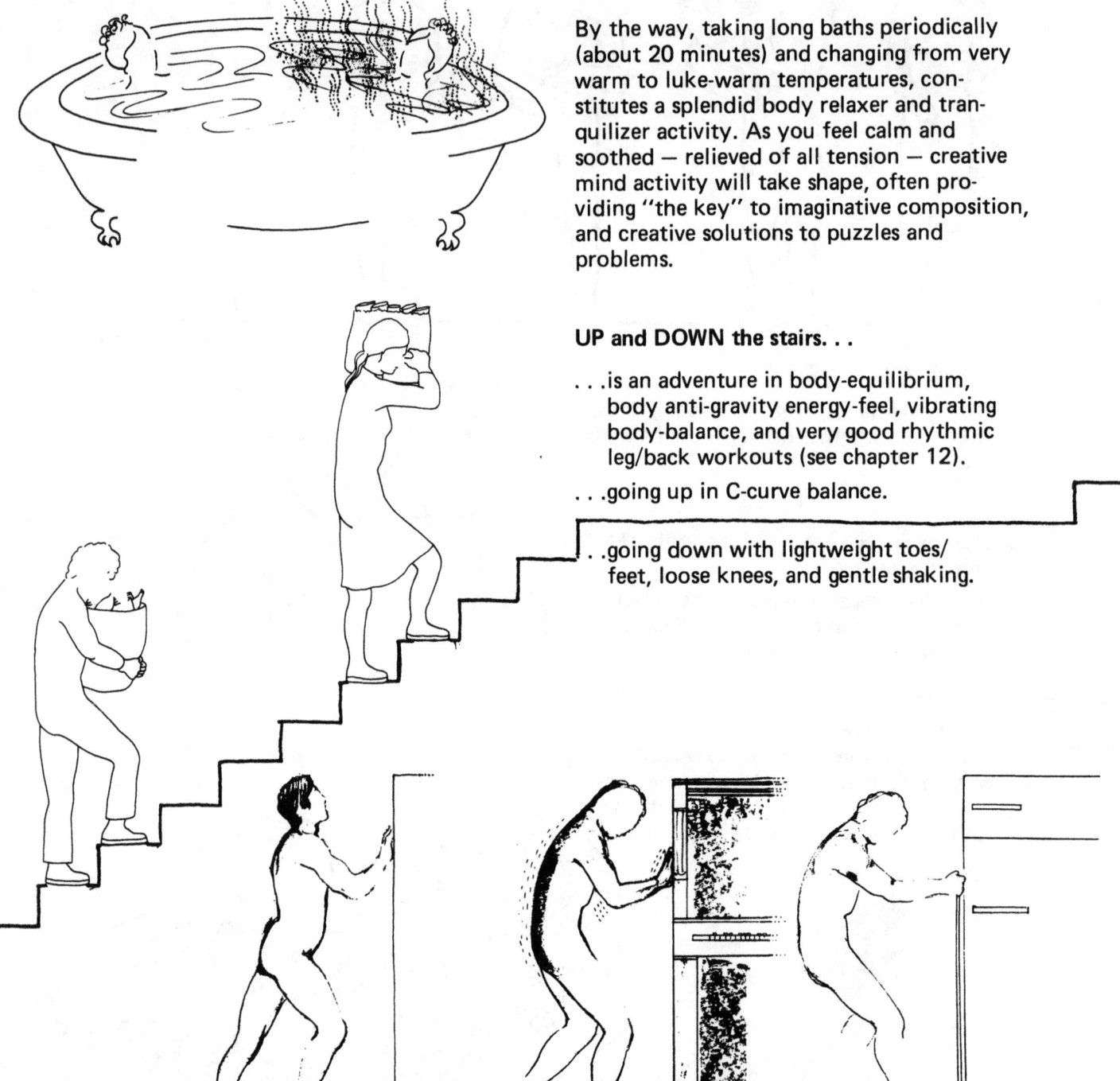

By the way, taking long baths periodically (about 20 minutes) and changing from very warm to luke-warm temperatures, constitutes a splendid body relaxer and tranquilizer activity. As you feel calm and soothed — relieved of all tension — creative mind activity will take shape, often providing "the key" to imaginative composition, and creative solutions to puzzles and problems.

UP and DOWN the stairs...

...is an adventure in body-equilibrium, body anti-gravity energy-feel, vibrating body-balance, and very good rhythmic leg/back workouts (see chapter 12).

...going up in C-curve balance.

...going down with lightweight toes/feet, loose knees, and gentle shaking.

wrong back curve

...always with rounded back, in C-curve balance with bent knees and muscle-yawn stretch.

When fatigue overtakes you at home, don't flop on your sofa out of heavy exhaustion — instead, turn on some music . . . take a few pleasant "sigh-breaths" . . . turn on your "humor-sensing" device . . . and start your body on a rhythm exploring trip, into: creative body exercise . . . ballroom dancing . . . rock/disco dancing . . . or interpretive or free expression dancing.

Under any circumstances . . . sing, **every day,** for at least six 5-minute intervals (other than shower-singing) . . . dance, **every day,** for at least 30 minutes total in any style, form, or exploration that pleases you . . . respond to smiles; take notice of little children and tall trees; interpret expressions on people's faces with positive curiosity; listen to music (but not to noise — musical or otherwise). . .avoid any body-anesthesia whenever possible by experiencing the "dance-feel" when you walk, and the "tone-feel" when you talk!

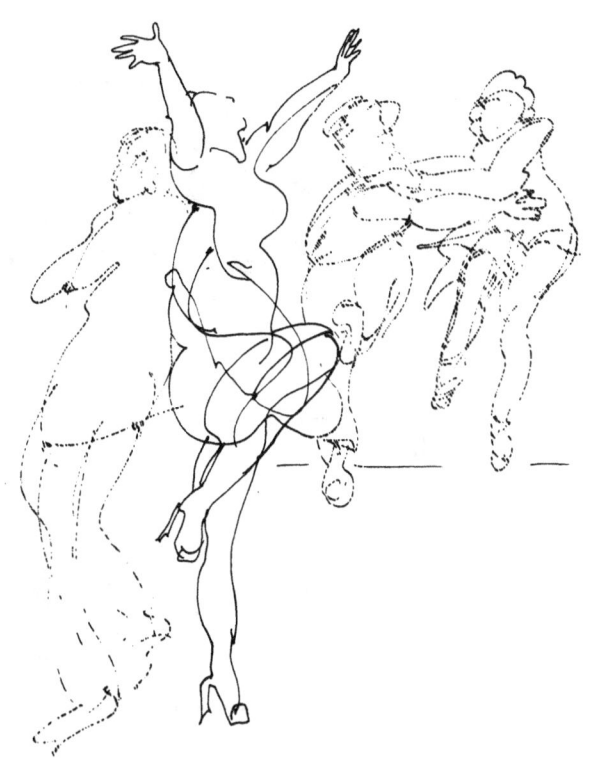

   . . .it used to be the unwed mother, but whatever reason a woman might have for concealing her pregnant condition, it can only lead to better posture, better positioning of the baby, to a more comfortable time during pregnancy and to a generally easier time in childbirth. By contrast, an ostentatious non-concealment leads to an exaggerated or increased curvature of the lower spine and hence to an overall shortened spine, bringing with it a crippling backache which often becomes chronic. In this position the abdominal muscles are overstretched and they become hypersensitive for the ensuing labor.

   . . .through the use of the "C-curve" posture the knees are loose, the buttocks turn gently inward thus flattening the abdomen and **reducing** the curvature of the lower spine.

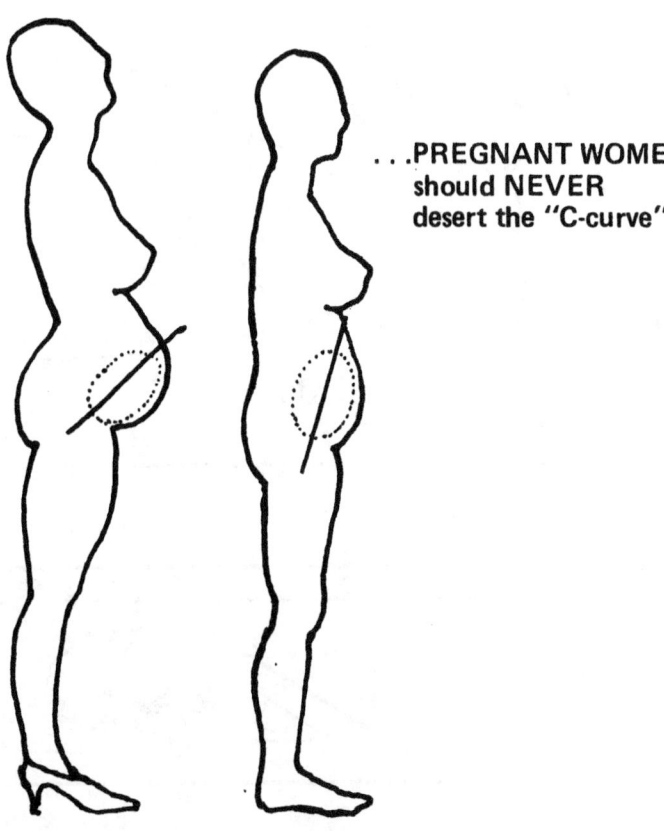

. . .PREGNANT WOMEN should NEVER desert the "C-curve" . . .

Wrong way: Premature body exhaustion and potential backache.

Proper Way: Body balance is correct naturally; locomotion of mother's body is freer and easier.

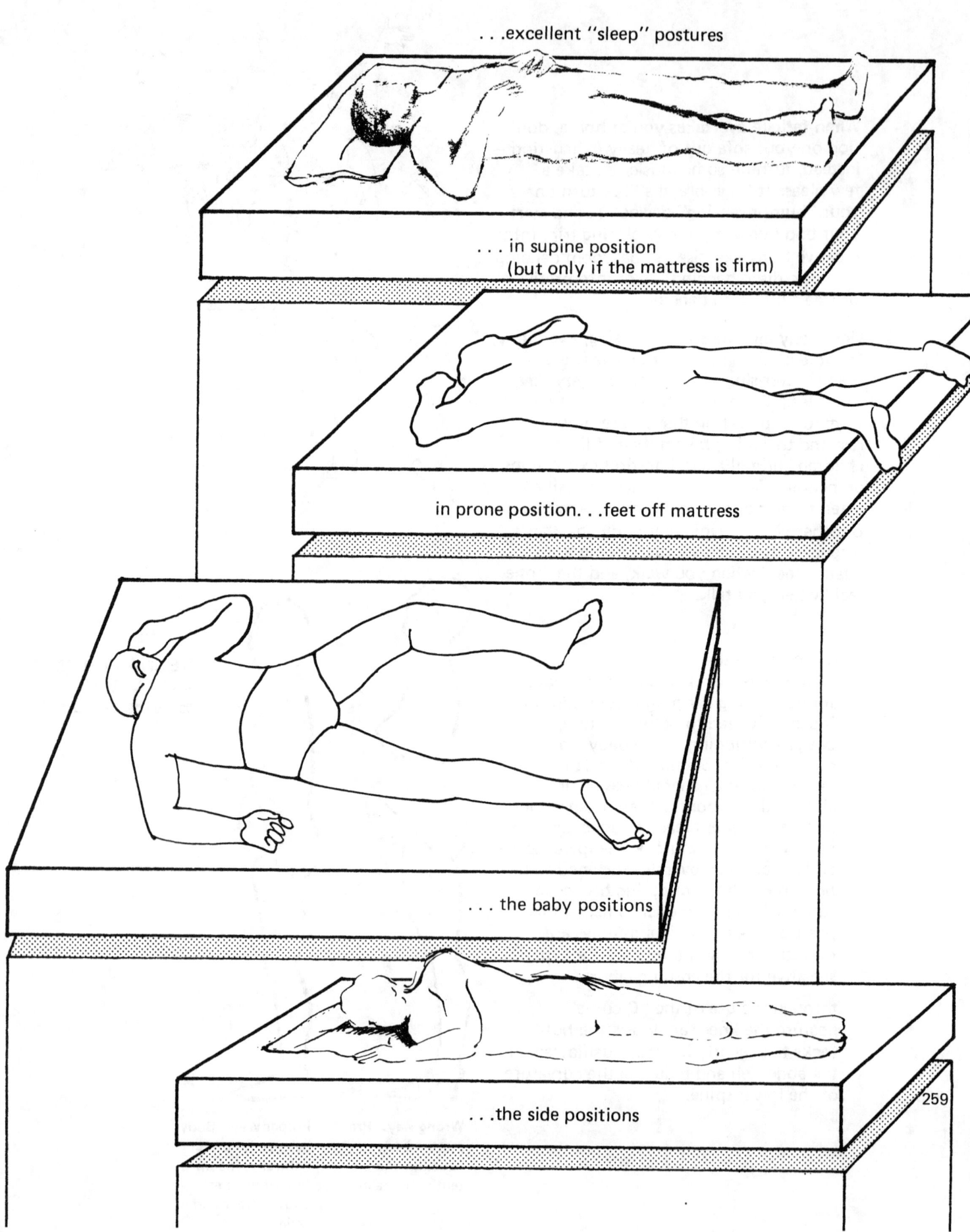

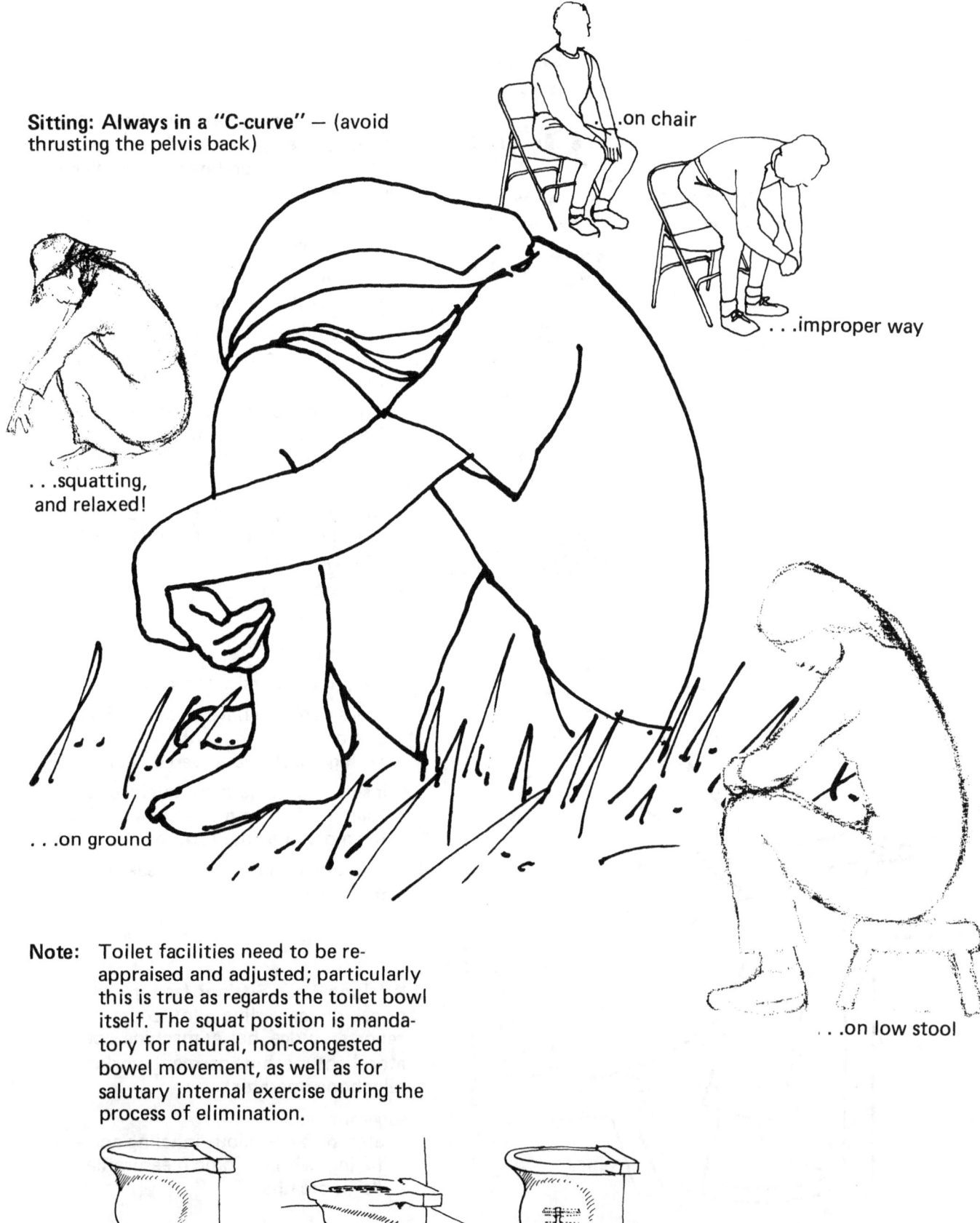

Sitting: Always in a "C-curve" — (avoid thrusting the pelvis back)

...on chair

...improper way

...squatting, and relaxed!

...on ground

...on low stool

Note: Toilet facilities need to be reappraised and adjusted; particularly this is true as regards the toilet bowl itself. The squat position is mandatory for natural, non-congested bowel movement, as well as for salutary internal exercise during the process of elimination.

...regular bowl is too high

...low toilet bowl

...regular bowl fitted with adjustable squatting foot ledge.

You and Your Body at Work

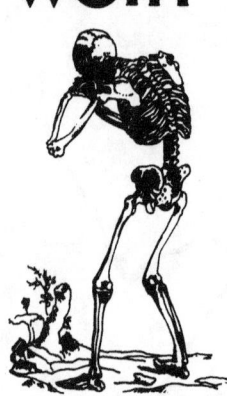

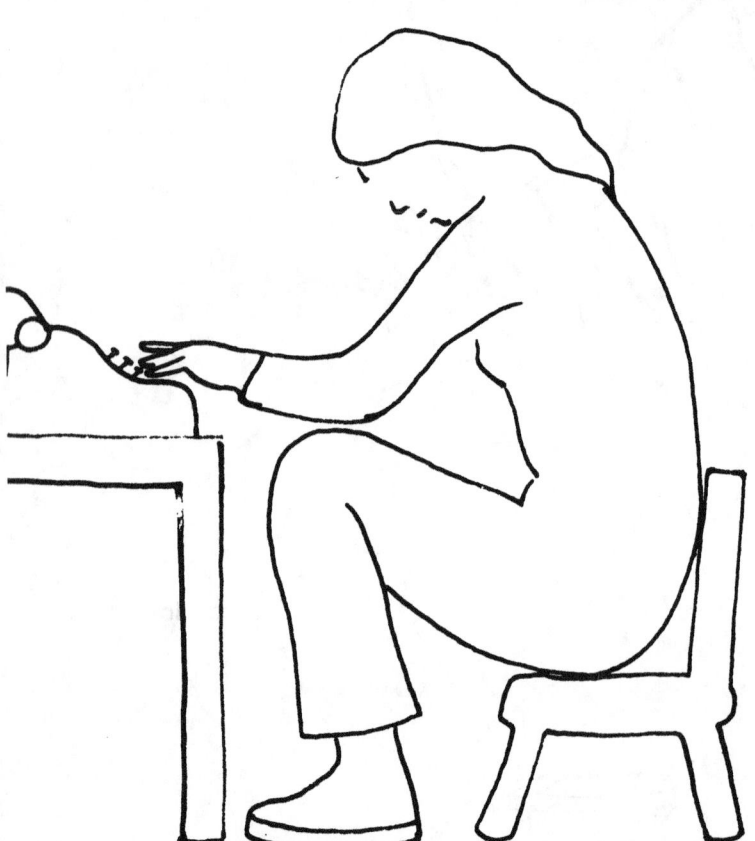

...**Working on Your Feet?** (as clerk, police, waiter, barber, guard, cook, house-painter, production-line worker, elementary school teacher) suggestions:

— no leaning of your body weight on your heels

— keep your knees always unlocked, loose, and movable

— even while resting on one foot the knee of the other leg must never be locked

— whenever you think of it you must learn how to shake and vibrate calf and thigh muscles; also ankle and knee joints

— when sitting to rest always use low stools so as to be in a full or semi-squat position

— no tight collar

— no tight belts

— no tight pants

— no girdles or waist-trimmers

— shoes ought to have thick yet light bottom (soles) but totally level — no high heels, no lowered heels!

— inside your shoe there ought to be a foam-rubber, or matting, or leather lift molded to the form of your feet

— take one minute shake-breaks every half hour

...**Working While Sitting?** (as typist, truck or cab driver, airline pilot, court reporter, judge, heavy machine operator, light machine garment worker, telephone operator)

suggestions:
— attend to conscious inhaling and exhaling, with periodic pleasurable "sigh breaths"

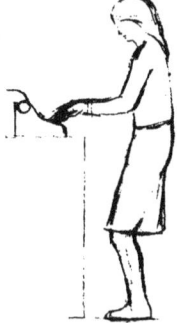

- typist-work ought to permit the alternate placing of notes and copy to both right and left sides
- even if, due to an emergency task, there is no time to stop for rest, the typist should work while standing for several minutes, then sit again with alternate note placement
- tables, chairs, desks, etc. in offices, factories or schools ought to be height-adjustable to fit the comfort and structure of each individual
- practice rhythmic swallowing of collected saliva
- yawn-stretch your body musculature every 20 minutes or so, for at least 15 second periods (particularly the shoulders, neck, back, and pelvic joint); take shake breaks as well as stretch breaks instead of smoke breaks

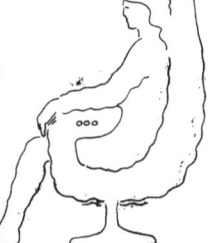

- devices provided by employers, such as vibrating chairs, vibrating belts or hand vibrators, should be used periodically to release fixations or impingements in the body due to long and fixed postures — vibrations should be applied particularly to areas such as face, neck, shoulders, back

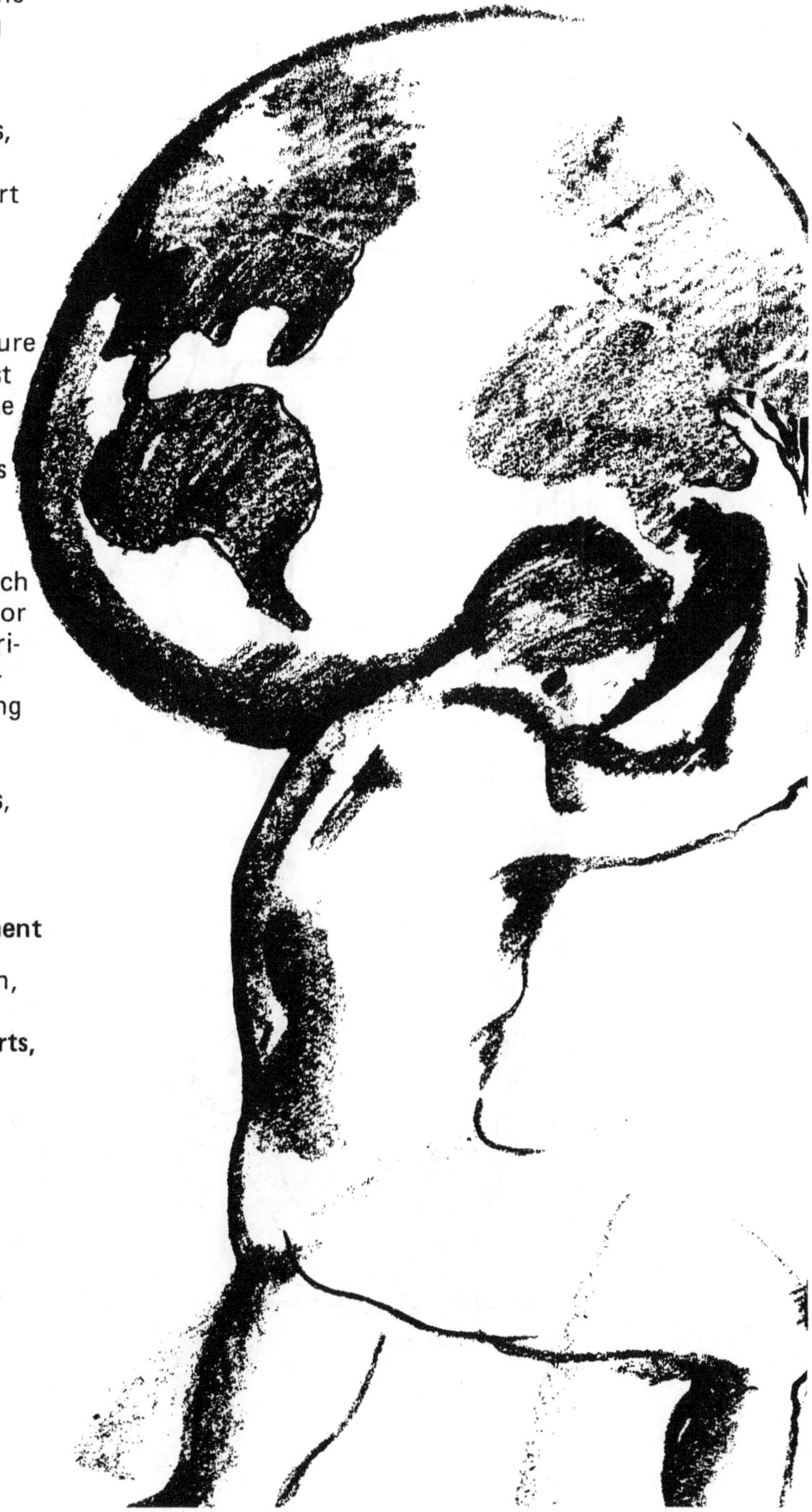

...To Labor Without Force or Punishment

For those who must lift, carry, dig, push, climb, pull, or press, the solution is the same, whether **at Home, at Play, in Sports, or in the Arts**; the activity must be accomplished with:

- bent knees
- broad expanded back
- lengthened spine
- balanced body

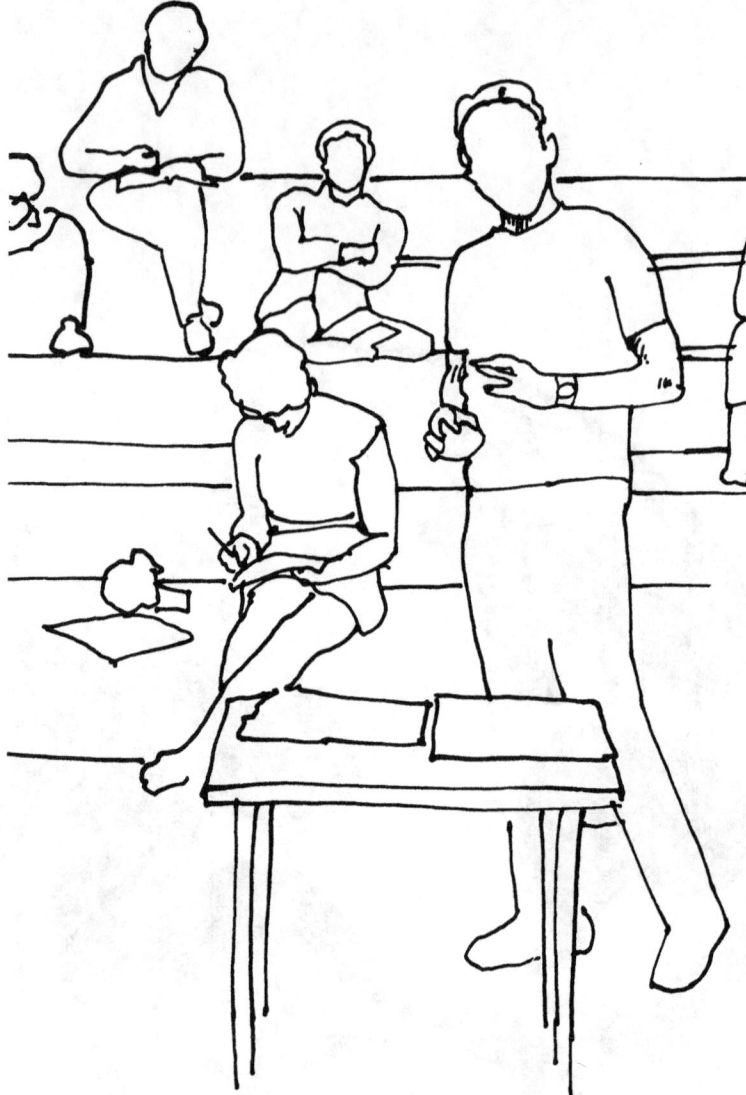

— balanced muscle tonicity (longer rather than shorter muscles)

— muscle-yawn stretching and grasping for optimal strength and flexibility

and by the:

— process of alternating weights or objects to both sides

— centering weights or objects on upper back and shoulder girdle, or in stomach area **without losing the spinal "C-curve"**

— Also, periodic "shake-breaks" and one-minute sessions with vibrating devices are extremely helpful

Up and down and saying something...
...in class

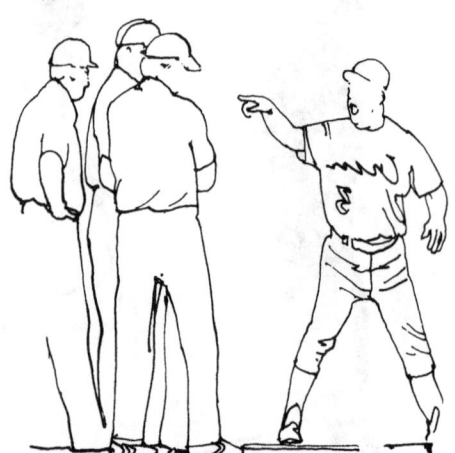

...in the baseball argument

...Up and Down and Saying Something

Lawyers, teachers, professors, demonstrators, lecturers, ministers, business executives, managers, coaches, guides, etc., all have greater latitude of physical movement — standing, sitting, walking, gesturing, etc.; in itself, this will less likely lead to fatigue than the more restricted work postures.

However, it is in this group that exhaustion and tensions are more likely to stem from: **the jaw, neck, throat, face** and **head areas** as the body exercises its vocal experiencing system in trying so hard to communicate, convince, persuade, inspire, sell, teach, supervise, and lead.

Experiencing the physical feel of the voice and periodic swallowing of saliva is important here.

Knowing how to "feel" and "perceive" your listening and responding to others is also extremely important here.

You and Your Body at Play

"Play" is hard to define!

The child does it naturally because it is its genuine means of instinctive activity without problems of either tension or awareness...the child does not need awareness since it does have the talent of curiosity, inquisitiveness, and naive questioning.

Is a game of baseball or basketball "play" when athletes are not paid, and is it work when they **are** paid?

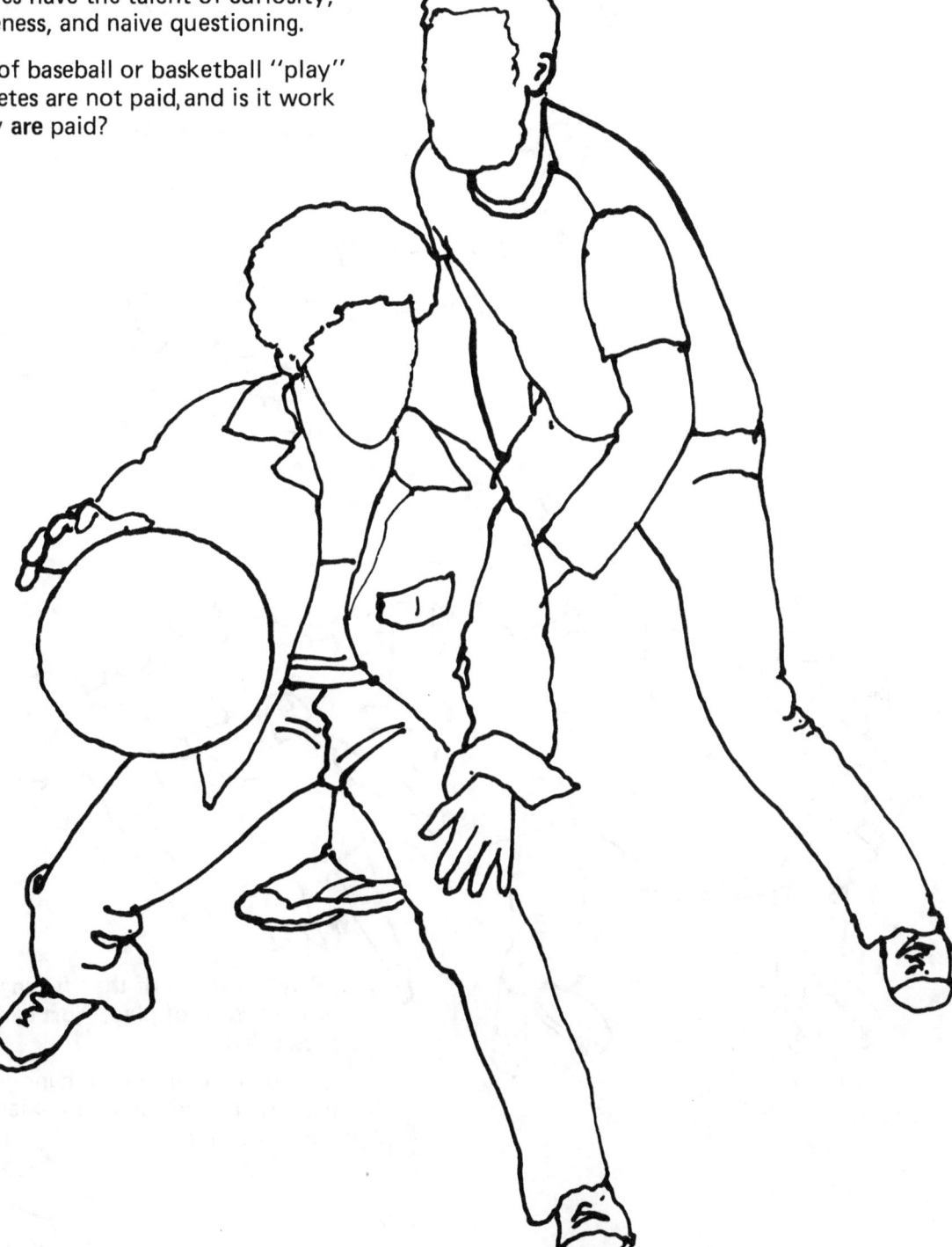

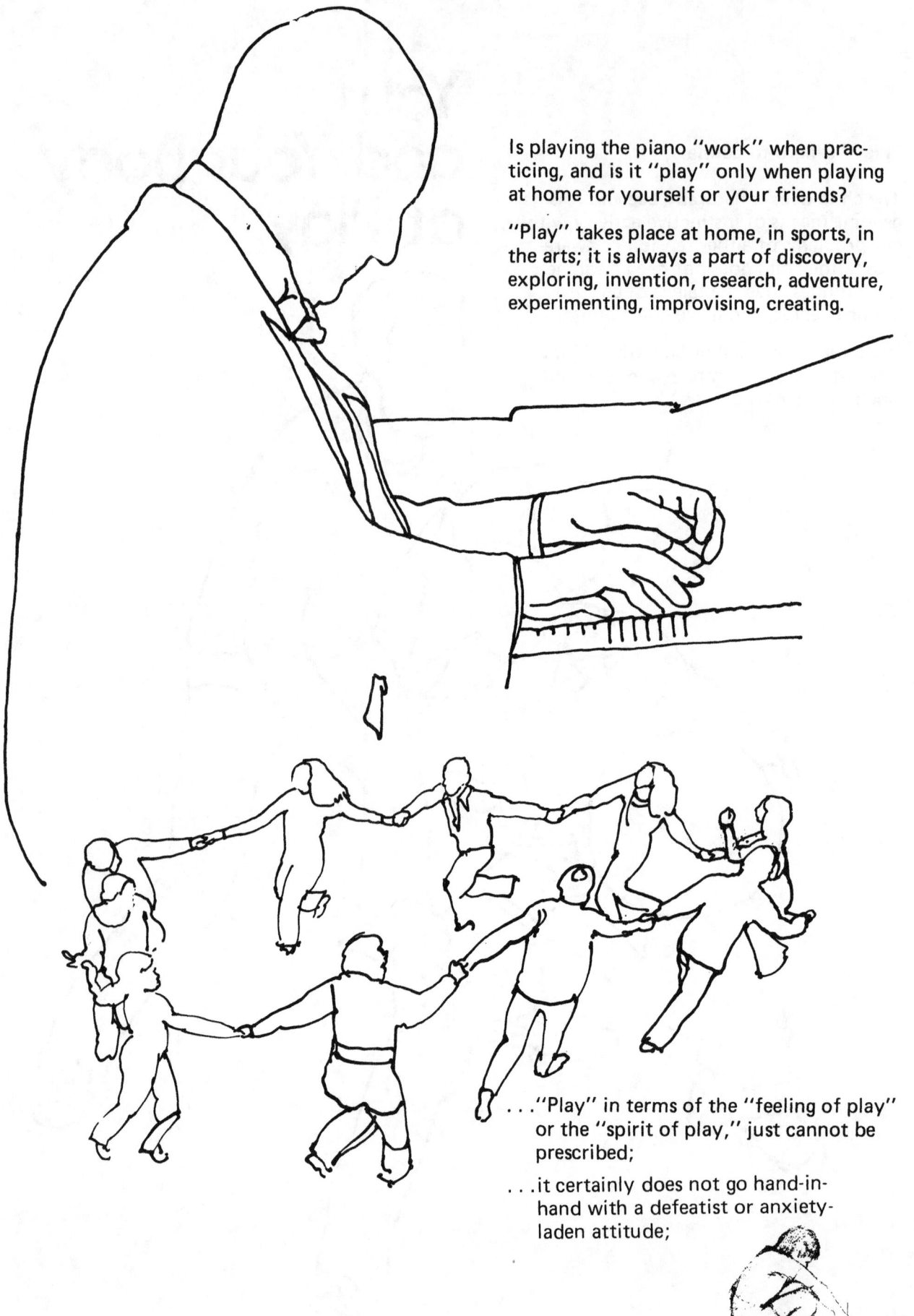

Is playing the piano "work" when practicing, and is it "play" only when playing at home for yourself or your friends?

"Play" takes place at home, in sports, in the arts; it is always a part of discovery, exploring, invention, research, adventure, experimenting, improvising, creating.

..."Play" in terms of the "feeling of play" or the "spirit of play," just cannot be prescribed;

...it certainly does not go hand-in-hand with a defeatist or anxiety-laden attitude;

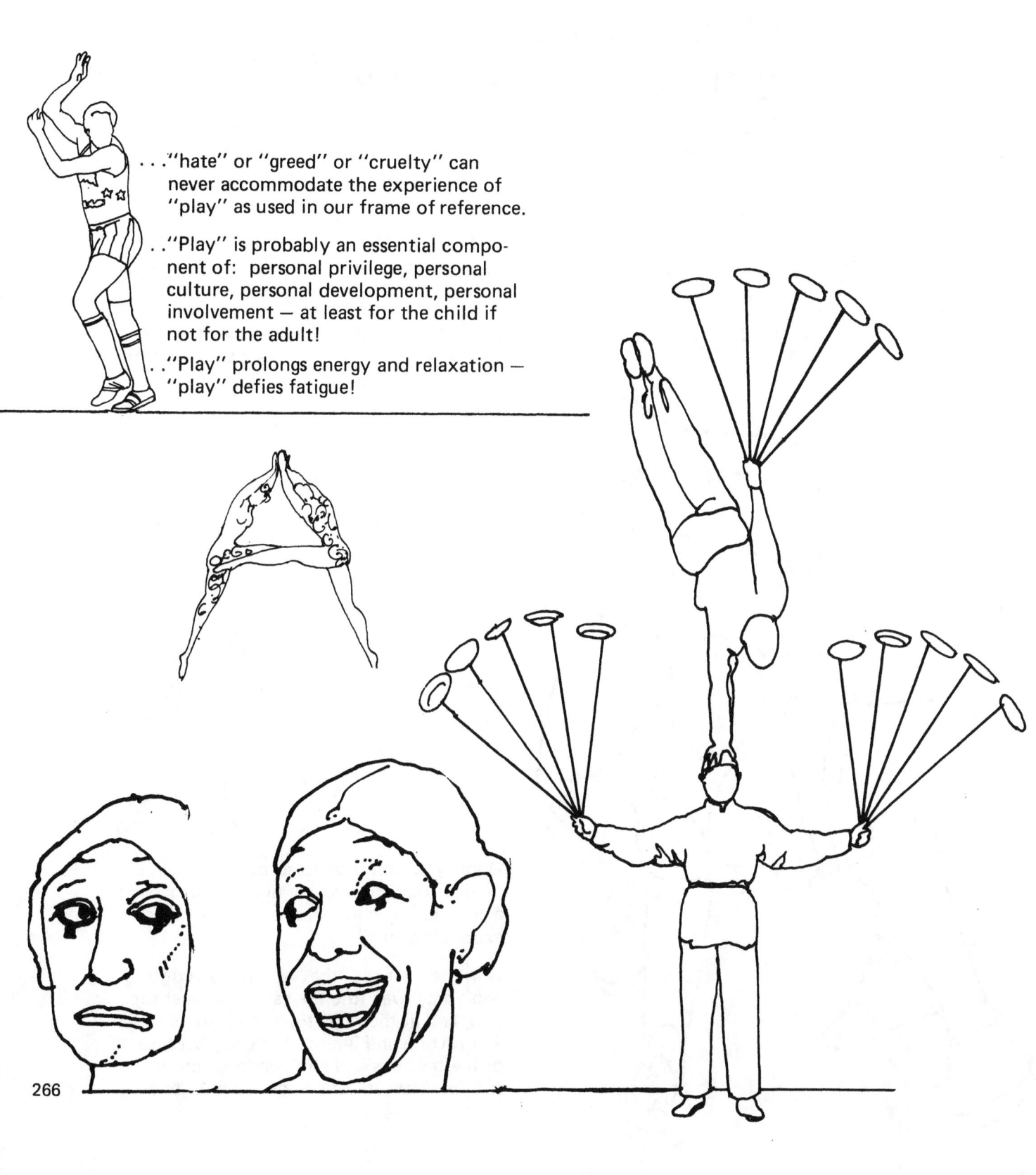

..."hate" or "greed" or "cruelty" can never accommodate the experience of "play" as used in our frame of reference.

..."Play" is probably an essential component of: personal privilege, personal culture, personal development, personal involvement — at least for the child if not for the adult!

..."Play" prolongs energy and relaxation — "play" defies fatigue!

You and Your Body in Sports

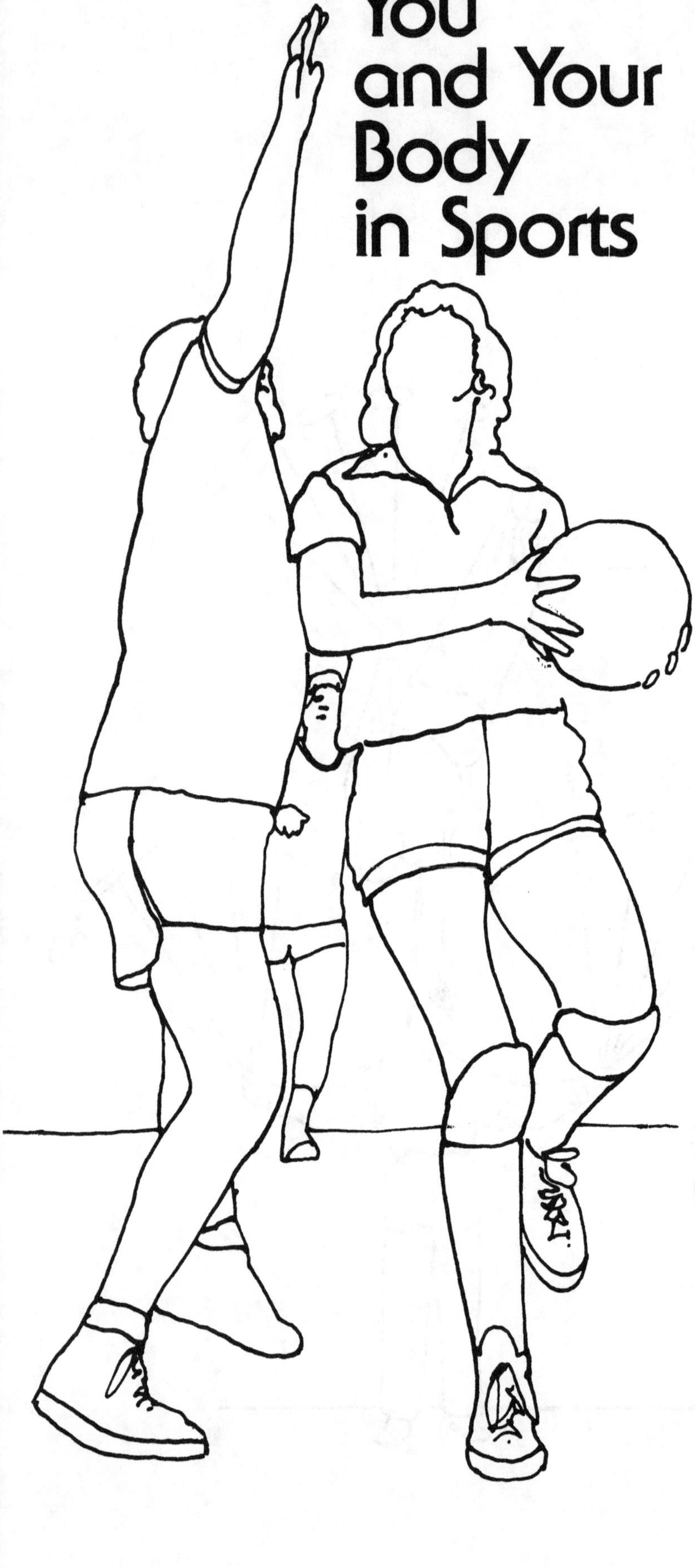

Psycho-somatically, your body will function quite differently:

...if you are out to win — **at all costs!**

...if you harbor a "fear of losing"!

...if you work hard at the sport, for pay!

...when you perform in your sport as a creative artist!

...when it is pure "play" for the joy of doing (and of teaching yourself)!

Only the last two follow the benefits and privilege of "body esthetics"; the first three always get tangled up with body anesthetics!

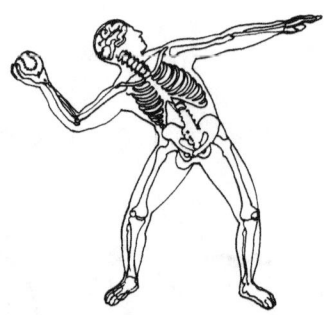

Don't you first have to surpass yourself, before you can have any hope of surpassing a competitor whose past performance has exceeded yours?

Is it not clear that the "absolute **need** to win" may even **lose** the game (or race) for you, and at the same time seriously punish and torture and injure your body because of the tensions and anxieties implicit in the "mental set" of competing **only** to win?

(It is quite possible that athletes and coaches (and even 'the fans') have their external eye glued on statistics and goals rather than on process and growth; they work, too hard perhaps, to emphasize the quantitative aspects of training and performance rather than the qualitative ingredients of body esthetics.)

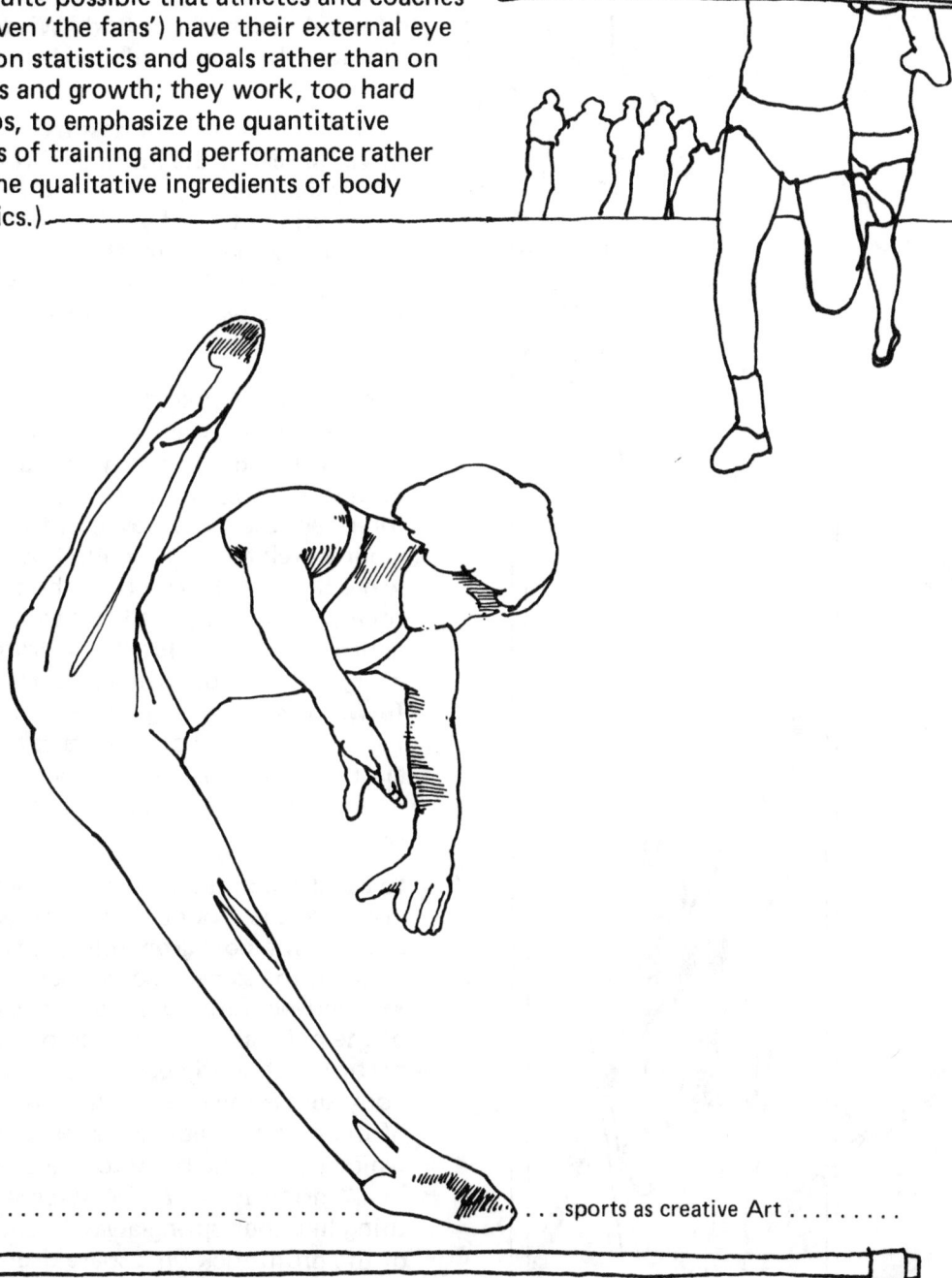

....sports as creative Art........

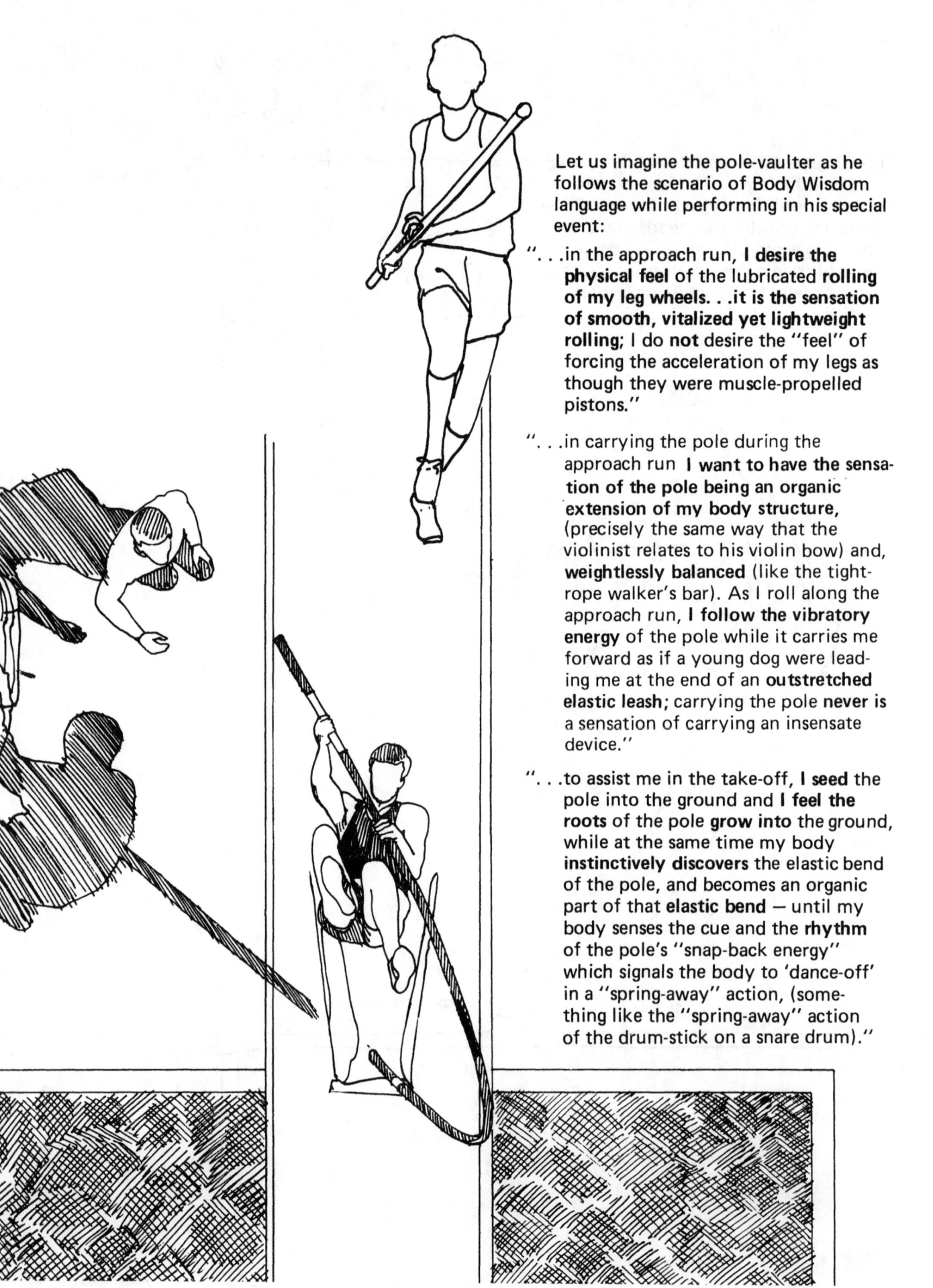

Let us imagine the pole-vaulter as he follows the scenario of Body Wisdom language while performing in his special event:

"...in the approach run, **I desire the physical feel** of the lubricated **rolling of my leg wheels**...it is the **sensation of smooth, vitalized yet lightweight rolling**; I do **not** desire the "feel" of forcing the acceleration of my legs as though they were muscle-propelled pistons."

"...in carrying the pole during the approach run **I want to have the sensation of the pole being an organic extension of my body structure**, (precisely the same way that the violinist relates to his violin bow) and, **weightlessly balanced** (like the tight-rope walker's bar). As I roll along the approach run, **I follow the vibratory energy** of the pole while it carries me forward as if a young dog were leading me at the end of an **outstretched elastic leash**; carrying the pole **never** is a sensation of carrying an insensate device."

"...to assist me in the take-off, **I seed** the pole into the ground and **I feel the roots** of the pole **grow into** the ground, while at the same time my body **instinctively discovers** the elastic bend of the pole, and becomes an organic part of that **elastic bend** — until my body senses the cue and the **rhythm** of the pole's "snap-back energy" which signals the body to 'dance-off' in a "spring-away" action, (something like the "spring-away" action of the drum-stick on a snare drum)."

"...I do **not** desire to feel the sensation of "digging in with the pole," or of "force-lift jumping," or of "body-hurling" over the bar, because under such circumstances it is extremely difficult to experience **the rolling, the gliding, the sailing, the free "follow-through,"** the feeling of being now, **the natural extension** of the pole itself; I want to feel the "passing by" of the air, or the "body sculpting and/or penetrating the space around me; or the sensation of body buoyancy and body balance, and the rhythms of the body music as my moving personal space sphere swims and sails through the outer environment openness."

Perhaps no pole-vaulter actually ever said these words on the way to a vault event; but I do know that many have felt them and some have subconsciously self-communicated them. And this is how "work" may become mature "play!"

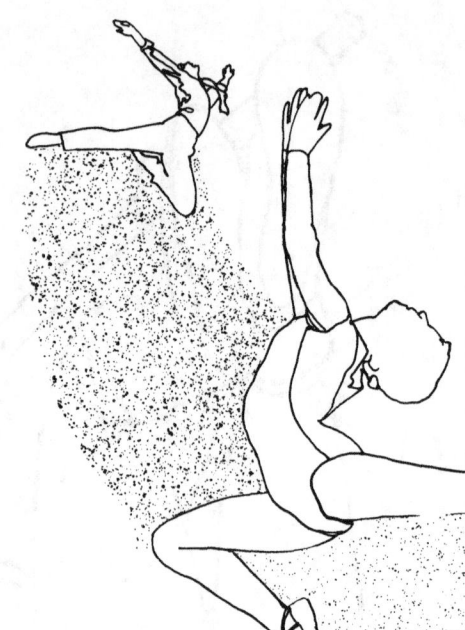

You and Your Body in the Arts

Just as the athlete must discover "the ART" and must perceive the "body esthetics" in his/her work...

...so must the artist discover and respond to the physical skills and the bio-dynamics of the whole organism in his/her work!

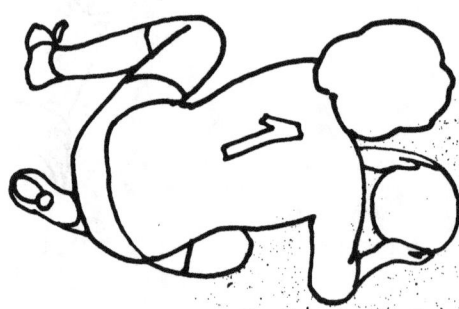

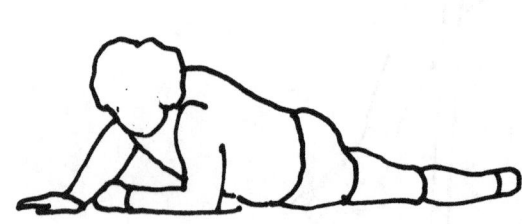

To what extent is the athlete a dancer?

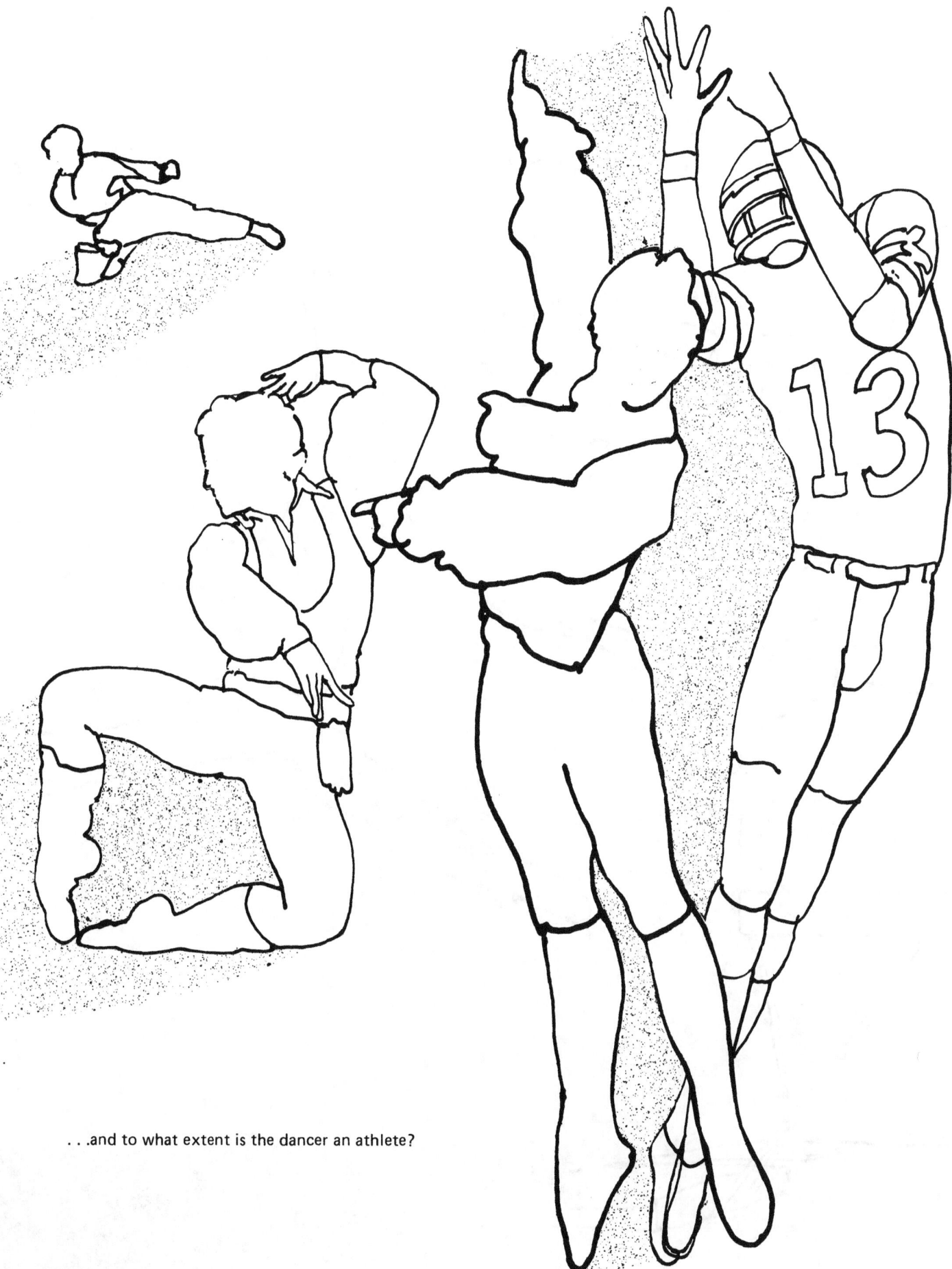

...and to what extent is the dancer an athlete?

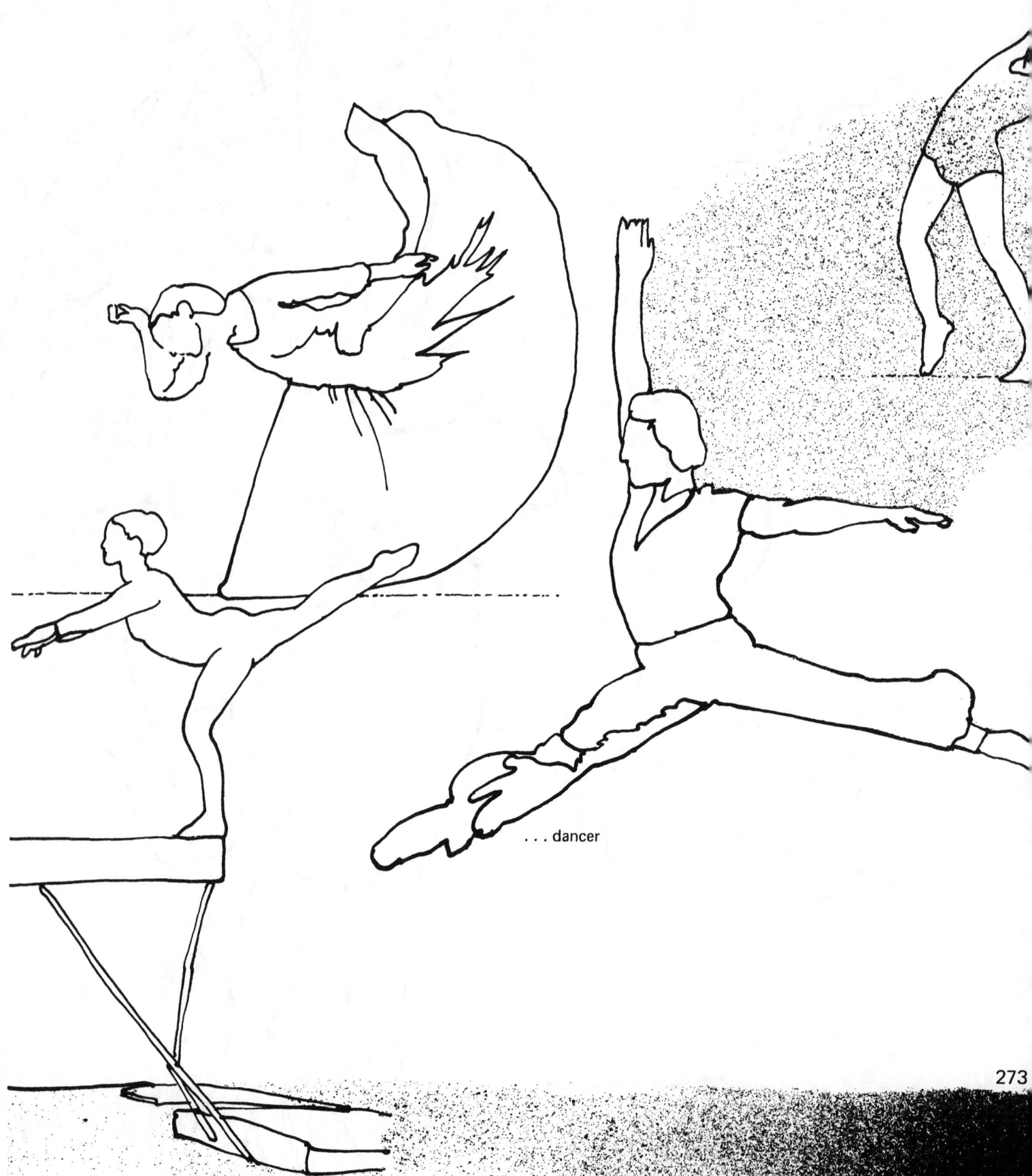
...dancer

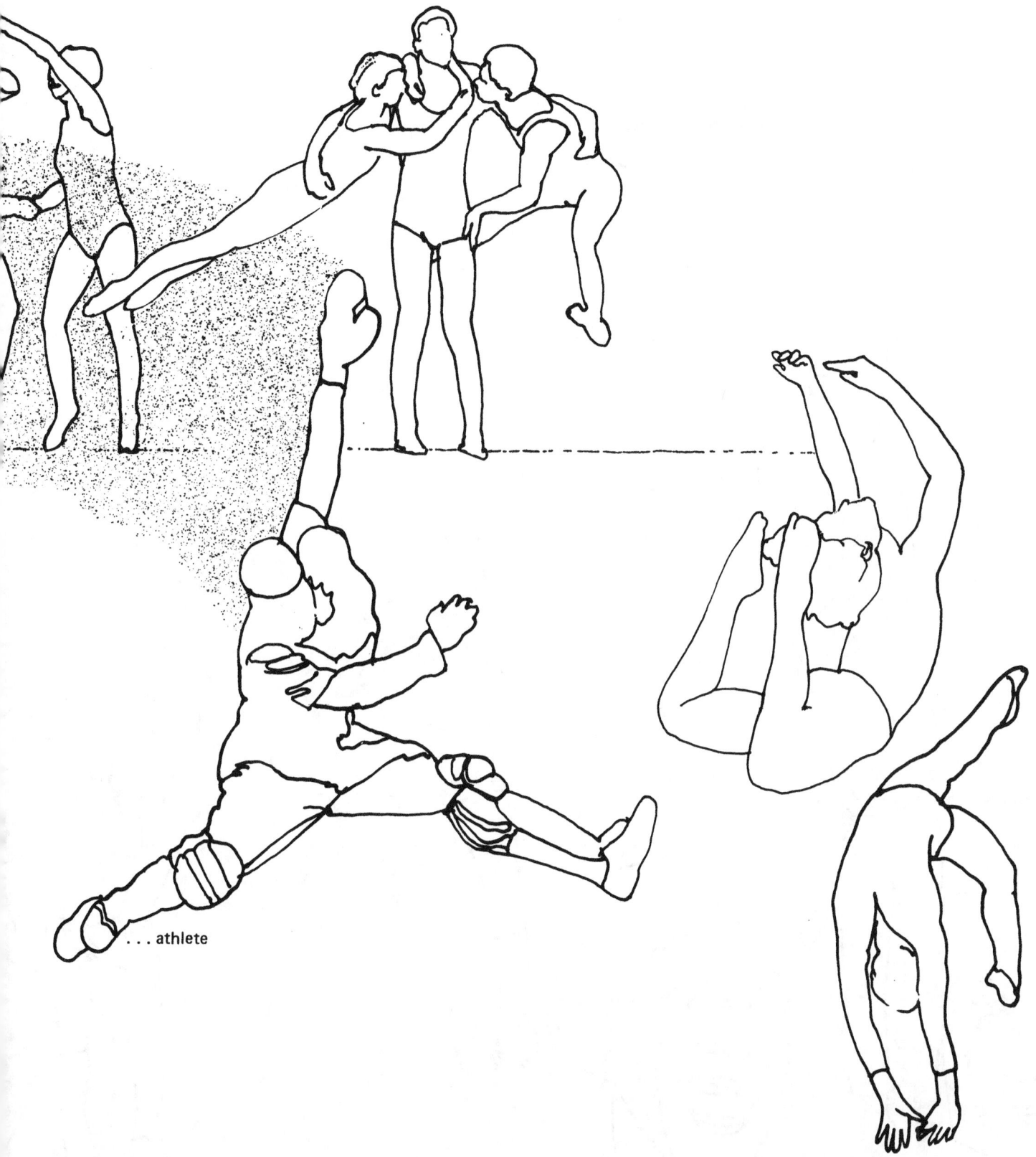
...athlete

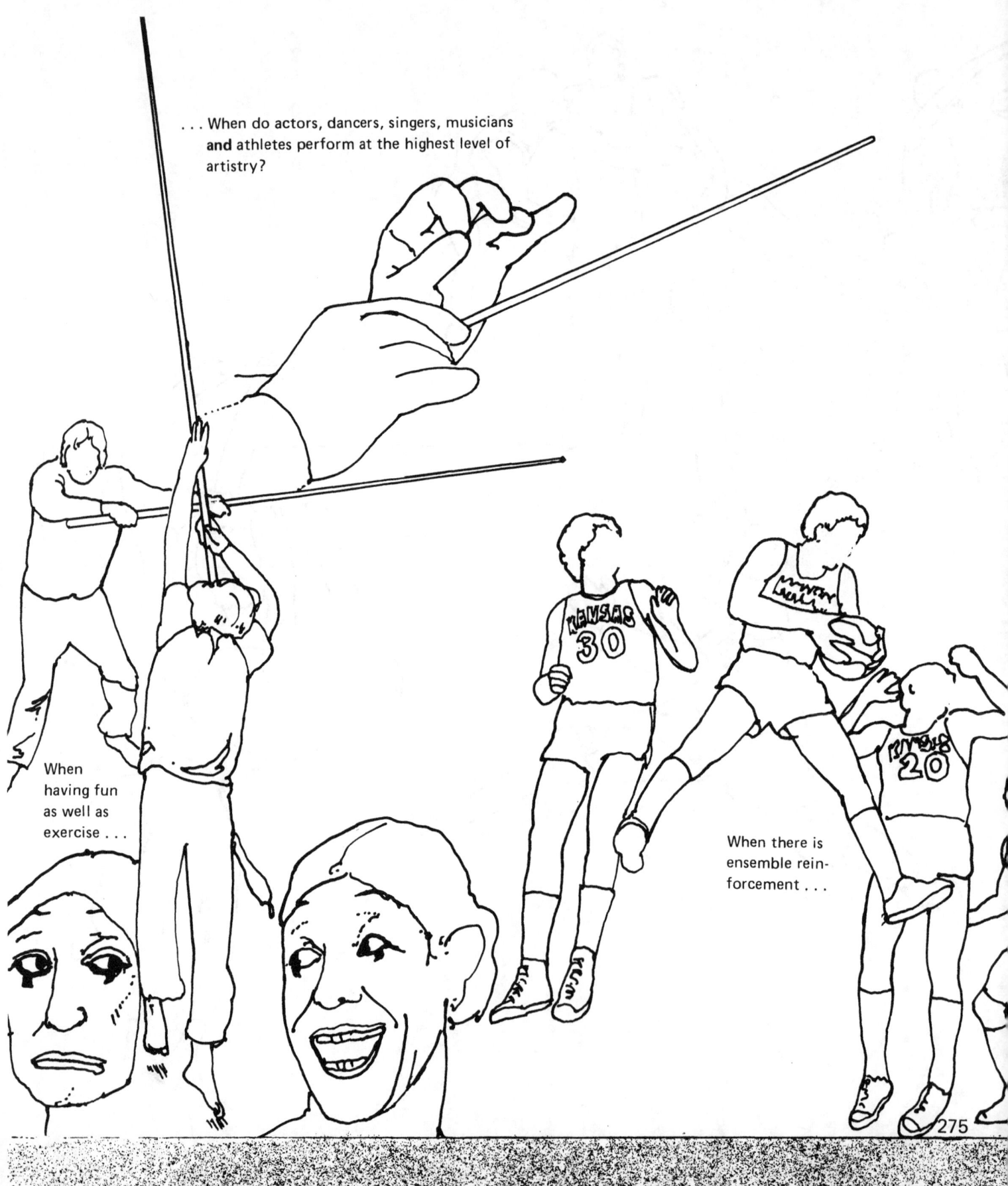

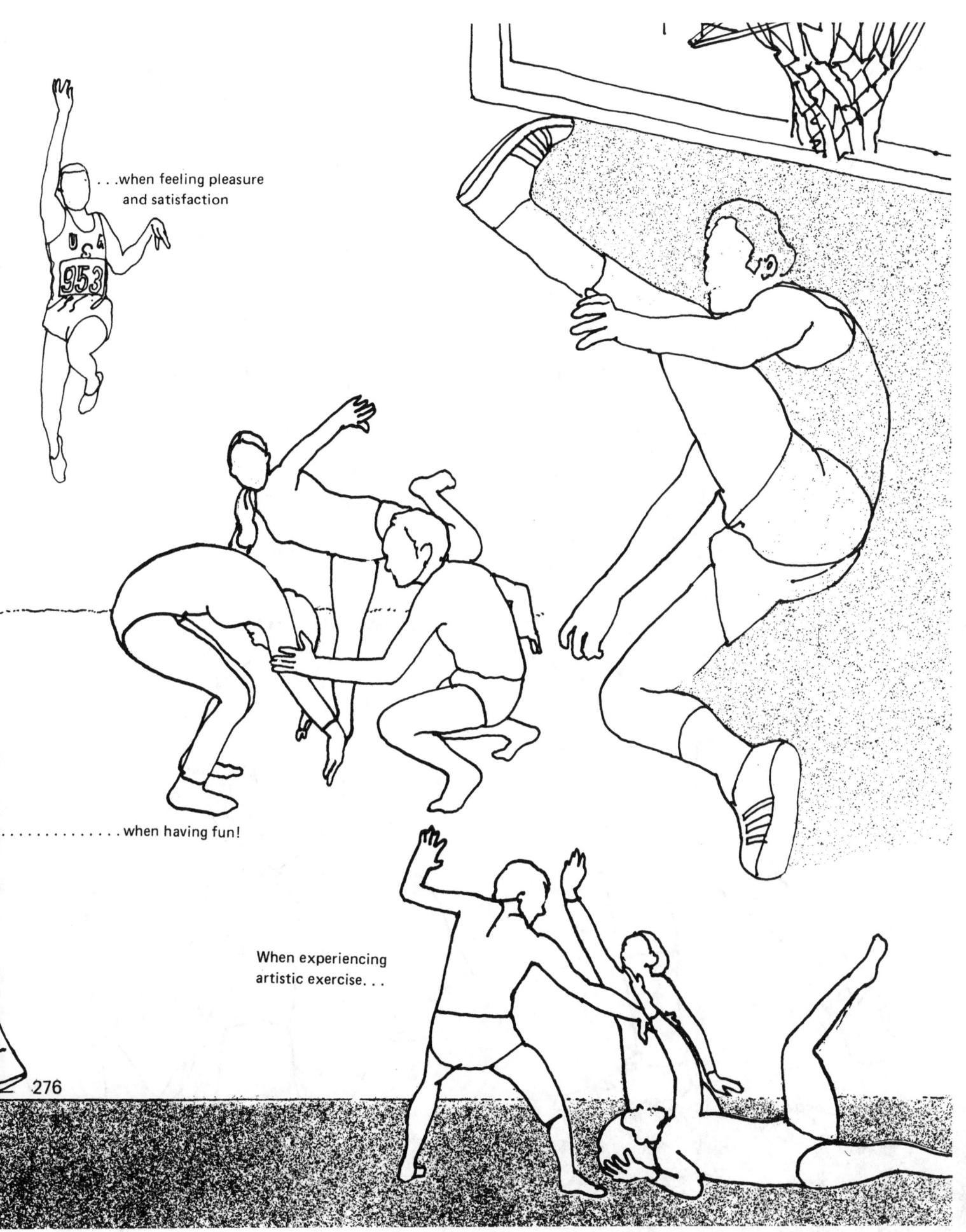

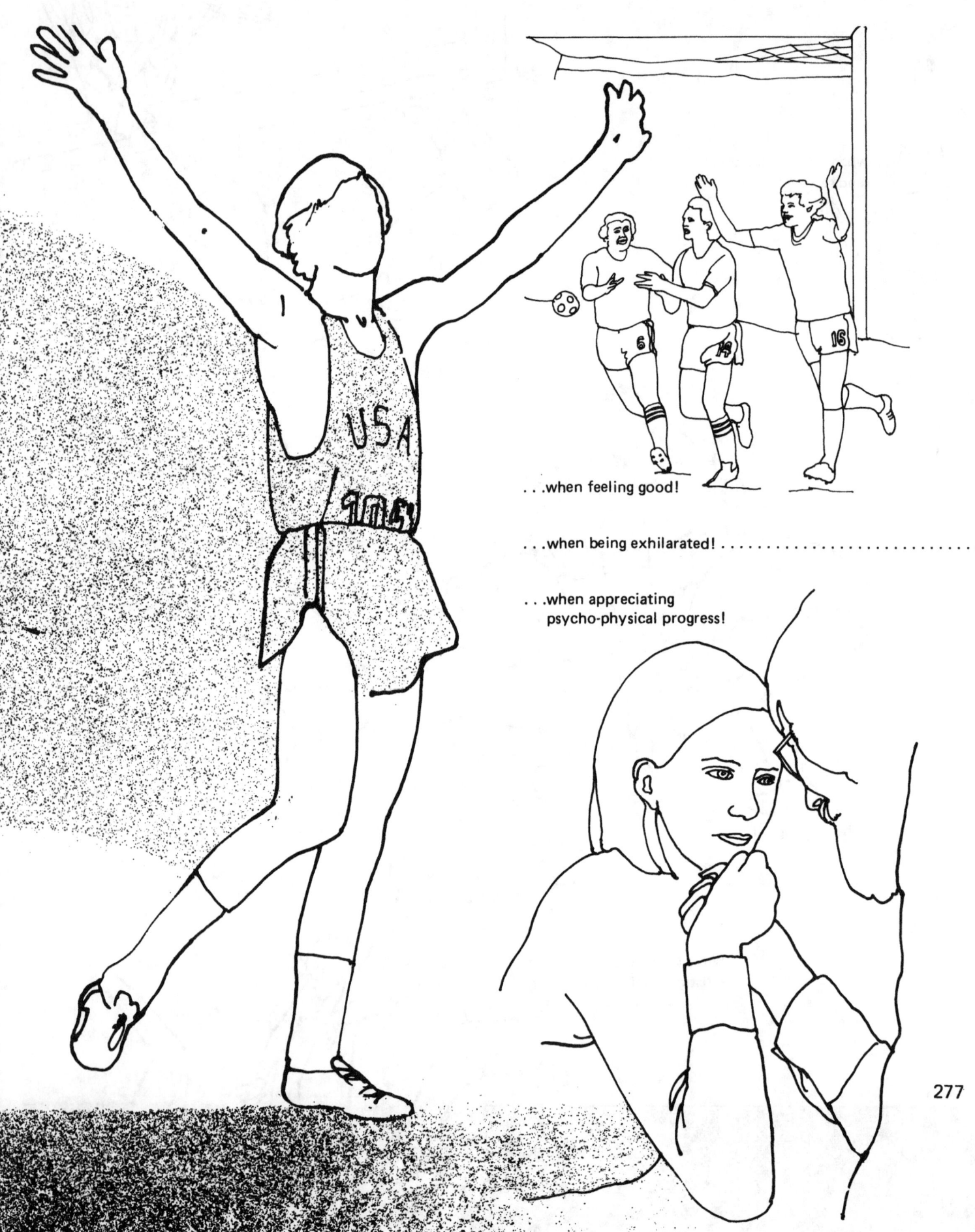

...when feeling good!

...when being exhilarated!

...when appreciating psycho-physical progress!

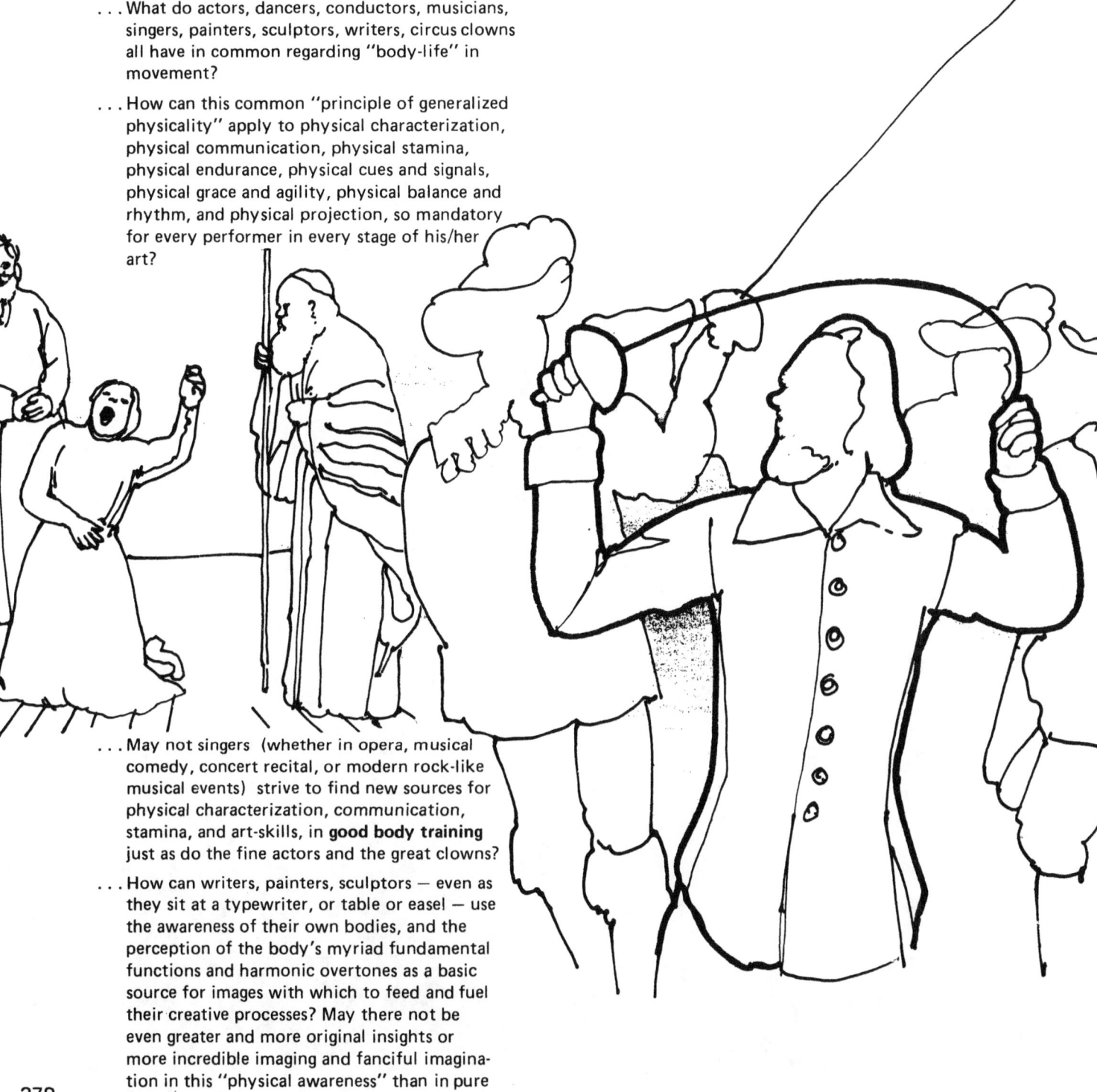

...What do actors, dancers, conductors, musicians, singers, painters, sculptors, writers, circus clowns all have in common regarding "body-life" in movement?

...How can this common "principle of generalized physicality" apply to physical characterization, physical communication, physical stamina, physical endurance, physical cues and signals, physical grace and agility, physical balance and rhythm, and physical projection, so mandatory for every performer in every stage of his/her art?

...May not singers (whether in opera, musical comedy, concert recital, or modern rock-like musical events) strive to find new sources for physical characterization, communication, stamina, and art-skills, in **good body training** just as do the fine actors and the great clowns?

...How can writers, painters, sculptors — even as they sit at a typewriter, or table or easel — use the awareness of their own bodies, and the perception of the body's myriad fundamental functions and harmonic overtones as a basic source for images with which to feed and fuel their creative processes? May there not be even greater and more original insights or more incredible imaging and fanciful imagination in this "physical awareness" than in pure cerebration?

...END of CODA

INDEX

INDEX

A

Acting   Preface ii-iii, Foreword vii, 253. See Applications of Body Wisdom in Wisdom in the Arts, Coda, Vocal Life

Active Rest/Restful Action   32-33, 57, 59, 67. See Energy and Relaxation

Aerobics   219

Aesthetics   26-27, 69. See Body Esthetics

Anaerobics   219

Anesthetics   See Body Anesthetics

Applications of Body Wisdom:

    At Home - 4, 25, 148, 184, 203, 241, 250-255 (Coda)

    At Work - 4, 25, 55, 123, 148, 184, 250-255 (Coda). See also Work and Relaxation, Work/Play

    At Play - 4, 25, 148, 184, 250-255 (Coda). See also Play, Work/Play, Child and Body Wisdom

    In Sports - Preface ii-iii, Foreword vii, 1-4, 11, 24-25, 32-33, 48, 69, 71, 77, 123, 135, 137, 141-143, 148, 179-180, 184, 192, 197-198, 204-205, 209, 217, 220, 223-224, 241-242, 250-255 (Coda). See also Athletic Coaching, Olympic Athletes and Body Wisdom, Exercise Classifications, Running, Jogging, Leaping, Rope-Skipping, Springing/Jumping, Sprinting, Tumbling, Diametric Exercising, Relaxer-Energizers, Body Energizers

    In the Arts - Preface ii-iii, Foreword vii, 1-4, 11, 25, 32, 48, 69, 71, 77, 123, 137, 143, 148, 153-156, 180, 205-206, 241-242, 250-255 (Coda). See also Acting, Dancing, Ensemble, Vocal Life, *Use and Training of the Human Voice.*

    In Everyday Life - 51, 148, 250-255 (Coda)

Architectural Principle of Body Wisdom   161

Arm Circles   176-177, 179-182, 187-188, 191, 228-229

Arm Training while running   210-211

Athletic Coaching and Body Wisdom   253. See also Applications of Body Wisdom in Sports

Atom-to-Atom Discovery   See Contiguous Continuity

Auditory Sense   27-29, 227

Auditory Space Sphere   214, 227, 233, 235-237, 238, 240, 243-244, 248

B

Back   77, 108, 112-113, 118, 125-126, 160, 166-167, 170, 175, 177-178, 180, 192, 199, 251. See also Lower Back Center, Upper Spine Center, Rocker-Rims

Back Brain   13, 16, 30, 180, 222-223. See also Split-Brain Research, Two Dominances

Back Orb   176

Backward Single Shoulder Roll   117-119, 122

INDEX

Backward Roll 100, 119, 121-122

Balance 4, 9, 14, 26, 38, 42-44, 46, 62, 74-75, 77, 81, 86, 92, 101-104, 113, 119-123, 127, 135, 148, 152, 159, 164, 169, 175, 177, 181, 184, 187, 189, 207-208, 218-219, 234, 248, 251, 253

Balance and Rhythm 4, 7, 59, 71, 74-77, 85, 90-91, 97, 101, 105, 110-112, 119, 135-136, 160-161, 173, 193, 195, 202, 207, 210-212, 215, 217-220, 224-225, 231, 234, 236, 238, 242

Balance in Movement/Movement in Balance 47, 74-75, 81, 92-93, 122, 139, 148, 180-182, 191, 194-196, 205, 218, 221

Balanced Muscle Tonicity 6, 42, 44, 51, 75, 110, 112, 135-136, 242, 251

Bannister, Roger 3

Beyond Wildness 17-19

Bilateral Body Development 173, 215, 220-223. See Sinistrality

Bio-feedback 28, 30, 254. See Feedback Principle

Bio-physical/Bio-neural Sensation 28-29, 171

Bio-plasmic Sensation 29

Bio-psychic Sensation 29

Body Anesthetics 2, 26ff, 47, 59, 77, 80, 136, 239, 251

Body Blocks 126, 170-172, 175

Body Building (Objectives and Exercises) 199, 215-216

Body Circles 71, 159, 174-175, 179. See also Leg-Wheels, Arm Circles, Double Figure-Eight, Body Curves in Movement

Body Curves in Movement 71-72, 76, 88, 90, 108, 124-125, 218, 227, 248. See Body in Movement, Evolving Body Curve, Body Circles

Body Deterioration 11, 14, 22, 30, 59, 159, 161, 216. See also Conditioning (Outer-Environment), Psychosomatic Illness, Breathing, Posture, Joints and Hinges

Body Energizers 34-58 (Chapter IV), 79, 223

Body Esthetics 3-4, 9, 25-33, 46-47, 57, 59-60, 73, 104-105, 135, 154, 161, 180, 190, 192, 198, 201, 213, 217-218, 220, 223-224, 236, 239, 242, 247, 253

Body Fatigue (Body Exhaustion) 26, 74, 94-95, 136-137, 194 note, 208, 216, 219, 225, 242, 250, 252-253

Body Fitness (Objectives and Exercises) 215-217

Body Flexibility (Objectives and Exercises) 55, 173, 175, 215, 217-218, 242, 251

Body Folklore 31

Body Heaviness 26, 35, 39, 50, 109, 112, 136, 170-171, 179, 191, 195, 202, 225

Body Height 170. See Structural Space Sphere

Body Loops 71, 124, 134, 159, 174-179

INDEX

Body Hygiene   144, 155 ff, 216. See also Psychosomatic Health, Preventive Medicine

Body in Movement/Movement in the Body   2, 4, 6, 9, 22, 33, 36-37 ff, 70, 72, 74, 77, 109, 135, 148, 161, 175, 182, 188, 193, 210, 217-218, 227-228, 243, 245, 246-248

Body Intelligence   13, 16, 20, 25, 30, 32-33, 60, 67, 69, 109, 115, 137, 171, 179, 198, 213, 217, 236, 252

Body Languages, Dialects and Idioms   Foreword vi, 1, 3-5, 13, 16, 24-25, 30-31, 32-33, 35, 47, 55-56, 67, 71, 204, 213, 252

Body Potential   See Instinctive Body Skills, Natural Talents

Body Power&Body Strength   See Potency

Body Reaching   35-43, 46, 50, 53-56, 67, 138, 221. See also Sustained Extension

Body Rhythms   See Rhythm Experience, Rhythm Feel/Dynamics

Body Rolls   90, 93, 95-100, 104-107, 117-120, 124, 127-130. See also Rocking and Rolling

Body Sphere in Movement   71 ff, 96, Chapters VII through XII, 218, 226, 235, See also Evolving Body Curve, Personal Space Spheres, Self-Image

Body Strength/Body Power   See Potency

Body Swiftness (Objectives and Exercises)   55, 215, 217-218. See also Speed

Body Time   17

Body Training   Preface i-iii, 3-4, 5, 22 ff, 25, 29, 30-31, 33-34, 55, 92, 98 note, 164 ff, 175, 186, 209-210, 215-225, 246, 254

Body Vibrations   See Vibratory Experience

Body Weight-Lifting   215-216

Body Wisdom   1-4 (premises and assumptions), 5-7 (scientific principles), 7-10 (pre-scientific principles) and passim

Body Wisdom and Design Engineering   Foreword iv-vii, 253 (Coda)

Body-Yawn Sit-Ups   54

Body-Yawn Stretch   34, 51-55, 68, 73, 76, 83, 102, 113-114, 116-117, 135-136, 144, 166, 194, 197, 204, 215, 217-218, 221. See also Potency

Bow and Wheel Exploration   136, 180-181, 183-184

Bow and Wheel (Penguin) Walk   196

Bow-Shaped Crescent Curve   66, 71, 108-108. See Parenthesis Curve

Breath Energy   35, 40-45, 55, 82, 85, 89, 106, 111, 113, 116-117, 157-158, 187, 196

Breathing   7-9, 11-12, 23, 35-45, 49, 51-56, 60-62, 66, 76-77, 89, 91, 97, 102-103, 109-110, 112, 125-128, 134, 139-142, 143-157, 173, 175-177, 187, 189-190, 192-194 note, 195, 199, 208-209, 215-216, 219, 225, 231, 235, 245, 247, 251, 253. See also Posture

Breathing Rhythms   61, 208-209

INDEX

Brooks, Alfred Preface i

Buddy Work (Exercises) 53, 84, 104-107, 122-123, 131-132, 173, 206-208, 215-216

Bug-Blade-Bead Association 68-69, 74. See also Transformation Process

Buoyancy 26, 34-47, 67, 79, 83, 88, 94, 101, 103-104, 110, 112-113, 128, 135, 137, 143-144, 150, 157, 177, 180-181, 186-187, 192, 196, 199-200, 209-210, 217, 221, 225, 229, 231, 234, 242

Buoyancy Feel 47, 49, 67, 73, 234

Buoy-Float Leg-Lift 116

Buoyancy Leg-Lift 116

Buoyancy Sit-Up 37-43, 55, 113-114 ff

C

C-Curve 9, 26, 42, 62, 66, 77, 83, 98 note, 109, 123-124, 127, 140-143, 162, 165, 167-168, 184-185, 188, 191, 193-195, 197, 199-200, 204, 206-207, 218, 225, 231, 252-253. See also Curvo-linear Principle

Carry-Over Experiences 46-47, 58, 75, 85-86, 88, 124, 136, 142, 206, 215, 242

Carefreeness Principle 6, 48, 72, 77, 90, 201-202, 251

Caruso, Enrico 3

Catapulting 207-208

Centering the Body 177-178

Chaplin, Charlie (Chaplinesque Body) 34, 48, 187. See also Radiancy

Chemical Energy 52, 137

Child and Body Wisdom 2, 12, 14, 20, 48, 61, 67, 71-72, 77, 88, 118, 161, 222, 252. See also Instinctive Body Skills, Natural Talents, Play

Chin-Ups (Body-Yawn) 52-53, 133, 135

Climbing on Wheels 124, 135, 137, 140, 161, 174-175, 179, 181-182, 212, 216, 242

Climbing Up Hills, Up Stairs, Downstairs 136, 175, 194-197, 204, 216, 225, 242, 252

Coda 250

Coil-Spring Sit-Up 50. See Nervous Energy

Coil-Spring Stretching 206-207

Communicating Skills and Body Wisdom 4, 11, 24-25, 56, 76, 115, 133, 139, 156, 227, 232, 235-236, 238, 245, 252

Combined Energy State Leg-Lift 117, 119

Complementary Opposites 32-33, 59, 61, 220. See Synergy, Cross-Quality Synthesis, Third-Force Unity

Conditioning (Outer-Environment) 3, 11, 13-19, 20-21, 27, 71, 136, 139, 158-159, 161, 216, 222, 224, 226, 245, 247-249, 251. See also Two Environments, Imitative Learning, Future Shock

INDEX

Conflict Resolution and Body Wisdom 252-253

Conical Rolls 124, 130, 140

Consonant Action 34, 58, 152-156, 220. See also Consonant Orchestra, Vocal Life, *The Use and Training of the Human Voice.*

Consonant Orchestra 58, 144-147, 220-221. See also Consonant Action, Vocal Life, *The Use and Training of the Human Voice.*

Contact Vanishing Point 38, 41, 47, 79, 83, 110 ff, 122, 126, 133, 135, 197-198

Contiguous Continuity (Atom-to-Atom Discovery) 77, 85, 91-92 ff, 96 ff, 99-100, 101, 103-104, 106, 110-112, 116, 118, 120, 123, 126-127, 135

Convex Back Curve 62, 66, 97-98 note, 124, 127, 160-161 ff, 167, 178. See C-Curve, Curvo-linear Principle

Creative (Contemplative) Calm 44, 46, 49

Crescent Curve See C-Curve, Curvo-linear Principle

Crescent Lying Down (Body As A) 77, 124-134 (Chapter X), 227

Crescent Push-Ups and Lift-Ups 131-132

Crescent Standing Up (Body As A) 77, 138, 139-174 (Chapter XI), 180-182 ff, 227

Criss-cross Squat 80 ff, 86, 106, 118-119, 141

Cross-cultural Quality of Body Wisdom 4, 231-232, 252-254 (Coda). See also Democracy Principle

Cross-quality (Holistic) Synthesis 9, 32-33, 56. See also Synergy, Complementary Opposites, Third Force Unity

Crying 77, 148-149, 153-155

Curvo-linear Principle 7, 26, 42, 62, 67, 76, 79, 109, 124, 127, 135, 160-161, 163, 177, 226-227, 245, 247-248, 253

Cylinder Rolls 124, 127-128, 140, 211

Dancing (Free-form Body Expressiveness) 40, 43-44, 46, 54, 66, 83, 123, 124, 149, 211, 217, 233, 241

Dancing on Wheels 103, 136-137, 149, 164, 173-174, 179, 183, 185-188, 194 note, 197-200, 212, 216. See also Rope Dancing

Dancing Relaxation 50. See Radiancy

Deaf and Hearing-Impaired 58, 180, 235-236

Deep Knee-Bend 79-80. See Squats

Democracy Principle and Body Wisdom 4, 16, 250-251 (Coda)

De-Patterning Principle 6

Design Engineering See Body Wisdom and Design Engineering

Destruct Patterns 11. See also Body Deterioration, Conditioning (Outer-Environment)

INDEX

Diagonal Shoulder Roll   100. See Shoulder Girdle Roll

Diametric Exercising   215, 219-222

Diamond-Shaped Shoulder Girdle Roll   120

Diminishing Fatigue Principle   9. See also Body Fatigue, Relaxer-Energizers, Body Energizers

Direct Images   40-41, 73, 75, 93. See also Organic Images

Distribution Principle   8. See Muscle-Sharing Responsibility

Dominance   See Sinistrality, Two Dominances

Double Figure-Eight   175-179, 181, 228. See also Body Circles, Body Loops, Rocker-Rims, Five Kinesthetic Energy Circuits

Downhill Running   195. See Running

Dualities   32-33, 59, 71-72, 74-76, 134, 188, 220

Dynamic Energy   7, 32-33, 34-58. See Energy and Relaxation, Relaxer-Energizers

Dynamic Relaxation   32, 35, 38. See Energy and Relaxation, Relaxer-Energizers

E

Ecology of the Human Body   4, 15, 212, 226. See Body Wisdom

Ecology of Human Potential   4, 11. See Body Wisdom, Instinctive Body Skills, Natural Talents

Electricity (Body Electricity)   26, 32, 47, 49-50, 111-114, 199. See Radiancy

Elongated Spine   66, 109, 124, 165, 167, 177. See also Spine, Back, C-Curve

Emo-tivated Breathing   148-158. See also Breathing, Inter-Involvement

Emo-tivated Leg-Lift   See Inter-Involvement Leg-Lift

Emo-tivated Sit-Up   See Inter-Involvement Sit-Up

Energetic Relaxation   33, 55, 75, 133, 136, 196, 204, 207, 224. See also Energy and Relaxation

Energy   5, 6, 9, 12, 20, 22, 29, 32-33, 34-58, 137, 148, 226, 228, 232, 235, 247. See also Energy States

Energy and Relaxation   32-33, 35-42, 52, 55, 57, 59, 67, 76, 94, 97, Part Three: Chapters VII - XII, 218, 220-221, 251. See also Relaxer-Energizers

Energy States (Derived)   34, 57-58

Energy States (Primitive, Non-Derived)   32-33, 34-58, 51 note, 67, 83, 105, 108-109, 122-123, 137, 143-144, 161, 164, 198, 208-213, 217-218, 230, 234, 242, 248, 251. See Buoyancy, Radiancy, Potency, Inter-Involvement

Energy Support Fields   35-47, 234

Endurance   52, 54, 71, 83, 135, 173, 187, 189-190, 192, 199, 201, 216, 251

INDEX

Ensemble Activities See Buddy Work, Acting, Applications of Body Wisdom in the Arts

Equilibrium 32, 46-47, 75, 79, 101, 111, 119, 148, 152, 180, 182, 186, 207, 219-220, 236, 238, 251

Esthetics See Body Esthetics

Esthetic Process 27

Esthetic Tap 251

Eurythmics 47, 199, 218

Evolving Body Curve 72, 76-77 ff, 94, 108-109, 122, 124 ff, 134, 139 ff, 159-160 ff, 174, 226, 250. See also Body Sphere in Movement

Executive Management Training 253

Exercise Classifications 34, 57-58 (Vocal Life), 164, 211, 214, 215-225 (Body Training)

Expanded Sphere (Body As An) 77, 104, 107, 108-123 (Chapter IX), 124

Expanded Sphere Leg-Lifts 116-117, 123

Expanded Sphere Sit-Ups 113-116, 123

Extended Reaching See Body Reaching, Sustained Extension

F

Falling 12, 42, 93, 99, 101, 106, 132, 191, 208. See also Fear of Falling

Familiar Event 22-23 ff, 32, 37-39, 42, 60, 95, 123, 140-143, 148, 173, 177, 184, 190, 223. See also Unique Event, Feeling Process, Organic Instructions

Fear-Diffusion 12, 67, 76, 81, 85, 91, 105, 136, 149, 152-153, 157, 180, 218, 242, 250-251

Fear of Falling 42, 47, 77, 81, 85, 91, 93, 97, 101, 132, 136, 179, 182, 251

Feedback Principle 8, 20 ff 39, 45, 136-137, 236, 239, 247

Feeling Process Preface ii, 1-3, 5 ff, 10, 20-28, 30-31, 60, 72, 92, 96, 108, 198, 213, 218, 226, 239, 245-246, 248, 250

Finger-Tip Control 83, 104-106, 110 ff, 122, 135

Five Kinesthetic Energy Circuits 175-179, 181, 228, 243. See also Double Figure-Eight

Five Outer Senses 21, 27-28, 45, 71, 180, 227, 248

Flat-Sole Squats 80 ff, 87, 141

Floating Buoyancy 32, 34, 36-47, 54-55, 75, 135, 143, 150, 155, 177

Floating Squats 79-87, 88, 141

Floating Sit-Up 37-43, 46

Foot Rocker Loops 175-176, 196, 203

Foot-Scooters 181-185

INDEX

Forward Roll 100, 118-119

Future Shock Foreword v, 18, 71, 251

G

Generalization of Energies 56, 220

Generalization Principle 8, 33, 56. See also Carry-over Experiences

Gentle Turbulence 6, 16, 29, 36, 42, 67 ff, 246

Gestalt Approach Preface ii, 5, 220

Gravity-free Feeling (Body as Center of Gravity) 39, 42, 66, 76, 79-81, 84, 97, 101-103, 136, 170, 213, 215, 217, 234, 242. See also Weightlessness, Zero Pressure

H

Habitual Awareness Principle 6, 9

Harmonic Overtone Sensory System 5, 21-22, 28-29, 33, 45, 55, 67, 70, 72, 180, 213, 222, 224, 227, 236, 247, 249

Head Loop 175

Healthy Compromise 15, 24, 136

Hiring an Image 44, 47, 74-75, 87-88, 125, 179, 185. See also Organic Images

Hopping (Body Hops) 124, 133, 198, 202-206, 216

Human Likeness Principle 5. See also Structural Space Sphere

Human Musical Instrument Principle 5, 57-58, 144-147, 220. See also Consonant Action, Consonant Orchestra, Vocal Life

Humming 64-66

Hysteresis 6

I

Images See Organic Images

Image Energy 36

Image Envelope 26

Images in Movement 72-73

Image Instruction 41. See also Organic Instructions

Imitative Learning (Imitative Behavior) 11-12, 14, 16, 18, 20-21, 72, 88, 159, 161, 226, 247-248. See also Conditioning, Two Environments

Incoming Sensation 28

Indirect Images 73, 75. See also Organic Images

Inner Environment 13-19, 27, 34, 39, 45, 71, 172, 215, 222, 226, 243-245, 247, 249, 253. See also Two Environments, Personal Space Spheres, Harmonic Overtone Sensory System

INDEX

Inner Input 15-16, 27, 72

Inspired Inhalation 45, 60, 85, 106, 126, 155

Inspirational Images 74-75

Instinctive Body Skills 3-4, 5 ff, 13, 22, 29-30, 123, 180, 218, 222, 250, 254. See also Natural Talents

Intelligence See Body Intelligence, Body Languages

Interdisciplinary Character of Body Wisdom 5 ff, 250-255 (Coda). See also Research and Development Institute

Inter-Involvement Energy 9, 32, 34, 55-56, 58, 67, 74, 76, 128, 135, 203, 209-210, 227, 233-234, 238

Inter-Involvement Leg-Lift 117

Inter-Involvement Sit-Up 56, 115

Internal Body Exercise 47

Internal Body Competition 26-27 ff, 59, 68, 72, 77, 136, 220-221

Internal Space 45-46, 85. See also Inner Environment, Personal Space Spheres

Isometrics 219

Isotonics 219

J

Joints and Hinges 2, 40, 44, 50, 80, 108-110, 116, 125-126, 128, 132, 139, 159-170, 172, 175, 193, 195, 197, 202, 217, 225

Jogging (A New Approach To) 136, 175, 177, 186-190, 192, 201, 209, 216, 220

Just Noticeable Difference 33, 98 note, 104-105, 110 ff, 122, 135

K

Key Signature 189-190, 192-193 note

Kinesensics 10, 18, 21, 23-24, 28, 32-33, 35, 57-58, 60, 67, 93, 108, 110, 135-136, 179, 187-188, 216-220, 235-236, 246-247, 253

Kinesensic Phonetics 57-58. See also Vocal Life, Consonant Orchestra, *The Use and Training of the Human Voice.*

Kinesensic Photo-Survey 93, 103, 162, 165

Kinesthetic/Nerve Energy Circuits 114, 157, 178. See also Five Kinesthetic Energy Circuits

Kinetic Energy 51, 76

L

Lambency 114, 114 note, 121, 166, 192, 194. See Radiancy

Language (Non-Linear) 13, 25, 30-31. See Body Languages

Laughing 62, 65-66, 77, 148-149, 153-155

INDEX

Laurel and Hardy 48

Leaping 103, 135, 161, 175, 198, 205, 209-211, 216-217, 220. See also Springing/Jumping

Leg-Lifts 37-42, 75, 116-117, 133

Leg-Lift Flip-Over 117

Leg-Wheels 71, 87, 116, 134, 159, 174-188, 190-197, 201, 210, 224, 228, 242. See also Running on Wheels, Dancing on Wheels, Climbing on Wheels

Lessac, Michael 11

Lift-Ups 131-133, 135, 140

Listening Within 45, 235-236. See also Synesthesic Activity

Live Rope 174, 200, 216

Live Weight vs. Dead Weight 46, 50, 79, 100-101, 135-137, 160, 169, 170-172, 179, 215-216

Long Distance Running 190, 192-193 note, 242

Loping Run 132, 190-192

Lowen, Walter Foreword iv

Lower Back Center (Lower Spine Energy Center) 66, 89, 97-98 ff, 103, 125-127, 132, 142, 156, 167, 176-177, 181, 185, 191-192, 194 note, 195, 225, 228

Major Key Rhythmics 64. See Shaking

Midword Break 135-138, 224

Minor Key Rhythmics 64. See Shaking

Movement and Relaxation 36-37. See Body in Movement/Movement in the Body, Restful Action/Active Rest, Energy and Relaxation

Movement Dynamics 46, 67

Moving Backward 179-180

Moving (Traveling) Balance 75, 85 ff, 102-104, 111, 122, 207

Moving Meditation 46. See Creative Calm

Muscle Dynamics 2, 6-7

Muscle Loosening 91, 94-95, 110 ff, 112, 117, 119, 138, 166, 193, 195-196, 199, 202, 220-221. See also Shaking, Quivering, Vibratory Experience

Muscle Power 51-53, 56. See Potency, Body Yawn-Stretch

Muscle Quieting 110, 112, 117, 119

Muscle Release 49-50

Muscle-Sharing Responsibility 42, 56, 80, 120, 123, 126, 137. See also Distribution Principle

INDEX

Muscle Tension 62, 123. See Tension, Tension-Relief, Stress and Strain, Relaxer-Energizers

Muscular Flabbiness 26

Natural (What Is Natural?) 10-13

Natural Healing Process 154. See also Psychosomatic Health, Preventive Medicine

Natural Talents 3-4, 13, 22, 29-30, 69, 71, 123, 180, 222, 250-251, 254. See Instinctive Body Skills

Nervous Energy 48-50, 69, 157, 187

New Learning Process 1-3, 5-10, 20-25. See also Organic/Sensory Learning, Feeling Process, Psychosomatic Learning

Non-Voluntary Sensation 29-30, 39-40, 59, 70

Olivier, Laurence 3

Olympic Athletes and Body Wisdom 3, 33. See Applications of Body Wisdom in Sports, Athletic Coaching

Optimal Functioning 26, 32-33, 52, 55, 71, 76, 139-140, 160, 191-192, 211, 216-218, 220, 224, 226, 242, 248, 253-254

Organic Cues and Signals 105-106, 137, 193, 236, 238. See also Buddy Work, Fear-Diffusion

Organic Images 9, 20, 23-26 ff, 36-42, 47, 49-50, 70-74, 88, 95, 110, 113, 116, 135-136, 137, 144, 149-153, 160, 162, 171, 175, 177, 182-183, 185-186, 193, 203, 206, 211, 215, 217-219, 223, 230, 234, 247

Organic Instructions Foreword vi, 20-23 ff, 26 ff, 33, 39-40, 44, 67, 69-70, 72-74, 76, 91, 95, 160, 162, 171, 175, 177, 188, 194, 224, 250

Organic Sensation 1-4, 20 ff, 211

Organic/Sensory Learning 27, 109, 218, 246. See Psychosomatic Learning, Feeling Process, New Learning Process

Outer Environment See Conditioning, Five Outer Senses, Two Environments, Future Shock

Owens, Jesse 3

Output Sensation 28

P

Paddle-Wheel Leg-Lift 116-117

Pain Therapy 47, 67-69, 72, 154

Parenthesis (Crescent) Curve 66, 124-126, 160, 162, 165, 167-168, 170, 176-179. See also C-curve, Curvo-linear Principle

Pavlova 3

INDEX

Pedestal Balance   75, 102-103, 122, 207

Peel-Ups   124, 128-130

Penguin Walk   183-184, 188. See Bow and Wheel Walk

Perceivable Rhythms   67. See also Rhythm Experience, Rhythm Feel/Dynamics

Perception of Being Upright   77, 139 ff, 138-139, 157-174, 182

Perception of Movement   76

Perception of the Mysterious   30

Perceptive Awareness   6, 20 ff, 27, 70, 96, 232, 236

Perceptual Awareness   6, 15

Personal Culture   15-16, 35, 47. See also Self-Image

Personal Mime   130-131. See also T'ai Chi, Dancing (Free-form Expressiveness), Plastique Body Movement

Personal Space Spheres   71, 174, 214, 226-245 (Chapter XIII), 248. See Structural, Auditory, Visual, Vocal, Traveling Space Spheres

Physics (Optimal Principle)   2, 6. See Hysteresis

Pin-point Balance   75, 102-103, 122, 207

Plastique Body Movement   44, 46-47, 54, 217, 233. See also Space-Sculpting, Dancing, Personal Mime

Play   6, 48, 71-72, 74, 77, 101, 106, 135, 148, 173-174, 184, 188, 210, 251. See also Child and Body Wisdom, Work/Play

Plumb-line Balance   181-182, 186, 191, 195, 197, 199

Pogo-Stick Spring and Jump   198-200-201

Postscript   215-225

Posture   11-12, 23, 26, 42, 57, 60-62, 76-77, 79-87, 88-107, 109, 124 ff, 134, 139-174, 174-214, 215-216, 225, 228-230, 249, 251. See also Breathing

Potency (Body Power/Body Strength)   32, 34, 51-55, 67, 83, 88, 101-103, 110, 112, 128, 135, 143-144, 175, 180-181, 192, 194, 209, 215, 218, 221, 234, 242, 251

Potency Sit-Up   114 ff

Potency Leg-Lift   116

Potent Power of Breath   47

Pre-conditioned Body   32. See also Energy States, Inner Environment, Child and Body Wisdom, Instinctive Body Skills, Natural Talents

Pre-scientific Principles of Body Wisdom   5, 7-10

Preventive Medicine   2, 4, 221, 251, 253

Primary (Endogenous) Images   26. See Direct Images

Psychology of Institutions   17

INDEX

Psycho-Kinetics 30

Psycho-Physical Body-Whole Preface i, 1-4, 11, 16, 20, 26, 46, 55, 76, 137, 139, 196, 222, 224, 226

Psychosomatic Health 15, 18, 21, 60, 70, 137, 155-158, 163, 212, 224, 246

Psychosomatic Illness 2, 17, 21, 59, 67, 208, 246, 251

Psychosomatic Learning 20-22, 25, 26 ff, 28, 137. See also New Learning Process, Feeling Process, Organic/Sensory Learning

Push-Ups 52-53, 75, 124, 131-133, 135, 140

Q

Quivering 94, 110, 112, 138, 149, 153. See also Radiancy, Vibratory Experience

R

Radiancy 32, 34, 47-51, 67, 83, 88, 94, 101, 103-104, 110, 112, 121, 128, 135, 137, 139, 143-144, 150, 164, 172, 180-181, 186-187, 192, 196-198, 200, 209-210, 217, 234

Radiancy Sit-Up 50, 114 ff. See Coil-Spring Sit-Up

Radiancy Leg-Lift 116

Relaxation in Action 6. See Energy and Relaxation

Relaxed Energy 33, 75, 95, 133, 136, 196, 204, 224

Relaxer-Energizers 3, 7, 32-33, 57, 59-66, 67 ff, 70, 94-95, 97-98 note, 112, 122, 125, 132, 135, 137-138, 142, 148-149, 154-155, 166, 175, 177, 186, 192, 195, 198, 204, 213, 217, 223, 251

Research and Development Institute 254

Reserve Safety Cushion 52, 55, 67, 85, 135-137, 164, 208, 215, 219, 223-225

Resident Sensation 28, 72

Restful Action/Active Rest See Energy and Relaxation, Relaxer-Energizers

Resting Component (of Energy) 32

Resting Up and Resting Down (at the same time) 33, 38, 75-76, 84, 110 ff, 122, 126, 135, 160, 171, 180, 188, 198, 218, 220

Rhythm Experience 4, 9, 26, 29-30, 33, 37-38, 44, 46, 50, 66-71, 76, 142, 156, 182, 187, 211-212, 247

Rhythm Feel/Rhythm Dynamic 32, 44-45, 67-68, 84, 86, 94-95, 97-98, 100, 102-104, 112-113, 122, 142, 151, 173, 183-186, 188, 190-193, 197-202, 205, 211-212, 218, 221-222, 235, 242

Rising Buoyancy 34, 36-47, 75, 135, 143, 150, 155, 160, 165, 177, 180-181

Robinson, Bill 48

Rocker-Rims 112-113, 130, 174-175 ff, 179, 182-183, 189, 193-195, 211, 228

Rocking and Rolling 62, 85-86, 90-93, 95-100, 103-107, 109-112, 117-120, 127-128, 135, 175 ff, 179, 183-184, 187, 196, 203, 217, 219, 228-230, 241

INDEX

Rolling Uphill 194. See Climbing on Wheels

Rolling Up Stairs 196-197. See Climbing on Wheels

Roll-Overs 112-113

Roll-Ups 128-129, 135, 140

Rope-Skipping/Rope-Dancing 164, 173-175, 198-201, 211, 216-217

Rope-Springing 199, 201-202

Rope-Swinging 164, 201-202

Rowing 164

Running Downhill 195, 216, 223

Running on Walls 212-214, 223

Running (on Wheels) 86, 103-104, 109, 124, 132-133, 135-136, 140, 161, 164, 169, 174-175, 177, 179-182, 185, 187-192, 201, 208-214, 216-217, 220, 225, 242

Running Uphill 194-195, 216, 223

S

S-Curve 109, 162, 165, 168

Safety Reserve Cushion See Reserve Safety Cushion

Science and Body Wisdom Preface i, Foreword v-vii, 7-8, 30

Scientific Principles of Body Wisdom Foreword v-vi, 5-7

Self-Defense 218

Self-Image 14-19, 71, 76, 218, 223, 227, 231, 241, 245-249, 250, 252

Self-to-Other Communication 20, 28, 34, 115, 239, 244-245, 254

Self-to-Self Communication 9, 13, 20 ff, 24, 28, 33, 55-56, 135, 186, 227, 233, 245, 254

Self-Realization Movements Preface i, 19

Self-Teaching and Body Wisdom 1-5, 16, 20, 31-33, 40, 71, 103, 132-134, 162-163, 214-215, 250-251

Semi-Direct Images 73, 75

Semi-Voluntary Sensation 29-30, 36, 39-40, 59, 70, 115

Sensation 20-25, 26, 31, 37, 89, 104. See also Feeling Process, Sense Memory, Sensory Perception

Sensation-Perception-Awareness-Response 20-23 ff, 26-27 ff, 61, 72-73, 89, 91, 104, 110-111, 135, 218. See Feeling Process, Sense Memory, Feedback Principle

Sense Memory (Muscle Recall) 36-37, 42, 45, 50, 73, 92

Sense Memory Exercises 38-40

INDEX

Sensing of Humor 30-31, 65, 69, 187, 210, 213, 217, 232, 251

Sensory Perception 20 ff, 23, 28-29, 76, 144, 223, 232

Settling-Down Buoyancy 34, 36-47, 75, 133, 135, 143, 150, 155, 177

Shaking 32, 50, 58, 64-66, 94-95, 98, 110, 112, 122, 127-128, 138, 153-154, 164, 172, 175, 195-197. See Vibratory Experience

Shivering 65, 94, 148-149, 152, 154. See Vibratory Experience

Shoulder Girdle Roll 119, 122

Silent Language 231

Singing 14, 58, 65, 149. See also Breathing, Vocal Life, Consonant Orchestra, Posture

Sighing 45, 60, 62, 64, 86, 147, 149, 151-152, 154-155, 157, 192, 208-209. See also Breathing

Sinistrality 5, 215, 221-223. See Two Dominances, Bi-lateral Body Development, Split-Brain Research

Sitting Postures 37-43, 79 ff, 88 ff, 97 ff, 107, 111-113, 116, 118, 140 ff, 177, 181, 243. See also Squats, Coda graphics

Sitting Walk 184-185

Sit-Ups 37-43, 50, 54, 56, 75, 113-116, 140

Skipping 194 note, 198-199, 216

Slow-Motion Movement 40 (in water), 44 (in air), 91-93, 95, 99, 101, 111, 118, 128, 133, 217, 219

Small Compact Ball (Body As A) 77, 79-87 (Chapter VII), 94, 102 ff, 108-109, 111, 124, 139, 179, 227

Small Sphere (Body As A) 77, 139, 88-107 (Chapter VIII), 179, 227

Small Wheel Dance-Walk 185-186

Smell 26, 62, 147, 149-151

Smiling 65-66

Social Health 17

Somersaults See Forward Roll

Space-Sculpting 49, 54, 217, 234. See also Plastique Body Movement, Dancing (Free-form Expressiveness)

Sparrow Spring-Away 203

Speech 57-58, 139, 156-157, 220, 249. See also Vocal Life, *Use and Training of the Human Voice.*

Speech and Voice Therapy 30, 57-58, 158, 250-255 (Coda). See Vocal Life, Speech, *Use and Training of the Human Voice.*

Speed 190-192, 195, 201, 211, 215, 217-218, 221, 225, 241-242. See also Body Swiftness

Spine 13, 16, 57, 66, 108-109, 124-125, 132, 159-161, 165, 167, 175-177, 180, 188-189, 191-193, 199, 202, 215, 218, 229, 236

INDEX

Split-Brain Research Foreword v, 3, 5, 30, 221-223, 254. See also Back Brain, Two Dominances, Body Intelligence, Body Languages, Non-Linear Language

Springing/Jumping 133, 140, 161, 174-175, 182, 197-198, 202-206, 209-210, 212, 216, 220

Sprinting 175, 182, 188, 190, 192-194, 209-210

Sprinting Run 192-194

Squats 79-87, 88-89, 106-107, 111, 118, 140-141, 202-207, 216, 243

Squat Jog (Squat Dance) 203

Stage Fright 69, 254 (Coda). See also Transformation Process

Stillness in Motion/Movement of Stillness 45, 74-75, 89, 93-94, 99, 101, 159-160, 177, 206

Stradivarius (Body As A) Foreword vi, 1-2

Strain and Stress 26, 55, 57-58, 65, 80, 98, 157, 195, 216, 225, 236, 238, 240, 251-252

Structural Action 34, 57. See Vocal Life, *Use and Training of the Human Voice.*

Structural Space Sphere 214, 227, 228-235, 238, 241-243, 248. See also Body Height

Sustained Extension 26, 34 ff, 43, 46, 55, 67, 109, 138, 211-212, 217, 221, 240. See Body Reaching

Swallowing 60, 62

Synergy 28, 32-33, 56, 59, 209, 221, 227, 246. See also Cross-Quality Synthesis, Complementary Opposites, Third Force Unity

Synesthesic Activity 26, 26 note, 28, 45, 221, 235-236, 240, 245. See Harmonic Overtone Sensory System

Systems Research Foreword v-vi

T

T'ai Chi (Personal T'ai Chi and Body Wisdom) 217. See also Personal Mime, Plastique Body Movement, Space-Sculpting

Taste 26, 28

Technology and Body Structure Forward vi-vii, 253 (Coda). See also Design Engineering

Tension Centers See Upper Back Center, Lower Spine Energy Center, Relaxer-Energizers, Structural Action, Tonal Action, Consonant Action, Swallowing, C-curve, Elongated Spine

Tension-Relief 62, 64-65, 98, 112, 165, 219, 242, 251. See Relaxer-Energizers

Therapy (Physical) and Body Wisdom 252-253. See also Speech and Voice Therapy

Third-Force Unity 32-33, 59, 74, 177, 215, 220, 246. See also Synergy, Complementary Opposites, Cross-Quality Synthesis

INDEX

Tight-Rope Dancing 28

Time-Lag Catch-Up Principle 9

Toe-Stretch Squat 80 ff, 87, 141

Toe-Tip to the Wall Sit-Up 115-116

Toffler, Eric 18. See Future Shock

Tonal Action 34, 58. See Vocal Life

Touch 27-28

Transformation Process 54, 67-69, 74, 242

Traveling Space Sphere 193, 228, 241-244, 248

Trembling 50, 94, 148-149, 152-154. See Vibratory Experience

Tripod-Headstand Balance 120-121, 123, 140

Tumbling 62, 92, 95, 99, 109, 135. See also Rocking and Rolling

Two-Bladed Squat 80 ff, 86-87, 141

Two Dominances 5. See Sinistrality, Bi-lateral Body Development

Two Environments Foreword iv-v, 13-19, 27, 243-244, 247-248. See also Inner Environment, Conditioning (Outer-Environment).

U

Unhealthy Compromise 14-15, 17, 253 (Coda)

Unique Event 8, 23, 32, 37, 45, 60, 123, 148, 184, 190. See also Familiar Event

Unique Event Principle 10

Upper Spine Center 66, 89, 98, 98 note, 100, 103, 124-125, 156, 166, 176-177, 186, 192, 228. See Tension Centers, Relaxer-Energizers

Upright Posture 43-44, 77, 104, 106-107, 109, 124, 127, 134, 139-142 ff, 175-214 (Chapter XII), 224, 243

Use and Training of the Human Voice Preface ii, 1, 5, 34, 57-58, 147, 220, 239. See also Vocal Life

V

Vanishing Contact Point See Contact Vanishing Point

Vibratory Experience (Body Vibrato) 32, 47, 50, 58, 64-65, 79, 81, 94-95, 101, 110, 112, 122, 127, 138, 153-154, 187, 196-197, 203. See also Shaking, Trembling, Shivering, Radiancy

Visual Sense 27-28, 227

Visual Space Sphere 214, 227-228, 233, 235, 237-238, 240, 243, 248

Vocal Life (Vocal and Verbal Energy) 1, 3-4, 9, 12, 22, 25-26, 29, 30, 34, 51-52, 57-58, 63-64, 76, 83, 96, 98 note, 112, 134, 137, 144-148, 152 ff, 157, 220-221, 239, 243, 249. See also *Use and Training of the Human Voice,* Speech and Voice Therapy, Tonal Action, Structural Action, Consonant Action, Consonant Orchestra, Derived Energy States

INDEX

Vocal Sound Stream Principle 7, 239

Vocal Space Sphere 214, 227, 238-241, 243-244, 248. See also Vocal Life

Vocal Tone 57-58, 76, 112. See Vocal Life

Voluntary Sensation 29-30, 39-40, 59, 68, 115

W

Wafting and Waving 36-47, 73, 79, 81, 85, 90-91 ff, 96, 100, 105, 110 ff, 115, 118-119, 126-128

Walking (on Wheels) 86, 104, 109, 132-133, 140, 161, 168-169, 174-175, 179, 181-186, 188, 204, 209, 216-217, 220, 230, 242, 249

Water Buoyancy 36-42, 73, 111, 113, 116

Wave Principle 9

Weightlessness (Body Lightness) 26, 29, 35-40, 42, 44, 48, 50, 79, 97, 109, 111, 113, 135, 161, 173, 181, 184, 187-189, 192, 198, 202, 205-207, 213, 218, 230, 242. See also Contact Vanishing Point, Gravity-Free Feeling, Zero Pressure

Whole Brain 30. See Back Brain, Split-Brain Research, Two Dominances, Bilateral Body Development

Wildness 18-19. See also Beyond Wildness

Work and Relaxation 6, 75. See Relaxer-Energizers, Play, Work/Play, Energy and Relaxation

Work/Play 67-68, 74. See Play, Work and Relaxation

Writhing 67-68, 74. See also Transformation Process

Y

Yawning 61-62, 63-64. See also Body Yawn-Stretch

Yeats, William Butler 29

Yoga Headstand Balance 121-123, 140

Z

Zero Body Pressure 38, 41, 47, 79, 133, 219, 241. See Contact Vanishing Point, Weightlessness, Gravity-Free Feeling